Goodheart's Photoguide of Common Skin Disorders

Diagnosis and Management

SECOND EDITION

Goodheart's Photoguide of Common Skin Disorders

Diagnosis and Management

Herbert P. Goodheart, M.D.

Assistant Clinical Professor
Department of Dermatology
Mount Sinai School of Medicine
New York, New York

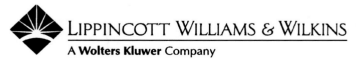

LIPPINCOTT WILLIAMS & WILKINS
A **Wolters Kluwer** Company

Philadelphia • Baltimore • New York • London
Buenos Aires • Hong Kong • Sydney • Tokyo

Acquisitions Editor: Beth Barry
Developmental Editor: Sonya Seigafuse
Production Editor: Sheila Higgins
Manufacturing Manager: Benjamin Rivera
Cover Designer: Wanda Kossak
Compositor: Techbooks
Printer: Walsworth Publishing Co.

© 2003 by LIPPINCOTT WILLIAMS & WILKINS
530 Walnut Street
Philadelphia, PA 19106 USA
LWW.com

Library of Congress Cataloging-in-Publication Data

Goodheart, Herbert P.
   Goodheart's photoguide of common skin disorders: diagnosis and management /
Herbert P. Goodheart.—2nd ed.
      p. ; cm.
   Rev. ed. of: A photoguide of common skin disorders / Herbert P. Goodheart. 1999.
   Includes index.
   ISBN 0-7817-3741-9
      1. Skin—Diseases—Handbooks, manuals, etc. 2. Skin—Diseases—Atlases. I. Goodheart,
Herbert P. Photoguide of common skin disorders. II. Title.
   [DNLM: 1. Skin Diseases—diagnosis—Atlases. 2. Skin Diseases—therapy—Atlases. WR
17 G652g 2003]
   RL74 .G66 2003
   616.5'0022'2—dc21   2002030006

Care has been taken to confirm the accuracy of the information presented and to describe generally accepted practices. However, the authors, editor, and publisher are not responsible for errors or omissions or for any consequences from application of the information in this book and make no warranty, expressed or implied, with respect to the currency, completeness, or accuracy of the contents of the publication. Application of this information in a particular situation remains the professional responsibility of the practitioner.

The authors, editor, and publisher have exerted every effort to ensure that drug selection and dosage set forth in this text are in accordance with current recommendations and practice at the time of publication. However, in view of ongoing research, changes in government regulations, and the constant flow of information relating to drug therapy and drug reactions, the reader is urged to check the package insert for each drug for any change in indications and dosage and for added warnings and precautions. This is particularly important when the recommended agent is a new or infrequently employed drug.

Some drugs and medical devices presented in this publication have Food and Drug Administration (FDA) clearance for limited use in restricted research settings. It is the responsibility of the health care provider to ascertain the FDA status of each drug or device planned for use in their clinical practice.

10 9 8 7 6 5 4 3 2 1

To my wife and best friend, Karen

What the mind
does not know,
the eyes
cannot see.
–Ancient proverb

CONTENTS

INTRODUCTION

PART ONE

Common Skin Conditions: Diagnosis and Management

PART TWO

Systemic Conditions and the Skin

PART THREE

Dermatologic Procedures

APPENDICES

Mary Ruth Buchness, M.D.

Associate Attending of
Dermatology and Medicine
Saint Vincent's Catholic Medical
Centers
New York, New York
Clinical Associate Professor of
Dermatology
New York Medical College
Valhalla, New York

Herbert P. Goodheart, M.D.

Assistant Clinical Professor
Department of Dermatology
Mount Sinai School of Medicine
New York, New York

Peter G. Burk, M.D.

Clinical Associate Professor of
Medicine (Dermatology)
Albert Einstein College of
Medicine
Attending Physician
Dermatology Service
Montefiore Medical Center
Bronx, New York

Kenneth Howe, M.D.

Assistant Clinical Professor
Department of Dermatology
Beth Israel Medical Center
New York, New York

FOREWORD

As a second-year medical student, I recall studying cardiology one evening when my brother Andrew asked me to look at a rash that developed on his trunk. I did not have a clue as to how to make *any* dermatologic diagnosis. So, after Andrew accused my father of wasting tuition money on my evidently inadequate education, I thought it proper to register for a dermatology elective in my fourth year. I reasoned that, regardless of whatever field I would ultimately choose, I would inevitably be confronted with some cutaneous dilemmas. It was with tremendous fortune that I subsequently trained at the Albert Einstein College of Medicine in the Bronx, New York, under the tutelage of Michael Fisher, M.D., who still heads an illustrious division of dermatology. It was during my training that I befriended the attending physician, Dr. Herb Goodheart. Herb always provided special insights, wisdom, and compassion in the evaluation of even the most rudimentary dermatologic disorders. He is a stellar teacher and dermatologist, who has compiled his years of perspicacity into this guide to dermatology.

As we begin the twenty-first century, the landscape of American medicine and dermatology is changing at an accelerating pace. Even though we can now comprehend many skin disorders at a molecular level and have advanced our therapeutic realm to include laser technology and immunobiology, the cornerstone of all dermatologic endeavors will always be careful clinical observation. As venues of practice shift toward a greater proportion of primary dermatologic care being delivered by nondermatologists, resources for these providers must be accessible, comprehensible, and practical. Dr. Goodheart's guide to dermatology is divided into common disorders, the interrelationship between the skin and systemic disease, basic and advanced dermatologic procedures, and a very useful appendix providing patient handout material in both English and Spanish. Importantly, it combines features of an atlas with Herb's pithy perspectives, as though he is standing over your shoulder in the dermatology clinic. Those who utilize this guide will come to appreciate many of the finer points and opinions that Dr. Goodheart provides and even more so when becoming more facile with the discipline. Use this guide as a primer, an atlas, a consultant, and as a supplement to more in-depth dermatology texts and medical literature. Your dermatologic knowledge base will flourish, your appreciation of the field will blossom, and most importantly, your patients will benefit from your expertise.

Warren R. Heymann, M.D.
Head Division of Dermatology
UMDNJ—Robert Wood Johnson School of Medicine at Camden
Newark, New Jersey

In dermatology, the naked eye is our primary tool, and because virtually every skin disorder is visible, the photographic image is an essential teaching aide.

Despite the commonplace occurrence of skin disorders, making a correct dermatologic diagnosis is a customary stumbling block for many health care professionals. It is rather unusual to find the nondermatologist who is comfortable diagnosing or managing most skin problems; in fact, many admit to using the frequent approach of "trial and error." Medical schools simply do not emphasize the teaching of dermatology. Skin diseases are generally considered less life threatening and are a lower priority than most of the conditions seen in teaching hospitals. Frequently, this can result in mistreatment, a delay in appropriate treatment, or a referral to a dermatologist.

This book is intended to be an accessible reference for nondermatologists such as family physicians, physician assistants, nurse practitioners, and medical students, who are often on the frontline in treating skin problems. Its focus has been limited intentionally to the diagnosis and management of the most common skin problems encountered in an outpatient setting. Wherever possible, "look-alike" photos are juxtaposed with photos of primary dermatoses to help the reader make the differential diagnosis.

Many changes have occurred in the four years since the first edition, *A Photoguide of Common Skin Disorders*, was published. This second edition has been expanded and extensively rewritten to reflect these changes. The treatment sections have been updated and offer more therapeutic options that also will serve as a resource for those in dermatology residency training. The photographs, on which this text is built, were enlarged for this second edition to achieve greater clarity and detail.

The English/Spanish patient handouts, in Appendix A, have been significantly revised and expanded in number. They can be photocopied and given to patients; they also can serve as an ongoing source of information for health care providers who use this book. A new feature that should be of benefit to international readers is Appendix B, "Brand Names of Dermatologic Medications in Various Countries," which will allow the reader to recognize dermatologic agents that often have different brand names in their respective countries.

I hope these changes will make this edition even more useful to those responsible for diagnosing and managing the common problems that account for the vast majority of dermatologic complaints.

Herbert P. Goodheart, M.D.

This second edition never would have been realized without the foresight and determination of Paul Koren at Lippincott Williams & Wilkins and also Beth Barry who carried this project to the finish line. My heartfelt appreciation goes to both of them.

My gratitude also extends to Jaquelyn Matos and Ellen Rosen at *Women's Health in Primary Care*, where my "Dermatology Rounds" appear on a monthly basis. *Women's Health in Primary Care* is a medical journal that brings the latest findings about the medical care of women. A great deal of material in this book has appeared in *Women's Health in Primary Care* with their invaluable editorial help.

Thanks go to my colleagues at Derm-Chat/Derm-Rx, who keep me up-to-date on the latest diagnostic and therapeutic issues in dermatology: Art Huntley at UC Davis, who founded and maintains this valuable on-line resource, as well as "heavy posters" such as Joe Eastern, Orin Goldblum, Diane Thaler, Ed Zabawski, Jerry Litt, Skee Smith, JoBohanon-Grant, Ben Treen, Chuck Fishman, Stu Kittay, Chuck Miller, Norm Guzick, Pat Condry, Kevin Smith, Steve Stone, Gail Drayton, Steve Emmet, Linda Spencer, and others who are too numerous to mention, have been my "on-line classmates."

Muchas gracias to Carlos Cohen and Monica Shapiro for the Spanish translations of my patient handouts. Appreciation also goes to Ross Levy whose hands and surgical skills are featured more than once in this book; Danielle Luquin of Blois, France, who provided the French brand names; Hans J. Kammler of Bonn, Germany, who supplied both German and French brand names; and Terry Marshall at Rotherham General Hospital, Yorkshire, England, who carefully researched brand names in the United Kingdom.

I am immensely pleased with the superb job my publisher, Lippincott Williams & Wilkins, has done in producing this edition. Special credit goes to Diana Andrews whose creative suggestions always respected the content of the material; Sonya Seigafuse, my developmental editor, who made excellent editorial and design contributions; and Sheila Higgins, the project editor, whose attention to detail has brought a complicated project to completion.

Illustrated Glossary of Basic Skin Lesions

Lesions

PRIMARY LESIONS

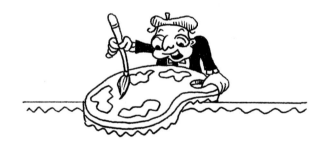

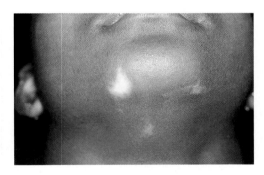

Macule. Vitiligo.

Macules are simply a change in skin color (you can't feel macules and, if you close your eyes, they "disappear"). They come in many shapes and sizes.

Examples include freckles, tattoos, hyperpigmentation, hypopigmentation, erythema, purpura, and vitiligo.

Patches are large macules.

Examples include melasma and vascular nevus ("salmon patch"). There is some confusion regarding patches; some dermatologists refer to a patch as a large macule, whereas others refer to patches as macules with overlying fine scale, for example, pityriasis rosea and mycosis fungoides.

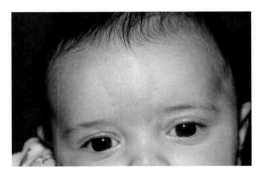

Patch. Vascular nevus ("salmon patch").

1

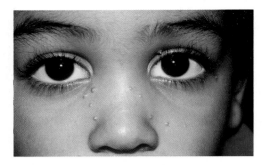

Papule. Molluscum contagiosum. Shiny papules.

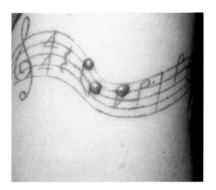

Macules and papules. Allergic reaction to the red dye of a tattoo. The macules are blue and yellow areas, and the papules are red bumps.

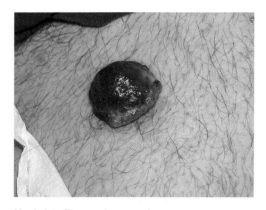

Nodule. Pyogenic granuloma.

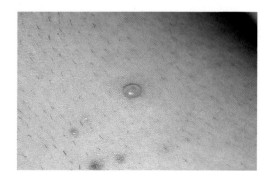

Vesicle. Chickenpox.

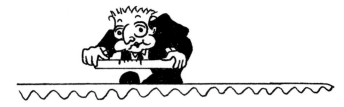

Papules are small, solid lesions that are generally 1 cm or less in diameter.

Examples include warts, nevi (moles), and molluscum contagiosum.

"Maculopapule" is a contradiction in terms, and the use of this term should be discouraged (an eruption may be described as being macular *and* papular, rather than "maculopapular").

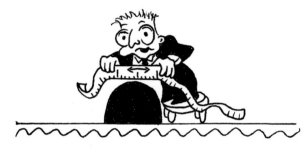

Nodules are solid palpable lesions that are generally 1 cm or more in diameter. They may be seen as an elevation or can be palpated within the skin. A **tumor** is a large nodule.

Examples include erythema nodosum, basal cell carcinoma, lipoma, and pyogenic granuloma.

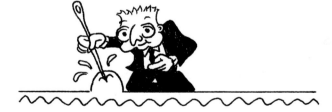

Vesicles (small blisters) are fluid-filled lesions generally 1 cm or less in diameter.

Examples include herpes simplex, acute tinea pedis, and chickenpox.

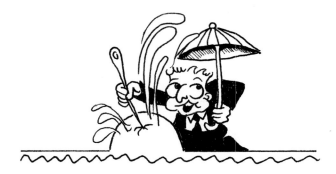

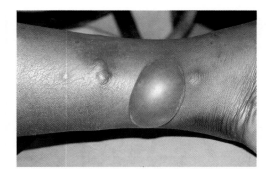

Bulla. Bullous insect bite reaction.

Bullae (large blisters) are fluid-filled lesions generally 1 cm or more in diameter.

Examples include herpes zoster, second-degree burns, and insect bite reactions.

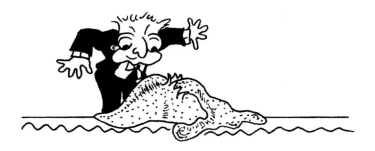

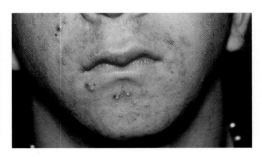

Pustule. Acne vulgaris.

Pustules are lesions that contain purulent, cloudy material (sometimes they may contain a hair and are then called follicular pustules).

Examples include acne and folliculitis.

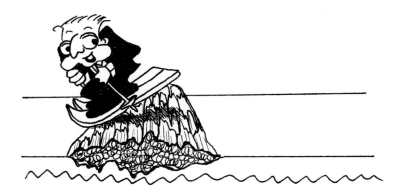

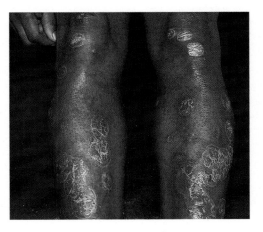

Plaque. Psoriasis vulgaris. Silvery plaques.

Plaques are solid, elevated, flat-topped, plateaulike lesions that cover a fairly large area; they may arise from papules that join together or arise *de novo*.

Examples include chronic eczematous dermatitis and psoriasis.

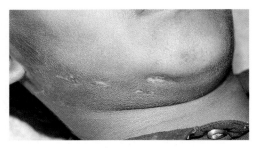

Atrophic plaque. Morphea (localized scleroderma).

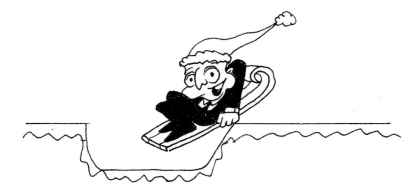

Atrophic plaques are depressed plaques.

Discoid lupus erythematosus and morphea often form atrophic plaques.

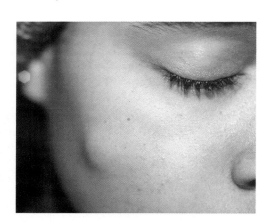

Wheal. Urticaria.

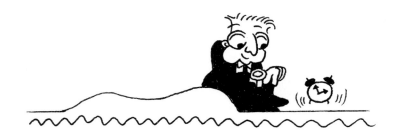

Wheals are raised flesh-colored or erythematous papules or plaques that are transient lesions. They generally last less than 24 hours, during which time they may change shape and size.

Wheals include urticaria (hives) and angioedema.

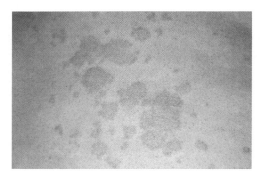

Cyst. Epidermoid cyst.

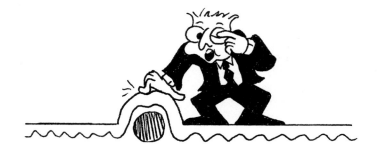

Cysts are walled-off lesions containing fluid or semisolid material. (They feel like an eyeball.)

Examples include pilar and epidermoid cysts.

SECONDARY (MODIFIED) LESIONS

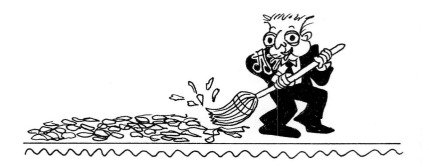

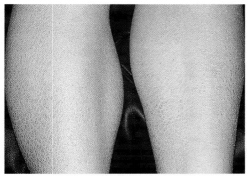

Scale. Ichthyosis vulgaris.

Scales (desquamation) comprise the outer layer of epidermis, which is imperceptibly shed daily. In many dermatologic conditions, abnormal accumulation or shedding of visible epidermis is called scale.

Examples include dandruff, psoriasis, and ichthyosis.

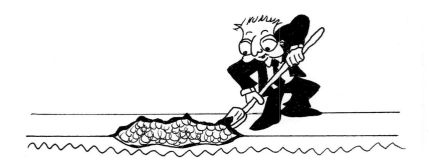

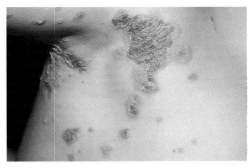

Crust. Bullous impetigo.

Crusts (scabs) are formed from blood, serum, or other dried exudate. Honey-colored crusts (impetiginization) are a sign of superficial infection.

Examples include excoriated or infected insect bites and resolving bullous lesions of impetigo.

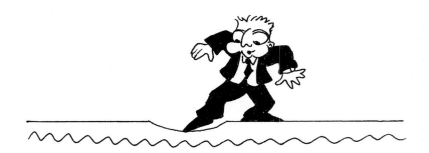

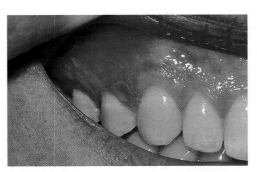

Erosion. Aphthous stomatitis ("canker sore").

Erosions are shallow losses of tissue involving only the epidermis ("topsoil"). They are nonscarring and often evolve from blisters and pustules.

For example, the secondary lesions of herpes simplex, herpes zoster, and lesions of aphthous stomatitis are erosions.

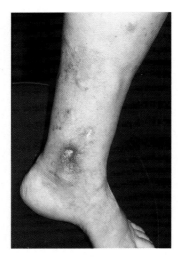

Ulcer. Venous stasis ulcer.

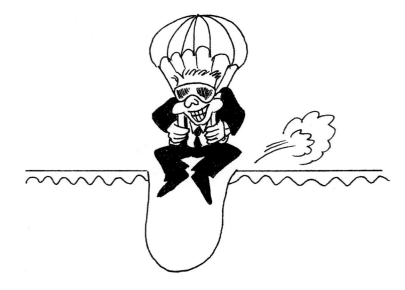

Ulcers are defects deeper than erosions. Ulcers involve the dermis or deeper layers and usually heal with scarring.

Examples include pyoderma gangrenosum and venous stasis ulcers.

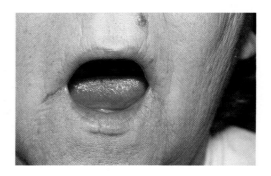

Fissure. Angular stomatitis (perlèche).

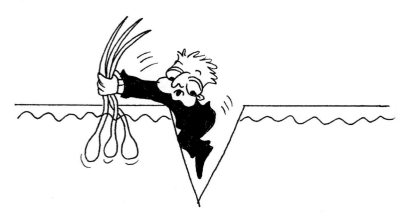

Fissures are linear ulcers or cracks in the skin. They are often painful.

They are seen in eczematous dermatitis of the fingers and at the angles of the mouth (perlèche).

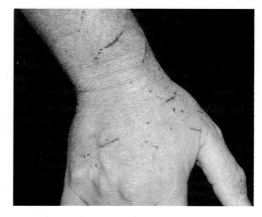

Excoriation. Cat scratches.

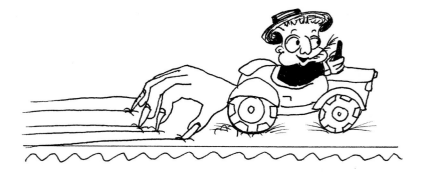

Excoriations are linear or punctate erosions induced by scratching.

Excoriations are seen as a result of scratching or picking at acne lesions, insect bites, or cat scratches.

Reaction Patterns, Shapes, and Configurations

Diseased skin has a limited number of clinical manifestations, and many skin disorders tend to occur in characteristic shapes, distributions, arrangements, and *reaction patterns* that often serve as diagnostic clues.

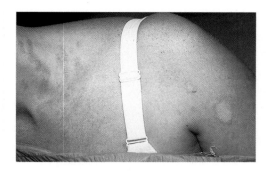

Papulosquamous reaction pattern.
Pityriasis rosea.

REACTION PATTERNS

The system of using reaction patterns is often inexact, and there is a great deal of overlap. However, using reaction patterns to describe individual skin lesions or eruptions often helps greatly in formulating a differential diagnosis.

Papulosquamous (maculosquamous) reaction patterns refer to eruptions in which the primary lesions consist of macules with scale (following the strict definition, a macule with scale is a plaque).

Thus, a papulosquamous reaction pattern suggests a diagnosis from a list that includes the following differential diagnoses: *psoriasis, tinea corporis, tinea versicolor, lichen planus, parapsoriasis, mycosis fungoides, and pityriasis rosea.*

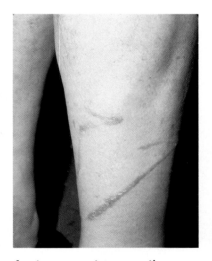

Acute eczematous reaction pattern. Poison ivy.

Eczematous reaction patterns are a little more difficult than papulosquamous patterns to describe (see Chapter 2, "Eczema"), because they may have various presentations and, at times, may be impossible to distinguish from papulosquamous patterns.

- **Acute and subacute eczema.** *Examples include erythematous "juicy" papules or plaques and/or weeping vesicobullous lesions such as seen in an acute contact dermatitis such as poison ivy.*

- **Chronic eczema.** The hallmark lesion of chronic eczematous dermatitis caused by scratching is lichenification, a plaque with an exaggeration of the normal skin markings that looks like the bark of a tree. *The lesions seen in atopic dermatitis and lichen simplex chronicus are the classic examples.*

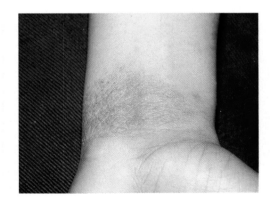

Chronic eczematous reaction pattern.
Atopic dermatitis.

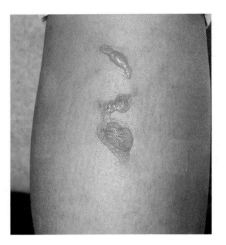

Vesicobullous reaction pattern.
Second-degree burn resulting from
spilled coffee.

Vesicobullous reaction patterns consist of blisters. However, lesions noted at an early stage may be erythematous macules or papules that later become filled with fluid.

A second-degree burn is a good example.

Dermal reaction patterns are characterized by lesions or eruptions that are confined to the dermis.

Examples include granuloma annulare and cutaneous sarcoidosis.

Subcutaneous reaction patterns are characterized by lesions or eruptions that are confined to the cutis (subcutaneous tissue).

Examples include erythema nodosum and lipomas.

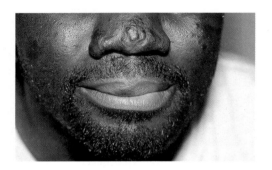

Dermal reaction pattern. Cutaneous sarcoidosis.

Vascular reaction patterns refer to erythema or edema resulting from changes in the vasculature, such as vasodilatation.

Examples include first-degree burns, viral exanthem, urticaria, erythema multiforme, and drug rashes.

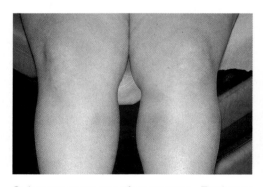

Subcutaneous reaction pattern. Erythema nodosum. Very tender red lumps.

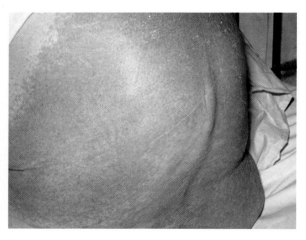

Vascular reaction pattern. Drug rash.

SHAPE OF LESIONS

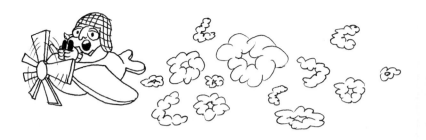

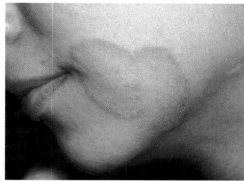

Annular and **arciform** are terms used to describe lesions that are ring-shaped or semiannular.

Examples include annular and arciform lesions frequently noted in urticaria, granuloma annulare, and tinea corporis (ringworm).

Annular lesion. Tinea faciale. Annular lesion.

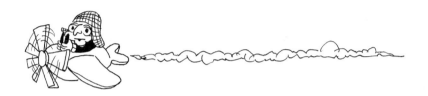

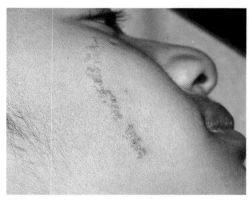

Linear shapes may result from exogenous agents, excoriations, and congenital growths.

Examples include poison ivy, dermographism, and epidermal nevus.

Linear lesion. Linear epidermal nevus.

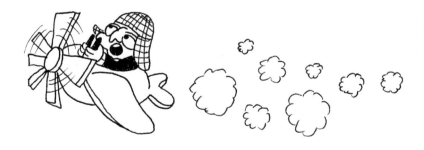

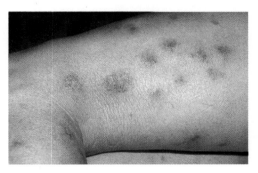

Nummular is a term that describes coin-shaped lesions.

Examples include lesions seen in discoid lupus erythematosus, psoriasis, and nummular eczema.

Nummular lesions. Coin-shaped lesions of nummular eczema.

The arrangement (configuration) of lesions is the interrelationship of multiple lesions.

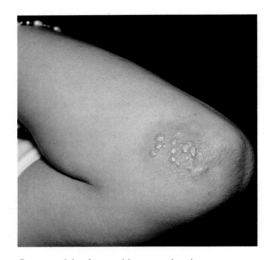

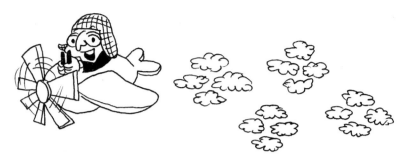

Grouped lesions are noted in "herpetiform" and "zosteriform" vesicles. *Examples are seen in herpes simplex and herpes zoster infections. Grouping is also noted in insect bites.*

Grouped lesions. Herpes simplex. Grouped vesicles.

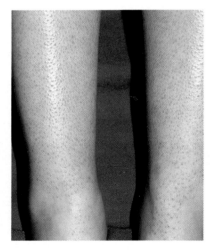

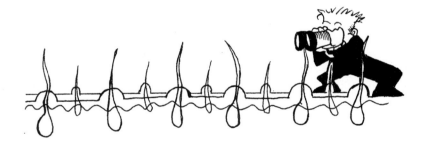

Follicular arrangement of lesions involves hair follicles. Lesions are often papular or pustular, with a central emerging hair. Lesions are spaced at fairly equal distances apart in a gridlike pattern *Keratosis pilaris and folliculitis are examples.*

Follicular lesions. Folliculitis resulting from leg waxing. Note the gridlike pattern.

Topical Therapy and Topical Steroids

Overview

Topical therapy, the mainstay in the treatment of many dermatologic conditions, traditionally has been the bailiwick of dermatologists. Thus, it is no surprise that an understanding of the appropriate use and abuse of these agents has been either neglected or misunderstood among the remainder of health care professionals. The following is an attempt to provide a practical overview of topical therapy. The primary focus is on the use of topical steroids.

General Principles of Topical Therapy

BASICS

- Topical therapy is generally safer than systemic therapy.
- Creams are generally more popular than ointments because they are less greasy; however, they are usually less potent than ointments.
- The application amount of a topical preparation does not affect its penetration or potency. The more thickly a preparation is applied, the more of it is wasted: Only the thin layer that is in intimate contact with the skin is absorbed; the remainder is rubbed off. More is not always better!
- Once- or twice-daily applications are usually sufficient with most preparations. (Sunscreens and some moisturizers are applied more frequently.)

Vehicles

- The active drug is combined with a vehicle, or base; these vehicles vary in their ability to "deliver" to the target site in the skin.
- The rate of penetration and of absorption of a topical preparation into the skin depends on how occlusive its vehicle is (discussion to follow) and on how readily the vehicle releases the active chemical.
- The vehicle should be cosmetically acceptable and nonsensitizing; it also must hold the drug in a stable solution.

Wet Dressings

- There is some validity to the old adage: "If it's dry, wet it; if it's wet, dry it."
- Wet dressings help to dry wounds, and they aid in the débridement of wounds by removing debris (e.g., serum, crusts). They also have a nonspecific antifungal and antibacterial effect, especially when chemicals such as aluminum sulfate, silver nitrate, acetic acid (vinegar is a dilute acetic acid), and potasium permanganate are added to them.
- Application of **Burow's solution** (aluminum sulfate and calcium acetate) helps to dry out lesions that are weeping and oozing (e.g., poison ivy, tinea pedis, herpes simplex, herpes zoster) or impetiginized (e.g., impetigo, infected stasis ulcers). It is available without a prescription. However, plain unsterilized tap water may serve as a less expensive, readily available—although probably less effective—alternative, if Burow's solution is not available (see the appropriate handout in Appendix A, "Patient Handouts").

Topical Steroids

MECHANISM OF ACTION

Topical steroids have two basic mechanisms of action: antiinflammatory and antimitotic.

- Antiinflammatory properties are of particular importance when they are used to treat eczematous and other primarily inflammatory conditions.
- Antimitotic properties of topical steroids help to reduce the buildup of scale, as in the treatment of psoriasis, a condition that is both inflammatory and hyperproliferative (has rapid cell division).

GENERAL PRINCIPLES

- Topical steroids are used to treat most inflammatory dermatoses. They are the cornerstone of therapy in dermatology, and, when used properly, they are quite safe.
- The unwanted effects of topical steroids are directly related to their potencies.
- When possible, the lowest-potency steroid should be used for the shortest possible time. Conversely, one should avoid using a preparation that is not potent enough to treat an intended condition.
- Occlusion (discussed later) increases hydration and hydration increases penetration, which, in turn, increases efficacy.

- Tachyphylaxis (tolerance) occurs when the medication loses its efficacy with continued use. It is most often seen in the treatment of psoriasis and other chronic conditions when very strong topical steroids are used for prolonged periods.
- To help minimize tachyphylaxis, dosing may be cycled (**pulse dosing**). The preparation is applied until the dermatosis clears and then is resumed on recurrence. A preparation may also be used intermittently (**intermittent dosing**), such as on weekends. Another option is to use a lower-potency topical steroid for maintenance.

Potencies
- Fluorinated topical steroids are generally more potent than other topical steroids. For example, triamcinolone acetonide, which contains a fluoride ion, is 100 times more potent than nonfluorinated hydrocortisone.
- When one is treating children and elderly patients, extra measures should be taken to avoid the use of potent fluorinated compounds, when possible.
- Even without an added fluoride ion, certain molecular structural changes can increase potency in corticosteroids. For example, hydrocortisone valerate, which contains no fluoride ion, is almost as potent as triamcinolone acetonide.
- Only nonfluorinated, mild topical steroids should be applied to the face and, ideally, only for short periods of time, to avoid atrophy and steroid-induced rosacea. (However, this rule can be broken. For example, for the treatment of severe acute contact dermatitis of the face, a superpotent topical steroid used briefly may be preferable to a mild, ineffective topical agent or systemic drugs.)
- Thin eyelid skin requires the least potent preparations for the shortest periods of time. The intertriginous (skin touching skin) areas similarly respond to lower potencies because the apposition of skin surfaces acts like an occlusive dressing. The axillae and inguinal creases are particularly prone to higher absorption and resultant steroid atrophy.
- It is necessary to become familiar with only one or two agents from each potency group to manage most dermatoses.
- For severe dermatoses, a very potent steroid may be used to initiate therapy, and a less potent preparation may be used afterward for maintenance ("downward titration").
- Every potency group has a generic preparation that is generally more economical than the trade name preparation. There is some concern about the bioequivalence between trade and generic formulations, however.

Delivery (Percutaneous Penetration)
Topical steroids and other topical preparations are ineffective unless they are absorbed into the skin. Percutaneous penetration varies among individual patients, and it can be manipulated by changing the drug, the vehicle, the length of exposure, or the anatomic surface area to which the drug is applied. It also depends on whether the skin is inflamed and therefore is less of a barrier to penetration (e.g., eczematous skin). Penetration also varies with the presence or absence of occlusive dressings.

- The barrier to cutaneous penetration is the stratum corneum. The thicker the stratum corneum—as on the palms, soles, elbows, and knees—the harder it is for the topical agent to penetrate the skin.

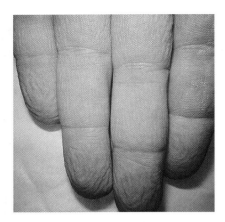

FIGURE I.1 Hydration. These fingers have been immersed in water for a prolonged period to increase the penetration of a topical drug. The corrugated appearance is probably the result of water absorption.

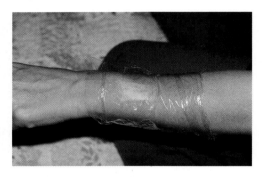

FIGURE I.2 Occlusion. A topical steroid cream has been applied, and a "nonbreathing" polyethylene wrap is used to cover it.

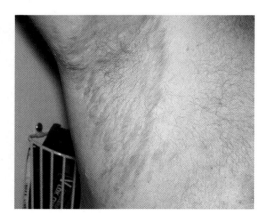

FIGURE I.3 Skin atrophy. Axillary striae. Linear atrophic scars may develop after repeated use of a potent topical steroid, particularly in an intertriginous (naturally occluded) area.

Hydration of the stratum corneum may be accomplished by two methods:

- **Soaking** or **bathing** an affected area before the application of a topical agent, generally a topical steroid. The wrinkling that develops after a hand or foot is immersed in water for a prolonged period results from the skin's increasing its surface area to accommodate the water it absorbs (Figure I.1).
- **Occlusion.** A "nonbreathing" polyethylene wrap such as Saran Wrap or Handi-Wrap, held in place by tape, a bandage, a sock, or an elastic (Ace) bandage, can provide occlusion to an area where topical steroids have been applied (Figure I.2). The wrap may be left on while the patient sleeps or worn several hours while the patient is awake. Specific areas may be occluded as follows:
  - A plastic shower cap can be used when the scalp is treated.
  - Cordran tape, which is impregnated with the steroid flurandrenolide, is helpful for occlusive therapy when relatively small areas are treated. However, it is expensive and can be uncomfortable when it is removed from hairy areas.
  - Rubber or vinyl gloves or finger cots may be used for the hands and fingers.
  - Small plastic bags such as Baggies may be used for the feet.
  - Occlusive garments (sauna suits) can be worn when extensive areas are involved.

A Cream, an Ointment, a Gel, or a Lotion?

- Creams are often preferred by patients for aesthetic reasons. Their water content, however, makes them more drying than ointments (oil-in-water preparations).
- Generally, ointments and gels are more potent than are creams or lotions, but their inherent greasiness often makes them cosmetically unacceptable. Ointments are helpful for dry skin conditions because of their occlusive properties. They are also more lubricating and tend to be less irritating and less sensitizing.
- Lotions, gels, aerosols, foams, and solutions are useful on hairy areas.
- They are easier than other preparations to apply to large areas.

Potential Side Effects

Possible adverse reactions to topical steroids are as follows:

- **Skin atrophy.** Epidermal atrophy is a local reaction demonstrated by shiny, thinned skin and telangiectasias. It rapidly reverses when the topical drugs are discontinued. Striae, or linear atrophic scars, may occur after repeated use of a potent topical steroid in one area. These permanent scars are seen most often in intertriginous areas, such as the axillae and groin, where the skin is generally thin, moist, and occluded (Figure I.3).

- **Acneform eruptions** of the face may occur (Figure I.4). Lesions resembling rosacea and perioral dermatitis may result from the regular use of topical fluorinated steroids on the face. These eruptions manifest as persistent erythema, papules, pustules, and telangiectasia. The condition often flares once the steroid is withdrawn *(rebound rosacea),* and it may not clear entirely for several months.
- **Ecchymoses** can occur. Purpura may be noted on the dorsal forearms after prolonged topical steroid use, particularly in elderly patients (Figure I.5).
- **Tinea incognito,** a superficial fungal infection, may be misdiagnosed because its clinical signs may be obscured by the use of topical steroids, which reduce inflammation and itching without killing the fungus.

Less Common Side Effects

- **Hypersensitivity reactions.** Allergic contact dermatitis to the steroid molecule may occur and may easily be overlooked. The hypersensitivity can be evoked by the steroid, the vehicle, or both, and it is often not suspected clinically. A clue to its presence is a lack of the expected antiinflammatory effect of the topical steroid.
- Other possible local effects of topical steroids are hypopigmentation, excess facial hair growth, and delayed wound healing.
- Extensive use of and occlusion with potent topical steroids may cause systemic adverse effects. Fortunately, these events rarely occur; in fact, hypothalamic-pituitary-adrenal axis suppression is quickly reversible and is unlikely to cause the same side effects as systemic steroid use.

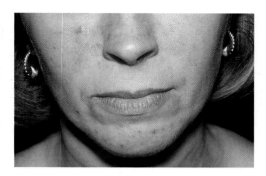

FIGURE I.4 Perioral dermatitis resembling rosacea. This reaction was caused by long-term use of a potent fluorinated topical steroid.

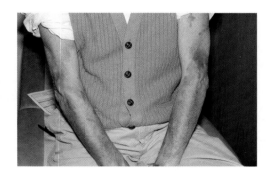

FIGURE I.5 Ecchymoses. Purpura on the dorsal forearms in this elderly patient occurred after prolonged topical steroid use.

POINT TO REMEMBER

- Intertriginous areas are naturally occluded, so less potent preparations are used in these areas to avoid atrophy.

HELPFUL HINTS

- Large amounts of triamcinolone cream and ointment may be purchased in 16-oz. (1-lb) jars, at considerable savings.
- Become familiar with only one or two agents from each potency group; that should be enough to treat most skin conditions that are responsive to topical steroids.
- How much cream, ointment, or lotion should one apply? Application should be thin, not thick—a little works as well as a lot.

Topical Immunomodulators

Concern exists about the long-term use of potent topical and oral corticosteroids in patients who have chronic dermatoses involving an extensive body surface. In addition, when a condition involves the face or intertriginous areas, high-potency steroid use may be an unwise choice that further limits therapeutic options.

- **Protopic (tacrolimus),** a potent nonsteroidal cytokine inhibitor, has been shown to be highly effective in the treatment and reducing the symptoms of atopic dermatitis. Its potential as a "topical steroid-sparing agent" may prove to be a great benefit in the management of other dermatoses as well. Protopic ointment in a 0.1% concentration has been approved for treatment in adults. A lower 0.03% concentration is designated for treatment in children (ages 2 years and older) and in adults for short-term and intermittent long-term therapy.
- **Elidel cream (pimecrolimus)** in a 1% formulation is another topical immunomodulator. It is approved for use in patients aged 2 years and older.

TOPICAL STEROIDS ("THE SHORT LIST")

The following agents should provide more than enough treatment options for the conditions discussed in this book. The table is by no means intended to be comprehensive.

POTENCY	GENERIC NAME	BRAND NAME
SUPERPOTENT	Clobetasol propionate cream/ointment 0.05%	Temovate
	Clobetasol propionate lotion	Temovate, Cormax scalp application
	Diflorasone diacetate ointment 0.05%	Psorcon
	Halobetasol propionate cream/ointment 0.05%	Ultravate
	Flurandrenolide (24- and 80-inch rolls)	Cordran tape 4 μg/cm^2
VERY STRONG	Desoximetasone cream/ointment 0.25%/gel 0.05%	Topicort
	Fluocinonide cream/ointment/solution/gel 0.05%	Lidex
STRONG	Triamcinolone acetate ointment 0.1%, cream 0.5%	Aristocort A
MEDIUM-STRONG	Hydrocortisone valerate ointment 0.2%, NF	Westcort
MILD-MEDIUM	Hydrocortisone valerate cream 0.2%, NF	Westcort
	Alclometasone dipropionate cream/ointment 0.05%, NF	Aclovate
	Desonide cream/ointment/lotion 0.05%, NF	DesOwen
MILD	Hydrocortisone cream/ointment/lotion 0.5%, 1.0%, 2.5%, NF	Hytone

Most preparations available in tubes of 15, 30, or 60 g; lotions are available in bottles of 20 to 60 mL.
NF, nonfluorinated.

Many topical steroids are available. However, all of them in the same group have roughly the same potency; they differ primarily in vehicle and price.

GENERIC NAME	BRAND NAME
GROUP I: SUPERPOTENT	
Betamethasone dipropionate gel/ointment 0.05%	Diprolene
Clobetasol propionate cream/ointment 0.05%	Temovate, Cormax, Clobevate
Clobetasol propionate lotion	Temovate, Cormax scalp application
Clobetasol propionate foam 0.05%	Olux foam
Diflorasone diacetate ointment 0.05%	Psorcon
Halobetasol propionate cream/ointment 0.05%	Ultravate
Flurandrenolide	Cordran tape
GROUP II: VERY HIGH-POTENCY	
Amcinonide ointment 0.1%	Cyclocort
Betamethasone dipropionate ointment 0.05%	Diprosone
Desoximetasone cream/ointment 0.25%/gel 0.05%	Topicort
Diflorasone diacetate cream 0.05%	Psorcon
Fluocinonide cream/ointment/gel 0.05%	Lidex
Halcinonide cream/ointment 0.1%	Halog
GROUP III: HIGH-POTENCY	
Betamethasone dipropionate cream 0.05%	Diprosone
Betamethasone valerate ointment 0.1%	Valisone
Diflorasone diacetate cream 0.05%	Florone, Maxiflor
Triamcinolone acetate ointment 0.1%, cream 0.5%	Aristocort A
GROUP IV: MID- TO HIGH-POTENCY	
Desoximetasone cream 0.05%	Topicort LP
Fluocinolone acetonide cream 0.2%	Synalar-HP
Fluocinolone acetonide ointment 0.025%	Synalar
Hydrocortisone valerate ointment 0.2%, NF	Westcort
Triamcinolone acetonide ointment 0.1%	Kenalog, Aristocort
Mometasone furoate cream 0.1%	Elocon
GROUP V: MID-POTENCY	
Betamethasone dipropionate lotion 0.05%	Diprosone
Betamethasone valerate cream/lotion 0.1%	Valisone
Fluticasone propionate 0.1% cream	Cutivate
Fluocinolone acetonide cream 0.025%	Synalar
Flurandrenolide cream 0.05%	Cordran SP
Hydrocortisone butyrate cream 0.1%, NF	Locoid
Hydrocortisone valerate cream 0.2%, NF	Westcort
Triamcinolone acetonide cream/lotion 0.1%	Kenalog
Triamcinolone acetonide cream 0.025%	Aristocort
GROUP VI: LOW-POTENCY	
Alclometasone dipropionate cream/ointment 0.05%, NF	Aclovate
Betamethasone 17-valerate lotion 0.1%	Valisone
Desonide cream 0.05%, NF	Tridesilon, DesOwen
Fluocinolone acetonide cream/solution 0.01%	Synalar
Mometasone furoate cream/ointment 0.1%, NF	Elocon
GROUP VII: WEAKEST-POTENCY	
Hydrocortisone cream/ointment/lotion 0.5%, 1.0%, 2.5%, NF	Hytone, Cortaid, Cortizone

NF, nonfluorinated.

PART ONE
Common Skin Conditions: Diagnosis and Management

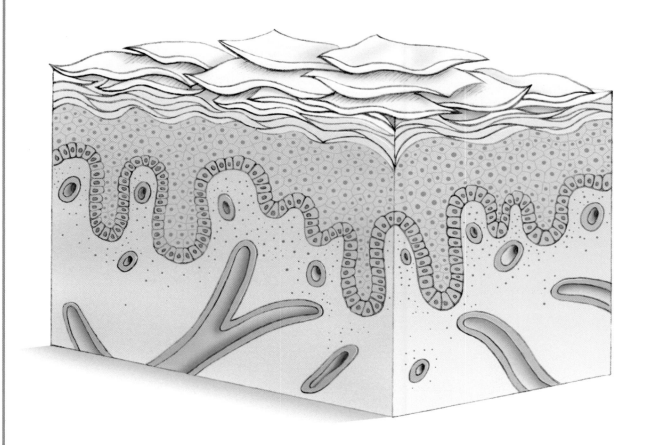

CHAPTER 1

Acne and Related Disorders

Overview

Acne, the most common skin disorder in the United States, is an embarrassing problem for many teenagers, but it is not limited to that age group. It may develop before puberty in either sex, or it may first be seen in adulthood, particularly in women.

Acne is a disorder that involves the hair-oil (pilosebaceous) apparatus of the skin. Acne vulgaris or common acne (referred to herein as adolescent acne) begins in the teen or preteen years and is readily diagnosed; its management, however, is frequently complex.

In general, acne becomes less active as adolescence ends, but it may continue into adulthood. Acne that initially occurs in adulthood is designated postadolescent acne or adult-onset acne. Despite the clinical similarities and occasional overlapping of adolescent and postadolescent acne, the pathogenesis and treatment of each type are somewhat different. Acnelike disorders, such as neonatal acne, drug-induced acne, rosacea, and other so-called acneiform conditions, are also considered separate entities because of differences in pathogenesis and treatment.

That being said, no clear lines separate the various types of acne; much of acne's features overlap and lie along a continuum. However, readers may find the following classifications useful for diagnostic and therapeutic purposes.

Classification

Adolescent Acne (Acne Vulgaris)

This includes preteen acne and adolescent acne that may persist into adulthood.

Postadolescent Acne

- Female adult-onset acne
- Male adult-onset acne (uncommon)

Acnelike Disorders

- Rosacea
- Perioral dermatitis
- Neonatal acne
- Drug-induced acne
- Endocrinopathic acne
- Physically induced and occupational acne
- Folliculitis
- Hidradenitis suppurativa
- Pseudofolliculitis barbae (see Chapter 10, "Hair and Scalp Disorders Resulting in Hair Loss")
- Acne keloidalis (see Chapter 10, "Hair and Scalp Disorders Resulting in Hair Loss")

ADOLESCENT ACNE (ACNE VULGARIS)

BASICS

This form of acne has a strong tendency to be hereditary and is less likely to be seen in Asians and dark-skinned people. It is a disorder of the sebaceous follicles. Lesions begin during adolescence when androgenic hormones cause abnormal follicular keratinization, which then blocks the sebaceous duct. This blockage results in a microcomedo (the microscopic primary lesion of adolescent acne). The microcomedo enlarges to become the visible comedo, which is the non-inflammatory blackhead or whitehead.

Alternatively, the microcomedo may become an inflammatory lesion, such as a papule or pustule. The development of inflammatory lesions is theoretically as follows: Androgenic hormones stimulate sebaceous glands to increase in size and function and thus to produce more sebum (oil).

The skin becomes oilier, and the microcomedo becomes more hospitable to the anaerobe *Propionibacterium acnes*. *P. acnes* then produce lipases that digest the lipids into fatty acids and cause a rupture of the microcomedo that incites a sterile inflammatory cell response in those adolescents who are genetically predisposed. Despite traditional beliefs, no evidence indicates that diet or a dirty face causes, or contributes to, adolescent acne.

Before our exploration of acne begins, it is helpful to dispel many of the myths and misconceptions about acne.

Acne Myths Versus Facts

Myth: Blackheads are caused by dirt.

Fact: They are black because of oxidized melanin. Blackheads, or open comedones, are collections of sebum and keratin that form within follicular openings and that, when exposed to air, become oxidized and turn black.

Myth: Frequent facials are beneficial.

Fact: Professional facials and at-home scrubs, astringents, and masks are generally not recommended because they tend to aggravate acne.

Myth: Cosmetics, particularly oil-based preparations, "clog pores" and cause acne.

Fact: Cosmetics probably pose much less of a problem to women's skin than was previously thought. Their use rarely, if ever, causes adult acne. More commonly, cosmetics can be irritants and may cause contact dermatitis.

Myth: Acne should disappear by the end of adolescence.

Fact: Some women have acne that persists well past adolescence. Others have an initial episode in their 20s or 30s. (Men who did not have acne in their teens rarely develop it after adolescence.)

Myth: Acne is caused or worsened by certain foods, such as chocolate, sweets, and greasy junk food.

Fact: Despite occasional personal anecdotes and persistent cultural myths, acne is probably not significantly influenced by diet.

Myth: A dirty face exacerbates acne; therefore, scrubbing the face daily will help to clear it up.

Fact: Scrubbing and rubbing a face that has acne, particularly inflammatory acne, will only irritate and redden an already inflamed complexion. Instead, the face should be washed daily with a gentle cleanser.

DESCRIPTION OF LESIONS

Acne lesions are designated as inflammatory or noninflammatory (comedonal), or a combination of the two.

Inflammatory Lesions
- **Papules:** Superficial red "pimples" that may have crusted, scabbed surfaces caused by picking or squeezing.
- **Pustules:** Superficial raised lesions containing purulent material, generally found in the company of papules (Figures 1.1 and 1.2).
- **"Cysts" (nodules):** Large, deep papules or pustules. Acne "cysts" are not really cysts. True cysts are neoplasms that have an epithelial lining. Acne cysts do not have an epithelial lining; they are composed of poorly organized, variously shaped and sized conglomerations of inflammatory material (Figure 1.3).
- **Macules:** The remains of formerly palpable inflammatory lesions that are in the process of healing from therapy or spontaneous resolution (Figure 1.4). They are flat, red or sometimes purple (violaceous) blemishes that slowly heal and may occasionally form a depressed (atrophic) scar.

Noninflammatory (Comedonal) Lesions
A comedo is a collection of sebum and keratin that forms within follicular ostia (pores).

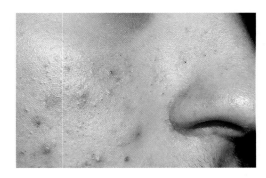

FIGURE 1.1 Adolescent acne. The face of this teenager shows oily skin, open and closed comedones, papules, and pustules.

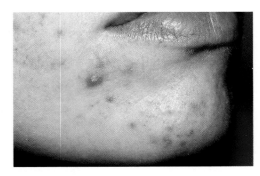

FIGURE 1.2 Inflammatory acne lesions. Papules, pustules, and closed comedones are all present on this patient.

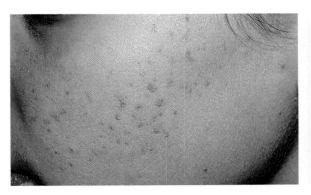

FIGURE 1.4 Mild to moderate inflammatory acne lesions. This patient exhibits small reddish purple macules—evidence of improvement resulting from treatment. The lesions are flat, red or sometimes purple (violaceous).

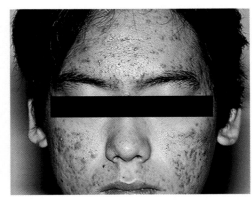

FIGURE 1.3 Severe cystic acne. This patient was subsequently treated with isotretinoin (Accutane).

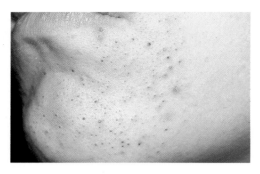

FIGURE 1.5 Noninflammatory lesions. The combination of open and closed comedones, as seen here, is most common in younger patients.

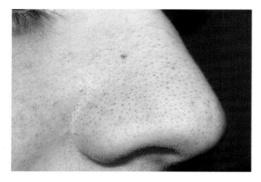

FIGURE 1.6 Follicular prominence. These are blackheadlike, dilated ostia (pores) that are frequently seen on the nose and cheeks in patients with acne.

- **Open comedones (blackheads):** Lesions with large ostia that are black not from dirt but from melanin (Figures 1.2 and 1.5).
- **Closed comedones (whiteheads):** Lesions with small ostia. A combination of both inflammatory and comedonal acne is most commonly seen in adolescent acne.
- **Follicular prominence:** Blackheadlike, dilated pores are frequently seen on the nose and cheeks in patients with acne (Figure 1.6).

Severity

Acne may be further classified as mild, moderate, or severe.

- **Mild acne** consists of comedones and/or occasional papules and pustules.
- **Moderate acne** is more inflammatory, with relatively superficial papules and/or pustules (papulopustular acne); comedones may also be present. Lesions may heal with scars.
- **Severe acne** (cystic or nodular acne, acne conglobata) has a greater degree, depth, and number of inflammatory lesions: papules, pustules, nodules, "cysts" (cystic acne), and possibly abscesses. Sinus tracts, significant scarring, and keloid formation may also be evident.

DISTRIBUTION OF LESIONS

- Acne most commonly erupts in areas of maximal sebaceous gland activity: the face, neck, chest, shoulders, back, and upper arms.
- In the more severe cases of acne, lesions tend to occur on the trunk as well as on the face.

CLINICAL MANIFESTATIONS AND SEQUELAE

- The more severe inflammatory lesions of acne are prone to heal with atrophic or pitted ("ice-pick") scars on the face and with hypertrophic scars or keloids on the trunk (Figure 1.7).
- Postinflammatory hyperpigmentation may occur, particularly in patients with darker skin (Figure 1.8).

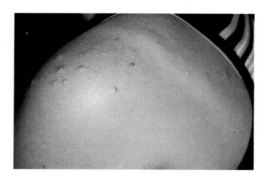

FIGURE 1.7 Acne scars. Hypertrophic scars are seen on the shoulder of this patient.

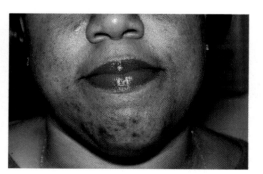

FIGURE 1.8 Acne. Postinflammatory hyperpigmentation is seen in this African-American patient.

- Moderate to severe involvement of the chest and back predict that the patient will have a poorer prognosis and will be more difficult to treat (Figure 1.9).
- Paramount are the negative psychologic effects of acne (e.g., lowered self-esteem) and their impact on limiting employment opportunities and social functioning.

DIAGNOSIS

- Adolescent acne is easy for the patient and practitioner to recognize; however, specific underlying causes of acne (e.g., polycystic ovarian syndrome) should be considered in certain female patients (see later).

 DIFFERENTIAL DIAGNOSIS

Keratosis pilaris (see Chapter 2, "Atopic Dermatitis")
- Lesions are small, follicular, horny spines. The tiny papules may resemble acne when they are inflamed (Figure 1.10).
- Lesions of keratosis pilaris are most often seen on the upper outer arms, back, thighs, and lateral face.
- In children, the lateral sides of the cheeks are frequently involved.
- Keratosis pilaris is more common in atopic patients.

Folliculitis and rosacea (see later)

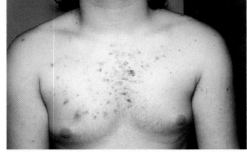

FIGURE 1.9 Severe cystic acne. This patient's severe acne shows early signs of significant scarring.

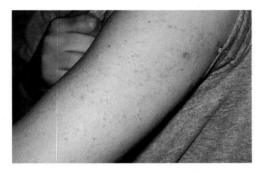

FIGURE 1.10 Keratosis pilaris. These are acnelike lesions seen on the upper outer arms.

MANAGEMENT

Goals
The three main therapeutic goals are as follows:

- To prevent scarring
- To help to improve the patient's appearance
- To make every effort to control acne with topical therapy alone

General Principles
- Treatment of acne should be individualized and frequently involves a "trial and error" approach beginning with those agents that are known to be most effective, least expensive, and having the fewest side effects.
- Acne is a multifactorial disease. Therefore, appropriate therapy often involves the use of more than one agent, each of which targets a different pathogenic factor.
- Mild acne can often be managed successfully with over-the-counter remedies.
- Every effort should be made to control acne topically if possible or to try tapering oral medications as soon as control is achieved.
- The patient should be advised not to squeeze or pick lesions.

Topical Treatment Modalities for Acne: Principles
Notwithstanding the testimonials seen on late-night television infomercials for acne preparations, no "one-size-fits-all" treatment for acne exists. In fact, the active ingredients in these advertised preparations can usually be obtained less expensively in other over-the-counter products. Over-the-counter products effectively manage many cases of mild acne, but prescription medications may be required for severe cases.

First-Line Topical Agents
When one is choosing a treatment for the various types of acne, the modes of action of each agent should be considered. Dermatologists generally employ these preparations in various combinations and in conjunction with oral antibiotics, if necessary.

Benzoyl Peroxide
Potent antibacterial agents, benzoyl peroxide preparations (Table 1.1) improve both inflammatory and noninflammatory lesions (comedones).

- They dry and peel the skin, and they help to clear blocked follicles.
- Benzoyl peroxide may be used alone to treat mild acne, but for more severe cases, it should be used in conjunction with topical retinoids, as well as topical or systemic antibiotics.
- Lower-strength (e.g., 2.5%) preparations are less irritating than, and probably are as effective as, the 5% and 10% concentrations.
- The addition of zinc to benzoyl peroxide in several newer products, such as Triaz, may enhance efficacy.
- Benzoyl peroxide is also available in combination with erythromycin (Benzamycin) and clindamycin (BenzaClin).

Benzoyl peroxide is an ingredient of many brand-name over-the-counter products, such as Clearasil and Oxy 5 and 10, as well as less expensive generic products. These products include both water- and alcohol-based vehicles; some are soaps, medicated pads, and washes. The soaps and washes may not be as effective as the lotions, creams, or gels, which will not wash off the skin as readily. Some patients prefer tinted formulations that can be used as concealers.

Prescription benzoyl peroxide formulations are probably no more effective than over-the-counter products. Bear in mind, however, that generic products may vary from batch to batch in terms of quality control and inert ingredients.

How to Use Benzoyl Peroxide
- Beginning with a lower-strength preparation, benzoyl peroxide is applied sparingly once or twice daily, in a thin layer across the acne-prone areas.
- Irritation and burning are not uncommon, but they usually resolve in 2 to 3 weeks.

Topical Retinoids
- The retinoids (Table 1.2) are primarily comedolytic (i.e., they treat comedones); they also have antiinflammatory effects.
- In addition, retinoids facilitate the penetration of, and may be used in combination with, other topical antiacne agents.
- These agents help to "plump up" the skin and make enlarged pores (follicular prominence) less obvious.
- All retinoids may produce sun sensitivity.
- These prescription drugs should not be used during pregnancy or breast-feeding (although no studies have shown them to be harmful to the fetus).

Retin-A is the standard to which other retinoids are compared because it was the first one available. The retinoid adapalene, found in Differin cream and gel, is as effective as tretinoin and appears to be better tolerated. In addition, the tretinoin products Retin-A Micro and Avita have been formulated to reduce the potential for irritation by incorporating tretinoin into new delivery vehicles.

(continued)

MANAGEMENT (*continued*)

How to Use Topical Retinoids
Topical retinoids are applied once daily, usually at bedtime.

- Patients who exhibit sensitivity may use it every other day, or less frequently, until they develop tolerance.
- The area of application should first be washed and thoroughly dried.
- Treatment usually starts with a lower-strength tretinoin 0.025% or adapalene 0.1% cream; in time, higher concentrations of tretinoin can be used as tolerated.
- Side effects may include erythema, dryness, and peeling. These usually resolve after 3 weeks.
- Use of a sunscreen should be advised, because tretinoin and adapalene may cause photosensitivity in some patients.

Topical Antibiotics
Preparations that contain the topical antibiotics clindamycin and erythromycin (Table 1.3) are active against *P. acnes*.

- In addition to their antibacterial action, these drugs have an antiinflammatory action that helps to clear inflammatory acne lesions (papules and pustules).
- Topical antibiotics can also be used to treat rosacea, perioral dermatitis, folliculitis, shaving bumps, and other acnelike conditions.
- Clindamycin and erythromycin are considered equally effective.
- Drug resistance has been reported with these antibiotics.

How to Use Topical Antibiotics
- These agents are applied once or twice daily, in a thin layer across the acne-prone areas.
- Irritation and burning are uncommon and may be avoided by using an ointment-based erythromycin such as Akne-Mycin or clindamycin (Cleocin T) in a lotion preparation.
- Topical antibiotics are often used as maintenance therapy after an initial course with a systemic antibiotic.
- Topical antibiotics are available in a variety of vehicles, including creams, lotions, ointments, gels, and solutions. This variety allows physicians to prescribe according to patient skin type and preference.

Combination of Topical Antibiotic and Benzoyl Peroxide (Table 1.4)
- Erythromycin and clindamycin are the most commonly prescribed topical antibiotics that are effective against mild inflammatory acne.

- However, as with other antibiotics, *P. acnes* can become resistant to both erythromycin and clindamycin.
- By combining these agents with benzoyl peroxide, bacterial resistance can be avoided; furthermore, there appears to be a synergistic effect (the combination appears to be more effective than either drug used alone) when clindamycin and erythromycin are combined with benzoyl peroxide.

How to Use Combination of Topical Antibiotic and Benzoyl Peroxide
- These preparations are applied sparingly in the morning and evening to acne-prone areas.
- The same cautions apply as for benzoyl peroxide. Dryness, erythema, and pruritus appear in about 3% of patients.

Other Topical Prescription Drugs
- Other topical prescription antiacne or antirosacea drugs (Table 1.5) include newer agents, such as azelaic acid, and older preparations that contain sulfur and sodium sulfacetamide.
- These medications are used as alternatives or adjuncts to retinoids, benzoyl peroxide, and topical clindamycin and erythromycin. They are second-line therapy for acne.
- Formulations with metronidazole, whose mechanism of action is not understood, are first-line topical treatments for rosacea.

Systemic Acne Therapies: Principles
Most patients with acne are treated with topical agents; however, patients who have moderate to severe acne that is unresponsive to topical treatment alone, or acne that tends to scar, must usually be given systemic therapy (Table 1.6). Furthermore, significant acne that occurs on the chest or back generally requires oral antibiotics because it does not respond to topical therapy as readily as does facial acne.

- The oral retinoid 13-*cis*-retinoic acid is reserved for more severe, recalcitrant disease.
- Hormonal agents, such as oral contraceptives, and antiandrogenic drugs, such as spironolactone, may also be prescribed in carefully selected situations.

Compared with topical therapy, systemic therapy has a more rapid onset of improvement, which may enhance patient compliance. However, whenever systemic drugs are administered, the potential dangers—including side effects, drug allergy or intolerance, drug interactions, and fetal exposure in women who are or who may become pregnant—must be carefully considered.

(continued)

A risk-to-benefit calculation is particularly important whenever you are treating a benign condition, such as acne.

When systemic therapy is used for acne, oral and topical agents are often given simultaneously. The objective, if possible, is to discontinue or taper the oral agent based on the clinical response.

Antibiotics

Oral antibiotics are used in the management of moderate to severe acne and acnelike disorders, such as rosacea. Tetracyclines are the usual drug of choice; of the tetracyclines, minocycline is considered to be the most effective. Both tetracyclines and the less frequently used erythromycin preparations inhibit the growth of *P. acnes,* and this inhibition decreases free fatty acid production and pustule formation.

In addition, these antibiotics have a significant antiinflammatory action—they inhibit the chemotactic response of neutrophils. This action is evident when tetracycline and erythromycin rapidly clear rosacea, perioral dermatitis, and other dermatoses in which pathogenic microbes have not been identified.

Broad-spectrum antibiotics alter intestinal flora, and they have been reported to interfere with the absorption and, thus, the efficacy of oral contraceptives. However, this information is based primarily on anecdotal evidence, and a recent study concluded that the antibiotics used to treat acne probably do not interfere with the efficacy of oral contraceptives. Nevertheless, patients taking oral antibiotics should be advised of this controversy so they can decide whether they wish to use an alternative or additional form of birth control.

The safety of oral antibiotics is another source of concern. Because antiacne oral antibiotics are frequently used on a long-term basis (in some instances, for years), patients and their families are justifiably anxious about the consequences. Overall, these drugs have a long record of safety, and studies have indicated that routine laboratory supervision of healthy young people given long-term tetracycline therapy is not necessary.

When treatment extends for more than 1 to 2 years, however, some dermatologists recommend periodically monitoring liver function and measuring antinuclear antibody levels. The frequency of monitoring should be greater in patients with a history of hepatic, renal, or collagen vascular disease. In addition, patients with a history of candidal vulvovaginitis should be advised that broad-spectrum antibiotics could permit the vulvovaginitis to recur.

Less commonly used antibiotics for acne are the cephalosporins and penicillins, particularly ampicillin. The use of azithromycin as 4- or 5-day pulse therapy in women who have monthly premenstrual acne flares has gained some interest.

Clindamycin and oral sulfonamides are also quite effective oral antiacne agents. However, the former has been associated with pseudomembranous colitis, and the latter may precipitate severe hypersensitivity reactions. Thus, these agents are not recommended in most situations.

Tetracyclines

- Tetracyclines are the staples of systemic acne therapy.
- Tetracyclines have the disadvantage of staining teeth in children younger than 9 years and, in fact, they may temporarily stain the teeth of older patients, particularly those with orthodontic braces.
- When tetracyclines are prescribed, the importance of good dental hygiene, including flossing, should be stressed.
- Tetracyclines may also cause gastrointestinal irritation, phototoxic reactions (an increased tendency to sunburn), and vulvovaginitis.

Generic tetracycline and brand-name preparations such as Achromycin and Terramycin are the least expensive of the tetracyclines. These formulations should be taken on an empty stomach (1 hour before or 2 hours after meals) and not with dairy products or divalent cations, such as iron, magnesium, zinc, or calcium-containing compounds—all of which may interfere with absorption. Esophageal irritation may be avoided by taking tetracycline with a full glass of water.

Tetracycline has been implicated in the development of benign intracranial hypertension (pseudotumor cerebri), particularly when it is given concurrently with 13-*cis*-retinoic acid.

Minocycline

This tetracycline antibiotic is more expensive but more effective than plain tetracycline for treating inflammatory acne. Minocycline's excellent absorption allows it to be taken with food, and it causes few, if any, phototoxic problems. It also appears to be less likely to induce candidal vulvovaginitis than plain tetracycline. However, minocycline is more likely than plain tetracycline to cause such side effects as nausea, vomiting, and, in high doses (those that approach 200 mg/d), dizziness resulting from vestibular dysfunction.

Less common, long-term treatment with minocycline may cause a reversible bluish hyperpigmentation of the gums and/or skin. In rare cases, it is associated with benign intracranial hypertension and hepatitis. Also rarely, long-term treatment may engender a lupuslike syndrome that is antinuclear antibody positive

(*continued*)

and that clears on discontinuation of the drug. This syndrome, which occurs most often in young women, usually develops late in the course of therapy and has rarely proved fatal.

No data support the hypothesis that minocycline worsens the natural course of systemic lupus erythematosus.

Doxycycline

Somewhat less expensive and probably less effective than minocycline, doxycycline is well absorbed and may be taken with food. Its main disadvantage is its phototoxic potential—the highest of the tetracyclines. Patients should be advised regarding sun protection. Vestibular dysfunction, hyperpigmentation, and the lupuslike syndrome associated with minocycline have not been reported with doxycycline. Benign intracranial hypertension has been reported.

Erythromycin

This drug is a useful second-line alternative when tetracycline fails or is not tolerated, when the patient is younger than 10 years, or when the patient is pregnant. Although it is always best to avoid, whenever possible, the use of systemic drugs in a woman who is pregnant, trying to become pregnant, or breast-feeding, in exceptional circumstances, erythromycin can be given.

Hormonal Treatment

Oral contraceptives or systemic antiandrogens (e.g., spironolactone) are used in women in whom hormonal treatment may be an effective alternative or adjuvant to antibiotics and oral retinoids. Hormonal treatment is an option when conventional topical and systemic therapies are not working or when an endocrine abnormality is found (see Chapter 11, "Hirsutism").

Cyproterone

An acetate steroidal androgen receptor blocker and potent progestin, cyproterone acts as a competitive inhibitor of testosterone and dehydroepiandrosterone at the level of androgen receptors. Diane-35, an oral contraceptive that is very effective in the treatment of acne but is not available in the United States, contains a combination of cyproterone acetate and ethinyl estradiol.

Accutane (13-*cis*-Retinoic Acid)

Also known as isotretinoin, 13-*cis*-retinoic acid is an oral synthetic derivative of vitamin A that promotes long-term remissions in severe nodular acne. It should be reserved for patients with severe nodular acne unresponsive to conventional therapy. Related acnelike conditions, such as severe rosacea and hidradenitis suppurativa, may also respond to 13-*cis*-retinoic acid, but to a lesser degree than acne. The efficacy of 13-*cis*-retinoic acid in patients with previously unresponsive acne is often profound and long lasting. In the United States, the drug is generally taken for 20 weeks; in Europe, 13-*cis*-retinoic acid is given until a total dosage of 120 to 140 mg/kg is reached.

Side Effects

Although common, side effects with 13-*cis*-retinoic acid are usually tolerable. Most patients experience cutaneous and mucous membrane inflammation and desquamation. Cheilitis, conjunctivitis, and dry skin may lead to nose bleeds, dry eyes, and itching. In general, these reactions are well tolerated because the drug is so effective that patients want to continue taking it despite any side effects. Less commonly, a patient will experience musculoskeletal and joint pains. In rare cases, hair loss may occur, but hair almost always grows back.

Systemic abnormalities in lipid levels may be seen with the use of 13-*cis*-retinoic acid. Approximately 25% of patients experience serum triglyceride elevations, and 15% have decreases in high-density lipoprotein levels. Pseudotumor cerebri, inflammatory bowel disease, hyperostosis, and ophthalmic changes, including corneal opacities and sudden alterations in night vision, are less frequent complaints.

Rare but troubling reports of depression and suicidal thoughts and acts have been associated with this drug. Patients and their families should be notified to report any depressive or unusual mental behaviors. Most important, 13-*cis*-retinoic acid is a teratogen that is absolutely contraindicated before and during pregnancy and for several months after childbirth. Central nervous system malformations, skull abnormalities, cardiovascular conditions, and cleft palate are but a few of reported fetal abnormalities caused by this drug. Thus, any clinician who is considering administering this drug should consider consulting with or referring the patient to a dermatologist. Dermatologists require that female patients who wish to take this teratogen be advised about birth control methods, and they often also require that patients take oral contraceptives before starting treatment. Before and during the course of treatment, repeated pregnancy tests are performed.

Other Therapeutic Modalities
Comedo Extraction (Acne Surgery)

- This has been performed less commonly since the arrival of topical retinoids. Removal of open comedones does not seem to influence the course of acne.

(continued)

MANAGEMENT (*continued*)

Intralesional Corticosteroid Injection

- Intralesional injections of glucocorticosteroids, introduced with a syringe and a 30-gauge needle, can reduce the inflammatory response and can decrease the size of deep nodular lesions.

- The recommended dose is of a triamcinolone acetate suspension is given in a concentration of 2.5 mg/mL, to avoid local steroid atrophy. For patients with severe disease and considerable scarring, the concentration can be increased to 5 or 10 mg/mL.

Further Acne Facts

- Because acne is a visible disease, patients may suffer from anxiety, impaired self-image, depression, employment insecurities, social withdrawal, self-destructive behaviors, and even suicidal ideation.
- Acne tends to improve temporarily during summer. Exposure to the sun, in small doses, diminishes acne, and tanning promotes a blending of skin tones.
- Fall and winter acne flare-ups are quite common and are often influenced by mood swings.
- Adult acne is often more persistent than is teenage acne.
- Severe, unremitting, scarring acne is more prevalent among men.
- Acne, hirsutism, and irregular menstrual periods may be associated with hyperandrogenism and/or polycystic ovaries.

 POINTS TO REMEMBER

- Because topical antibiotics are most effective in preventing the formation of *new* acne lesions, the patient should be informed that a significant therapeutic response may require 6 to 8 weeks.
- Every effort should be made to try tapering oral medications as soon as acne is controlled.
- In darkly pigmented people, the severity of inflammation may be equivalent to, but not as apparent as, that in persons with fairer complexions. Consequently, African-American patients are often as concerned about the acne-related pigmentary changes as they are about the acne itself.
- If there is evidence of scarring, acne should be treated more aggressively (even mild acne can heal with significant scarring).
- Acne on the chest and back is more difficult to treat and often portends a worse prognosis.
- Skin care should be kept simple and gentle with the use of mild soaps; loofahs, Buff-Puffs, and harsh soaps are to be avoided.
- The two Hs—hormones and heredity—underlie teenage acne (one or both parents probably had acne), and not the proverbial bad diet and dirty face—the two Ds.

 HELPFUL HINTS

- Tazarotene may be applied for 2 to 3 minutes and then washed off. This short-contact treatment appears to work quite well and helps to avoid retinoid irritation.
- Retinoids may make acne appear to be worse; therefore, inflammatory lesions should be approached first because they are usually the first to respond, and their quick disappearance can be helpful in obtaining compliance in teenagers.
- "Rollercoastering," defined herein as titrating or fine-tuning the dosage of oral antibiotics such as tetracycline, minocycline, and erythromycin, may help to minimize potential side effects and the total dosage of the medication. For example, a dosage schedule can begin as 50 mg minocycline capsules—two in the morning and one in the evening. This regimen will allow for an increase of an additional 50 mg when the patient is next seen in a follow-up visit. If there is marked improvement, the dosage can be titrated downward.

 SEE PATIENT HANDOUT, PAGE 437

POSTADOLESCENT ACNE (ADULT-ONSET ACNE)

BASICS

Dermatologists regularly hear the lament "Acne, at my age!" expressed by women in whom acne suddenly appears or in whom acne has not resolved by the age of 20 years. The prevalence of female adult acne has increased significantly in the past several generations. Proposed hypotheses to explain this apparent increase include the following:

- The entry of women into the workforce and its attendant stresses
- The later ages at which women are having children
- The use of oral contraceptives
- The proliferation of food additives and the injection of hormones and antibiotics into livestock

There is little question that acne is influenced by hormones. For example, many women report premenstrual or (less commonly) midcycle flares of inflammatory acne. Pregnancy, oral contraceptives, and hormonal supplementation also appear to affect a woman's complexion and cause fluctuations in acne.

Acne that has its onset in adulthood in men has traditionally been unusual. When it does appear, it tends to involve the upper back and upper arms. It has been seen increasingly in men and some women who participate in athletic activities. The reason for the increased prevalence of this type of acne is unknown. It has been speculated to be caused by one or all of the following: sweating, mechanical friction, anabolic steroids, and creatine-containing dietary bodybuilding supplements.

DESCRIPTION OF LESIONS

Unless preexisting adolescent acne is a concurrent problem,

- Postadolescent acne is relatively comedo-free and consists of evanescent, inflammatory red papules and/or pustules.
- The lesions more closely resemble those seen in rosacea or perioral dermatitis.
- In general, patients have fewer lesions than in adolescent acne (Figure 1.11).

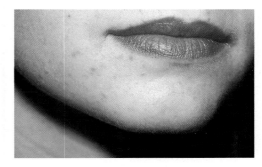

FIGURE 1.11 Postadolescent acne. Erythematous papules can be seen on the lower part of this woman's face.

DISTRIBUTION OF LESIONS

- In women, lesions occur on the face, most often in the perioral area, along the jaw line, or on the chin (Figure 1.12).
- In men, lesions tend to be limited to the trunk.

CLINICAL MANIFESTATIONS

- Lesions tend to appear and reappear like clockwork according to a woman's fluctuating levels of circulating hormones. They tend to recur premenstrually or at ovulation. They last for several days; sometimes they persist for a month or longer. In some women, the lesions occur irregularly.
- No such fluctuation occurs in men.

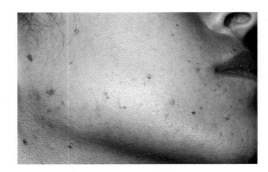

FIGURE 1.12 Postadolescent acne. Characteristic location of acne along the jaw line in a woman.

DIAGNOSIS

- The diagnosis is made clinically; however, in women whose acne is not responding to treatment, or in those who have other signs of hormonal excess such as male characteristics (e.g., facial hair) or irregular menstrual periods, hormonal tests are indicated.

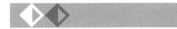

 DIFFERENTIAL DIAGNOSIS

Rosacea and Perioral Dermatitis (see later)
- These conditions are seen primarily in adults.
- They most often occur on the central third of the face (rosacea) or perioral area (perioral dermatitis).
- No comedones are present.

Folliculitis (see later and also Chapter 5, "Superficial Bacterial Infections")
- Papules and pustules with central hairs are the primary lesions (Figure 1.13).

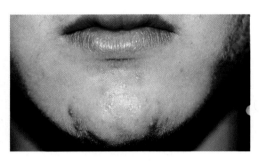

FIGURE 1.13 Folliculitis. This young man developed acne-like lesions that appeared under his football chin strap. Bacterial culture grew out coagulase positive staphylococcus aureus.

MANAGEMENT

Postadolescent acne in women may be treated with many of the same agents used for adolescent acne; however, retinoids and tetracycline should not be used during pregnancy or breast-feeding. In addition, women taking oral contraceptives and antibiotics should be advised to use an alternative or additional form of birth control, as discussed earlier.

In the treatment of women with acne, hormonal issues deserve further consideration. The rationale behind hormonal treatment includes the demonstration of elevated serum androgen levels in some patients. More often than not, however, these levels are normal, and it appears that these women may have an end-organ hypersensitivity to their endogenous androgens.

Patients with irregular menstrual cycles, hirsutism, a history of ovarian cysts, or infertility may also be candidates for hormonal therapy, although some of them should have an endocrinologic workup before hormonal treatment is initiated. Referral to an endocrinologist or a gynecologist should be considered.

Oral Antibiotics
Because it is very common for women to have premenstrual flares of acne, the dose of antibiotics can be increased 5 to 7 days before the patient's next menstrual period (see the earlier discussion of "rollercoasting").

Oral Contraceptives
By suppressing gonadotropins, reducing ovarian androgen secretion, and increasing sex hormone–binding globulin levels, oral contraceptives decrease serum testosterone concentrations. Oral contraceptives may be used in women older than 15 years who have no known contraindications to this form of therapy.

(continued)

Ortho Tri-Cyclen, a low-dose oral contraceptive, contains a norgestimate–ethinyl estradiol combination with minimal androgenicity, because the progestin used in this drug, norgestimate, has been shown to increase sex hormone–binding globulin levels and to decrease testosterone concentrations in healthy women. Other oral contraceptives that also have no substantial androgenicity, such as Alesse, Demulen 1/50, Yasmin, and Desogen, may also be tried.

Under supervision by dermatologists who are familiar with their use, other hormonal agents such as spironolactone and flutamide are used when conventional therapy fails. Cyproterone is an acetate steroidal androgen receptor blocker and potent progestin. Cyproterone acts as a competitive inhibitor of testosterone and dehydroepiandrosterone at the level of androgen receptors. Diane-35, an oral contraceptive that is very effective in the treatment of acne but is not available in the United States, contains a combination of cyproterone acetate and ethinyl estradiol.

 POINTS TO REMEMBER

- Every female patient with acne should be questioned about her menstrual history.
- A hormonal evaluation is appropriate for a few patients with acne, particularly women in their mid-20s or older who have treatment-resistant acne, virilizing signs or symptoms, irregular menstrual periods, or hirsutism. These patients should receive a complete endocrine and gynecologic evaluation.

BASICS

Rosacea is a disorder that is frequently mistaken for acne. In fact, as recently as 20 years ago, rosacea was referred to as *acne rosacea*. Both conditions look alike, they often respond to the same treatments, and they may coexist in the same patient.

Rosacea is a common condition. It arises later than does acne, usually when patients are between 30 and 50 years old. Rosacea occurs most commonly in fair-skinned people of northern European, particularly Celtic, descent; it is unusual among dark-skinned people. Women are reportedly three times more likely to be affected than are men.

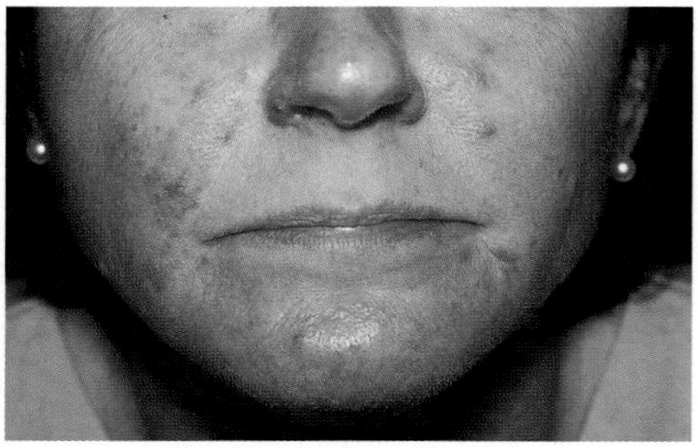

DESCRIPTION OF LESIONS

- Rosacea is a facial eruption that consists of acnelike erythematous papules, pustules, and telangiectasias.
- Rosacea lacks the comedones (blackheads or whiteheads) that are seen in acne vulgaris.
- In general, it does not scar or present with nodules or cysts, unless the patient has concomitant acne.

DISTRIBUTION OF LESIONS

- Lesions are most typically seen on the central third of the face—the forehead, nose, cheeks, and chin (the so-called flush or blush areas) (Figure 1.14).
- Rosacea lesions tend to be bilaterally symmetric, but they may occur on only one side of the patient's face.

CLINICAL MANIFESTATIONS

- Rosacea is primarily a cosmetic problem.
- Patients with rosacea may also have ocular involvement (Figure 1.15), which results most often in blepharoconjunctivitis. Episcleritis and keratoconjunctivitis sicca are rare complications.

Precipitating Factors that May Exacerbate Rosacea
- Sun exposure
- Excessive washing of the face
- Irritating cosmetics

There is no convincing evidence regarding whether the following environmental factors have any long-term deleterious effects on rosacea:

- Excess alcohol ingestion
- Emotional stress
- Spicy foods, smoking, or caffeine

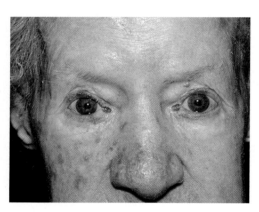

FIGURE 1.14 Rosacea. As seen here, rosacea is characterized by inflammatory papules and pustules and telangiectasias located on the central third of the face.

FIGURE 1.15 Occular rosacea. Note conjunctivitis. This patient also has facial lesions of rosacea.

Pathophysiology

Despite their similarities, acne vulgaris and rosacea seem to have quite different pathophysiologies. The microcomedo, the primary lesion of acne, arises in response to hormonal stimuli and bacteria in people genetically predisposed to the disorder. Rosacea emerges idiopathically, with no discernible inheritance patterns.

Several investigators have suggested that *Helicobacter pylori*, which is found in the stomach, may cause or exacerbate rosacea; others implicate the *Demodex* species of mite that is often found in the hair follicle of patients with rosacea. Evidence that either organism plays a central role in the pathogenesis of this disorder is lacking, however.

DIAGNOSIS

Rosacea is diagnosed clinically; however, a biopsy may be necessary in atypical cases.

 DIFFERENTIAL DIAGNOSIS

Conditions that may resemble clinical rosacea include adult acne, perioral dermatitis, seborrheic dermatitis, and the "butterfly" rash of systemic lupus erythematosus.

Adult Acne
- Comedones may be present.
- Facial flushing and telangiectasias are lacking.
- The distribution of lesions is wider than is seen in rosacea. *In adults, acne may coexist with, or may be indistinguishable from, rosacea.*

Seborrheic Dermatitis (see Chapter 2, "Eczema")
- Scale and erythema are present, but without acnelike lesions (papules and pustules).
- The distribution of lesions is in the nasolabial area, eyebrows, and scalp. *Because seborrheic dermatitis is a common scaly macular eruption, seborrheic dermatitis may coexist with rosacea* (Figure 1.16).

Systemic Lupus Erythematosus (see Chapter 25, "Cutaneous Manifestations of Systemic Disease")
- Papules and pustules are lacking.
- Antinuclear antibodies are present.
- Other characteristics of lupus are present.

CLINICAL VARIANTS

Variants of clinical rosacea include prerosacea, rhinophyma, topical steroid–induced rosacea, and perioral dermatitis.

Prerosacea
- The appearance of facial erythema and telangiectasias, without the inflammatory lesions of rosacea, is referred to as prerosacea. Many patients with *prerosacea*, with a "rosy-cheeked," ruddy complexion, may never develop the full clinical spectrum that is seen in patients with rosacea (Figure 1.17).

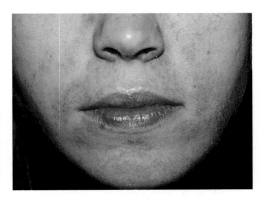

FIGURE 1.16 Perioral dermatitis and seborrheic dermatitis. Multiple acneiform papules can be seen on this young woman. Note also the scale and erythema characteristic of seborrheic dermatitis.

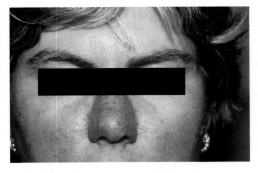

FIGURE 1.17 Prerosacea. This woman has "rosy cheeks" and telangiectasias. She may never develop the full clinical spectrum that is seen in patients with rosacea.

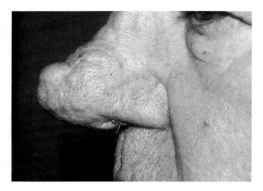

FIGURE 1.18 Rhinophyma.

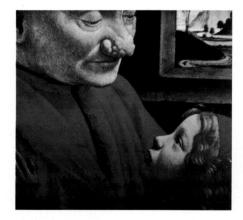

FIGURE 1.19 Rhinophyma. Ghirlandaio's portrait of an old man with his grandson (showing a tender human relationship, despite the appearance of his nose).

- The increase in medical and public awareness of rosacea has led to an overdiagnosis of prerosacea and rosacea by primary care clinicians and dermatologists alike.

Rhinophyma

- An extreme form of disfiguring sebaceous hyperplasia of the nose, rhinophyma seems to occur only in middle-aged men, many of whom also have typical facial and/or ocular rosacea (Figures 1.18 and 1.19).

Topical Steroid–Induced Rosacea

- Rosacea induced by topical steroids is often clinically indistinguishable from ordinary rosacea, but a history of long-term, indiscriminate misuse of potent topical steroids (a well-documented cause of rosacea) on the face helps to confirm the diagnosis (Figure 1.20).
- The condition typically worsens when the topical steroids are discontinued (an occurrence known as *rebound rosacea*). In an unfortunate cycle, the steroid is sometimes reapplied to diminish the erythema, and this only worsens the condition.

Perioral Dermatitis

- Also known as **periorificial dermatitis,** perioral dermatitis is an eruption resembling rosacea that is seen primarily in young women and occasionally in young boys and girls.
- It is usually found around the mouth, but it may be noted around the eyes and nose (hence the more inclusive term, periorificial) (Figure 1.21). As with rosacea, the origin of perioral dermatitis is unknown; potent topical steroids and fluoridated toothpaste have occasionally been implicated, but without any consistent evidence.

    Some features that distinguish perioral dermatitis from rosacea are as follows:

- Perioral dermatitis appears in women between the ages of 15 and 40 years.
- It manifests in small, erythematous papules or pustules without telangiectasia.
- It characteristically encircles the mouth and spares the vermilion border of the lips.
- Occasionally, there is superimposed scaling.
- Usually, this condition does not recur after successful treatment.

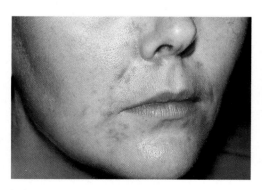

FIGURE 1.20 Topical steroid—induced rosacea. This woman had been applying a potent topical steroid everyday to her face for 8 months.

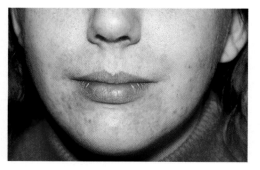

FIGURE 1.21 Perioral dermatitis. Multiple acneiform papules can be seen on this young woman. Note the characteristic sparing around the lips.

MANAGEMENT

Patients should be advised to avoid the sun or to apply sunscreen before sun exposure. They may also wish to avoid the environmental triggers discussed earlier.

Topical Therapy

If possible, long-term control of rosacea should be attempted with topical therapy alone, and oral antibiotics should be reserved for initial control and for breakthrough flares.

- Metronidazole 1% (Noritate) cream is used once daily.
- Twice-daily applications of 0.75% metronidazole cream (Metro-Cream), which is also available as a lotion, and gel preparations are also used.

Because it may take 6 to 8 weeks for an acceptable therapeutic response, an oral antibiotic such as a tetracycline (see later) is initially given in addition to topical therapy and is continued as the antibiotic is gradually stopped. In mild cases, topical therapy can be used alone.

- If metronidazole fails to control rosacea, less effective but still helpful treatments include topical clindamycin 1% lotion (Cleocin T) or erythromycin 2% solution in a nonalcohol base.
- A topical lotion containing sodium sulfacetamide 10% and sulfur 5%, such as Klaron or Sulfacet-R, a preparation that contains a cosmetic cover-up, is another treatment option.

Systemic Therapy

- Systemic antibiotics, such as tetracycline or, less commonly, erythromycin are used to treat the skin and ocular manifestations of rosacea and rosacealike disorders when topical therapy alone is unlikely to succeed.
- Attempts should be made to taper to the minimum drug dosage and to control the condition with topical therapy as soon as possible.
- Patients readily learn to titrate the dosage of oral antibiotics based on their disease activity.
- Treatment with tetracycline or erythromycin typically delivers a rapid therapeutic response, usually very effectively reducing acneiform lesions; this result pleases the patient and helps to confirm the diagnosis of rosacea.
- The mechanism of action of theses drugs is more likely anti-inflammatory than antibiotic, because no microorganisms have been definitively incriminated in the etiology of rosacea and rosacea variants.
- The "flat" telangiectasias and flushing erythema tend to persist and respond minimally, if at all, to antibiotic therapy.

Dosages

- Tetracycline is given in dosages ranging from 250 to 500 mg twice daily.
- The dosage is tapered when the acneiform inflammation has improved (usually after 3 to 4 weeks).

(continued)

- If tetracycline is ineffective, minocycline (50 to 100 mg twice daily), doxycycline (50 to 100 mg twice daily), or erythromycin (250 mg twice daily to 250 mg four times daily) may be tried.
- Isotretinoin (Accutane) has been used in patients with severe refractory rosacea.

Other Treatment Options for Rosacea and Its Variants
- Cosmetic foundations—to cover erythematous areas
- Electrocautery with a small needle—to destroy small telangiectasias
- Pulse dye lasers—for larger telangiectatic vessels
- Surgical reduction—to treat rhinophyma.
- Prerosacea generally does not require treatment, nor do any effective treatments exist. However, patients with prerosacea may be observed for signs of rosacea and encouraged to use sun protection.

 POINTS TO REMEMBER

- Rosacea is a chronic condition with no known cure.
- Acne, rosacea, perioral dermatitis, and topical steroid–induced rosacea all share similar clinical manifestations and overlapping management strategies, yet each has a distinctive course and prognosis; consequently, an attempt at making a specific diagnosis should be made.
- If possible, long-term control of rosacea should be attempted with topical therapy alone, with oral antibiotics used for breakthrough flares.
- The use of potent topical steroids on the face should be avoided.

 SEE PATIENT HANDOUT, PAGE 443

SYSTEMIC DRUG–INDUCED (OR DRUG-EXACERBATED) ACNE

Several drugs are known to provoke acneiform reactions.

- The management of drug-induced or drug-exacerbated acne includes the following choices: discontinuance of the causative drug, decreasing its dosage, or substituting it with another drug. Treatment of the acne is performed as described earlier in this chapter.
- Oral corticosteroids and adrenocorticotropic hormone produce acne lesions that are usually more monomorphic and symmetrical in distribution than those seen in adolescent and postadolescent acne. Lesions are located primarily on the trunk (Figure 1.22). The precise mechanism is uncertain.
- Acne may be exacerbated by lithium.
- Androgens (including anabolic steroids) and gonadotrophins may precipitate acne, especially in female patients and in athletes who take such drugs.
- Androgenic contraceptive pills that reduce sex hormone–binding globulin may also result in a deterioration of preexisting acne.
- Antiepileptic drugs, especially phenytoin, have been incriminated as causing or exacerbating acne; however, modern anticonvulsants appear not to have acne as a potential side effect.
- Patients taking isoniazid, especially those who slowly inactivate the drug, appear to be prone to develop acne.

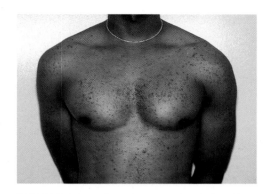

FIGURE 1.22 Systemic steroid–induced acne. This patient was taking prednisone for sarcoidosis.

Neonatal Acne

This self-limiting form of acne, seen mainly in male infants; it occurs from the stimulation of maternal androgens and requires no treatment.

Acne Excorieé des Jeunes Filles (Figure 1.23)

This type of acne is routinely picked at by the patient, who almost invariably is female.

- Many of these patients deny that they manipulate their skin, but it is rather obvious when there are no primary lesions present because all have crusts.
- Some of these patients may benefit from selective serotonin reuptake inhibitor drugs and psychotherapy.

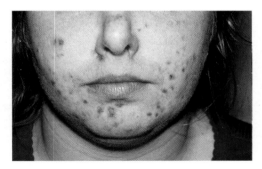

FIGURE 1.23 Acne excorieé des jeunes filles. This type of acne has obviously been picked at by the patient.

TABLE 1.1. BENZOYL PEROXIDE

OVER-THE-COUNTER PREPARATIONS

Oxy 5, Oxy 10	5% and 10% benzoyl peroxide
Clear By Design	2.5% gel benzoyl peroxide
Clearasil 10%	10% lotion benzoyl peroxide

PRESCRIPTION FORMULATIONS

Desquam-X 5, -X 10	5%, 10% benzoyl peroxide gel (water-based)
Desquam-E	2.5%, 5%, 10% benzoyl peroxide gel (water-based)
Brevoxyl-4, -8	4% and 8% benzoyl peroxide gel (water-based)
Triaz	3%, 6%, and 10% benzoyl peroxide gel (water-based)

ADVANTAGES	DISADVANTAGES

Available over the counter
  No reported bacterial
  resistance
 	
Available in many formulations,
  including cream and liquid
  (water-based gels less
  irritating than alcohol-based
  preparations)
	Often irritating (causes
	  stinging, redness, and scaling)
	  Contact sensitivity occasion-
	  ally occurs
	May bleach clothing and
	  bed linen

TABLE 1.2. TOPICAL RETINOIDS

BRAND NAME	GENERIC NAME	ADVANTAGES AND DISADVANTAGES	STRENGTHS
Retin-A cream, gel	Tretinoin	Available in various strengths and less expensive generic formulations; often irritating	Creams 0.025%, 0.05%, and 0.1% Gels 0.01% and 0.025%
Retin-A Micro topical gel	Tretinoin	Less irritating than Retin-A; one strength	0.1%
Avita cream, gel	Tretinoin	Less irritating than Retin-A; one strength	0.025%
Differin cream, gel, solution	Adapalene	Less irritating than Retin-A; less sun sensitivity than Retin-A; one strength	0.1%
Tazorac cream, gel	Tazarotene	Possibly more effective and faster acting than Retin-A; two strengths; irritating; expensive	0.05% and 0.1%

TABLE 1.3. TOPICAL ANTIBIOTICS

BRAND NAME	GENERIC NAME	SIZES	ADVANTAGES AND DISADVANTAGES
A/T/S solution, gel	Erythromycin 2%	60 mL	Effective for postadolescent acne, rosacea; irritation infrequent; often used in conjunction with benzoyl peroxide and/or retinoids; bacterial resistance possible
Akne-Mycin ointment	Erythromycin 2%	25 g	Least irritating topical antibiotic; excellent for atopic skin; somewhat messy to apply; bacterial resistance possible
Cleocin T solution, gel, lotion	Clindamycin 1%	60 mL	Effective for postadolescent acne, rosacea; lotion less irritating than solution and gel; bacterial resistance possible
Theramycin Z	Erythromycin 2% /zinc acetate	60 mL	Contains zinc; bacterial resistance possible

TABLE 1.4. COMBINATION OF TOPICAL ANTIBIOTIC AND BENZOYL PEROXIDE

BRAND NAME	GENERIC NAME	ADVANTAGES AND DISADVANTAGES	SIZES
Benzamycin gel	Erythromycin 3% and benzoyl peroxide 5%	Combination is more potent than either agent used alone (synergistic effect); no bacterial resistance; refrigeration necessary	50 g
Benzamycin Pak	Erythromycin 3% and benzoyl peroxide 5%	No refrigeration necessary	60 pouches per carton
BenzaClin gel	Clindamycin 1% and benzoyl peroxide 5%	Same as above, except no refrigeration necessary	25 and 50 g

TABLE 1.5. OTHER TOPICAL PRESCRIPTION AGENTS

BRAND NAME	GENERIC NAME	SIZES	ADVANTAGES AND DISADVANTAGES
Azelex cream	Azelaic acid 20%	30, 50 g	Used as an alternative to or in conjunction with retinoids or benzoyl peroxide; may lighten postinflammatory darkening resulting from acne; reduces both comedonal and inflammatory lesions; probably not as effective as other agents; irritation common
Sulfacet-R lotion, Novacet lotion	Sodium sulfacetamide 10% and sulfur 5%	25 g	Effective for rosacea; tinted preparation may be a good camouflage in fair-skinned patients with acne; not as effective as topical antibiotics
Noritate cream	Metronidazole 1%	30 g	Effective for rosacea; once-daily application
MetroGel	Metronidazole 0.75%	30, 45 g	Effective for rosacea; twice-daily application
MetroCream	Metronidazole 0.75%	45 g	Twice-daily application
MetroLotion	Metronidazole 0.75%	60 mL	Twice-daily application
Klaron lotion	Sodium sulfacetamide 10%	59 mL	Effective for rosacea; minimal reported irritation; clear, water-based lotion; probably not as effective as metronidazole for rosacea

TABLE 1.6. SYSTEMIC THERAPIES

ANTIBIOTICS	DOSES AVAILABLE	STARTING DOSES
Tetracyclines	250 mg, 500 mg	250 or 500 mg bid
Minocycline	50 mg, 100 mg	50 or 100 mg bid
Doxycycline	50 mg, 75 mg, 100 mg	50 mg, 75 mg, or 100 mg bid
Erythromycin	250 mg, 333 mg	333 mg tid or 500 mg bid

HORMONAL THERAPY

Hormonal treatments with oral contraceptives such as Ortho Tri-Cyclen, Alesse, Demulen 1/50, and Desogen. These agents are relatively low in androgen activity. Spironolactone and flutamide are antiandrogens that are sometimes used in recalcitrant female adult acne. *These agents should be prescribed only by those health care providers who are familiar with their potential side effects.*

OTHER THERAPY	DOSES AVAILABLE	STARTING DOSAGES
Accutane (13-*cis*-retinoic acid)	10 mg, 20 mg, 40 mg	0.5 to 1 mg/kg daily

This drug has severe teratogenic side effects in women and should be administered only by those who are familiar with its use.

Eczema

Overview

- Despite being the most common inflammatory skin condition, eczema is the most confusing skin ailment for both patients and their nondermatologic health care providers.
- Eczema is very difficult to define. United States Supreme Court Justice Potter Stewart once said that he could not define pornography, but he knew it when he saw it. Such is the case with eczema, a condition best understood through repeated viewing.
- The word *eczema* was coined by the Ancient Greeks to mean "a boiling out or over." Conceivably, Greeks viewed certain rashes as boiling out or erupting from under the skin. As a case in point, the acute eczematous eruption of poison ivy often manifests with a fiery red color and a linear, blistered appearance, suggesting an acute boiling, bubbling, second-degree burn.
- Terminologic confusion may also arise if the word *dermatitis*—a more generalized, often vague designation that refers to all cutaneous conditions with inflammation—is used synonymously with eczema or is coupled with it. In general, it is acceptable to use eczema and dermatitis interchangeably. Eczematous dermatitis, therefore, is somewhat redundant, although some could argue that the term is more inclusive than is either word alone.

The following clinical presentations of eczema or associated conditions are discussed in this chapter:

- Atopic dermatitis (atopic eczema)
- Nummular eczema
- Lichen simplex chronicus
- Prurigo nodularis
- Nonspecific eczematous dermatitis
- Asteatotic eczema
- Neurotic excoriations
- Chronic hand eczema and dyshidrotic eczema
- Contact dermatitis
- Seborrheic dermatitis
- Stasis dermatitis

Histopathology

- On a microscopic level, an eczematous epidermis contains intercellular and intracellular fluid that appears in a spongelike formation (spongiosis); vasodilatation of the dermis also occurs. These abnormalities result in the clinical manifestations of acute eczema: edema, erythema, vesicles, and bullae (e.g., from poison ivy).
- Later, the epidermis will thicken (acanthosis) and retain nuclei (parakeratosis), and an abundant cellular infiltrate will develop in the dermis. These changes account for the scale and lichenification of chronic eczema (e.g., chronic lichenified atopic dermatitis).

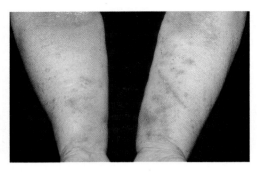

FIGURE 2.1 Acute allergic eczematous eruption of poison ivy. The fiery red color and linear blistered appearance suggest an acute "boiling," bubbling, second-degree burn.

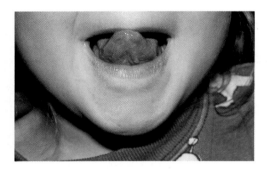

FIGURE 2.2 Acute irritant eczematous eruption. This child has irritant contact dermatitis caused by repeated lip licking.

Acute, Subacute, and Chronic Eczema

In reference to eczema, the designators acute, subacute, and chronic are somewhat arbitrary because they describe parts of a dynamic spectrum. A patient can present with lesions in any or all of the phases.

Acute eczema is manifested by itchy erythematous patches, plaques, or papules that may become "juicy" and develop into vesicobullous lesions (Figure 2.1). Alternatively, acute eczema may originate and continue as a less florid, nonvesicular, erythematous eruption (Figure 2.2).

Subacute eczema is an intermediate stage between acute and chronic eczema. The term has little clinical value. It is best simply to be aware that acute oozing lesions dry into crusts (scabs) (Figure 2.3), and they can later develop scales that overlie an erythematous base. Subacute eczema can become chronic, or it can resolve spontaneously or with treatment.

Chronic eczema is also known as chronic eczematous dermatitis. Its hallmark is lichenification—plaque with an exaggeration or hypertrophy of the normal skin markings. Lichenification resembles the bark on a tree trunk or, as implied, the lichen growth on the bark (Figure 2.4). In addition, scale and hemorrhagic crusts can result from scratched or drying vesicles. Older lesions may exhibit postinflammatory pigmentary alterations (hyperpigmentation and/or hypopigmentation) (Figure 2.5).

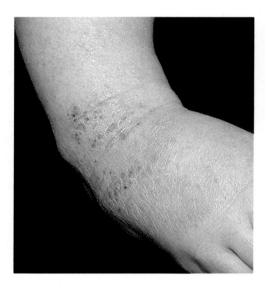

FIGURE 2.3 Subacute eczema. The crusts, scales, and erythema of subacute eczema are less intense than those seen in acute eczema. There is also lichenification, which suggests chronic eczematous dermatitis.

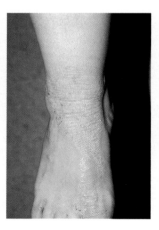

FIGURE 2.4 Chronic eczematous dermatitis. This patient shows lichenification, which was caused by repeated scratching.

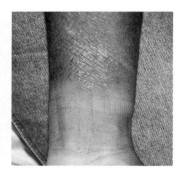

FIGURE 2.5 Chronic eczematous dermatitis. This lesion shows no evidence of active inflammation. Lichenification and postinflammatory hyperpigmentation are apparent.

BASICS

- Atopic dermatitis, also known as atopic eczema or endogenous eczema, is the most commonly seen type of eczema (Figures 2.6 to 2.8). Atopic dermatitis is a chronic, inflammatory, itchy skin condition with an unpredictable course of flares and remissions. An estimated 5% to 10% of the United States population has it. Atopic dermatitis is the most frequently seen skin condition among patients of Asian descent.
- By definition, atopic dermatitis occurs in association with a personal or family history of hay fever, asthma, allergic rhinitis, sinusitis, or atopic dermatitis itself. A probing history taking is often necessary to uncover symptoms of atopy. For example, patients should be asked whether they or their family members are allergic to pollen, dust, house dust mites, ragweed, dogs, or cats. Inquiries should be made about chronic recurrent symptoms that suggest atopy, such as nasal pruritus and rhinitis, rhinorrhea, paroxysmal sneezing, or itchy or irritated eyes. A personal or family history of allergies to multiple medications is also important. Furthermore, secondary relatives (aunts, uncles, cousins, and grandparents) may have an atopic predisposition.
- Most cases begin in childhood (often in infancy); however, atopic dermatitis may start at any age. The disease frequently remits spontaneously—reportedly in 40% to 50% of children—but it may return in adolescence or adulthood and possibly persist for a lifetime. Traditionally, patients and their families were advised that children "will grow out of eczema"; however, this optimistic prognosis is not always realized.
- Children with asthma—an increasing population in the inner cities of the United States—appear to have a higher prevalence of atopic dermatitis than do other children; atopic dermatitis often manifests in asthmatic children in a more extensive and chronic form. Severe eczema in childhood portends a worse prognosis in adulthood.
- Atopic dermatitis can present with a wide spectrum of severity. Some patients may have only a mild, recurrent, localized, itchy rash on "dry" or "sensitive" skin; others may experience a more severe, extensive eruption that can be accompanied by unremitting pruritus, sleepless nights, secondary cutaneous bacterial or viral infections, embarrassing alligatorlike lichenification, and, rarely, an exfoliative erythroderma. Many patients with atopic dermatitis have multiple accompanying atopic ailments, as mentioned earlier.
- In addition to the physical discomfort of atopic dermatitis, patients may suffer from embarrassment about the appearance of lesions. Psychosocial problems, such as poor self-image, anger, and frustration, may lead to depression and social isolation.

Pathogenesis

Atopic dermatitis is an inherited type I (Immunoglobulin E–mediated) hypersensitivity disorder of the skin. As compared with normal skin, atopic skin tends to be more prone to dryness, irritation, and infection; and it is more likely to be negatively influenced by emotional stress. The intense itching of atopic dermatitis is presumed to be produced by the release of vasoactive substances from sensitized mast cells and basophils in the dermis. The itching may be initiated by triggers, such as external agents (e.g., house dust mites) or nonimmunologic agents (e.g., certain foods; alcohol; and overexposure to dry, cold weather or to very hot, humid conditions that predispose to sweating).

There is considerable debate about whether atopic dermatitis is primarily an allergen-induced disease or, rather, an inflammatory skin disorder found in association with respiratory allergy or other atopic

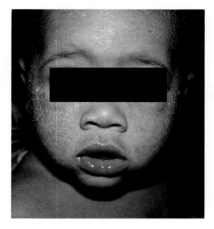

FIGURE 2.6 Atopic dermatitis in an infant.

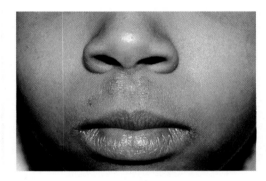

FIGURE 2.7 Atopic dermatitis in an 8-year-old child.

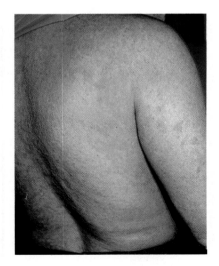

FIGURE 2.8 Atopic dermatitis in an adult.

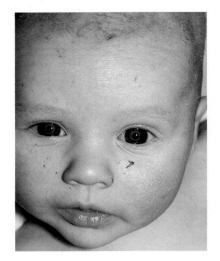

FIGURE 2.9 Infantile atopic dermatitis. This infant has typical erythema and scaling of her cheeks, as well as "cradle cap."

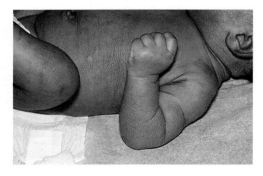

FIGURE 2.10 Atopic dermatitis. Widespread eruption has occurred in an infant.

symptoms. In support of the latter explanation is that a true allergic condition is permanent, whereas atopic dermatitis is often outgrown. Even though atopic dermatitis frequently remits spontaneously, patients, their families, and their health care providers—in particular, pediatricians and allergists—often relentlessly search for external sources that patients can avoid or eliminate from their environments. Avoidance of milk products and food preservatives and extreme dietary restrictions are not only very difficult to maintain on an ongoing basis, but they may also incite developmental problems in growing children—furthermore, they rarely, if ever, offer a cure.

DESCRIPTION OF LESIONS

Although the character and distribution of the skin rash tend to vary according to the patient's age, the different phases of atopic dermatitis are not always clearly distinct. Any or all manifestations of atopic dermatitis may exist in a single patient.

Infantile Phase
In patients aged 2 months to 2 years, the face (particularly the cheeks) (Figure 2.9) scalp, chest, neck, and extensor extremities are most often involved. The eruption may become generalized (Figure 2.10). In many cases, atopic dermatitis first manifests with severe "cradle cap" or severe recalcitrant intertriginous (groin, neck, axillae) rashes. As the patient approaches age 2 years, the flexor creases become involved. Lesions consist of scaly, red, and, occasionally, oozing plaques that tend to be symmetric (Figure 2.11).

Childhood Phase
Lesions seen in children aged 2 through 12 years tend to be less acute and exudative than those seen in infancy. In some patients, inflamed lesions become lichenified because of repeated rubbing and scratching. Lichenification occurs more commonly in Asian and black patients than it does in white patients.

Distribution of Lesions
Lesions tend to occur symmetrically, with characteristic distribution in the flexural folds: the antecubital (Figure 2.12) and popliteal fossae and the neck, wrists, and ankles. Lesions may also occur on the eyelids, lips, and scalp, and behind the ears.

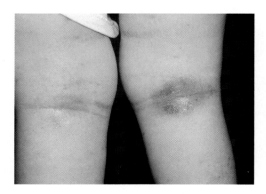

FIGURE 2.11 Atopic dermatitis. This is a toddler who demonstrates early flexural involvement.

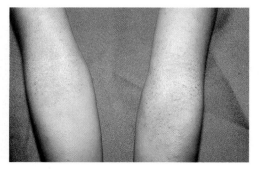

FIGURE 2.12 Atopic dermatitis in an older child. The crusting and lichenification involving the flexor crease were caused by repeated rubbing and scratching.

Adolescent and Adult Phase

In adolescents and adults, lichenified plaques are generally less well demarcated than are the plaques seen in psoriasis (Figure 2.13); these plaques tend to blend into surrounding normal skin. Postinflammatory hyperpigmentary and hypopigmentary changes may be seen, or the appearance of atopic dermatitis may change to poorly defined, itchy erythematous papules or plaques.

Distribution of Lesions

The distribution of lesions may be similar to that seen in childhood, that is, in the flexural folds. However, lesions may also be in extensor locations: the dorsa of the hands, wrists, ankles, and feet, and the nape of the neck. Alternatively, lesions may be limited to the lips *(atopic cheilitis)* (Figure 2.14), eyelids, vulvar (Figure 2.15) or scrotal areas (Figure 2.16), or hands (as in chronic hand eczema or dyshidrotic eczema, which may be the only features of atopic dermatitis that remain in some adults).

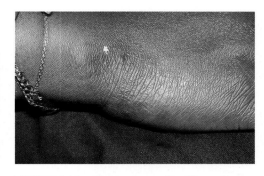

FIGURE 2.13 Atopic dermatitis. The extensor location on the dorsa of the hand shows postinflammatory hyperpigmentation.

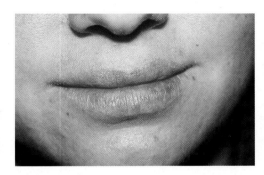

FIGURE 2.14 Atopic cheilitis (atopic dermatitis of the lips). Note the lichenification and the ill-defined outline of the vermilion border of the upper lip.

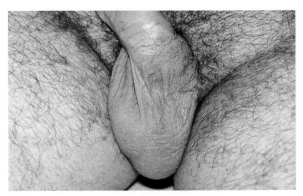

FIGURE 2.16 Atopic dermatitis (lichen simplex chronicus) limited to the scrotum. This patient was initially thought to have tinea cruris.

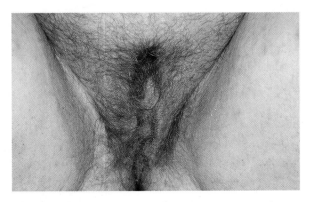

FIGURE 2.15 Atopic dermatitis limited to the vulvar and inguinal areas. This patient was initially thought to have tinea cruris.

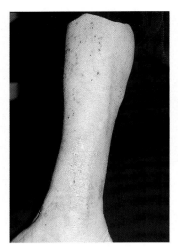

FIGURE 2.17 Xerosis. This elderly patient has a long history of xerosis and atopic dermatitis. Note the hemorrhagic crusts, scale, and lichenification.

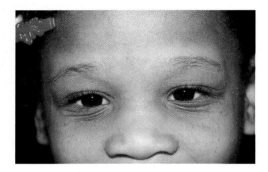

FIGURE 2.18 Eyelid atopic dermatitis. Note lichenification and the characteristic double-fold (Dennie–Morgan line) that extends from the inner to the outer canthus of the lower eyelid and the "allergic shiners," the darkening color of the periorbital areas.

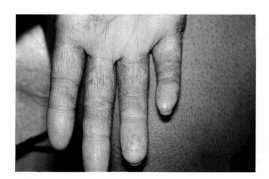

FIGURE 2.19 Chronic hand eczema in a patient with atopic dermatitis. Lichenification and hyperlinearity are evident on the palm.

OTHER CLINICAL ASPECTS

Additional associated features and findings that are clues to the diagnosis of atopic dermatitis include the following:

- Persistent **xerosis,** or dry, "sensitive" skin (Figure 2.17)
- **Dennie–Morgan** lines. These comprise a characteristic double fold that extends from the inner to the outer canthus of the lower eyelid (Figure 2.18).
- **"Allergic shiners."** This term refers to a darkened, violaceous or tan coloring in the periorbital areas. Along with Dennie–Morgan lines, this dark coloring may be an instant clue to the diagnosis of atopic dermatitis.
- **Hyperlinear palmar creases** (Figure 2.19)
- **Follicular eczema.** Eczema of the hair follicles is a common presentation in black patients (Figure 2.20).

Other associated dermatoses include the following:

- **Ichthyosis vulgaris.** This condition is frequently associated with atopy. Lesions, which are most apparent on the shins, resemble fine fish scales. Characteristically, the flexor creases are spared in this condition (Figure 2.21).
- **Keratosis pilaris.** These tiny, horny, rough-textured, whitish or red, follicular papules or pustules that occur during adolescence are also known as "allergic bumps." Most commonly, keratosis pilaris is noted on the deltoid and posterolateral upper arms, the upper back and thighs, and the malar area of the face. It is frequently confused with acne (Figure 2.22).

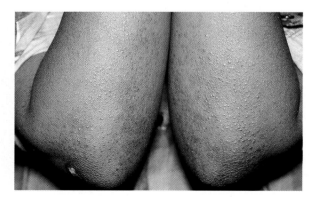

FIGURE 2.20 Atopic dermatitis of the hair follicles: follicular eczema. Note the gridlike pattern of follicular papules.

CLINICAL MANIFESTATIONS AND POSSIBLE COMPLICATIONS

- Pruritus may interfere with sleep. Itching is increased by repeated scratching and rubbing, which leads to lichenification, oozing, and secondary bacterial infection (impetiginization, or "honey-crusted skin").
- Secondary infection with *Staphylococcus aureus* may trigger relapses of atopic dermatitis.
- Secondary infections with herpes simplex virus may result in eczema herpeticum (Kaposi's varicelliform eruption), which is more commonly seen in childhood.

 DIFFERENTIAL DIAGNOSIS

The diagnosis of atopic dermatitis is generally not difficult, especially in patients with an atopic history in whom the following causes of eczema or eczemalike eruptions are excluded:

Contact Dermatitis (see later)
- Determine whether the patient was exposed to a substance that could cause contact dermatitis. The location of the lesions may suggest an external cause.

Scabies
- A history of exposure is important in diagnosing scabies.
- Characteristic distribution (e.g., in the webs between the fingers and on the flexor wrists) can mimic that of eczema.
- A positive scabies scraping is diagnostic of scabies.

Psoriasis
- Lesions are generally in extensor locations—on the elbows, knees, and other large joints—rather than in flexor creases (Figure 2.23).
- Patients may have a positive family history of psoriasis.
- Usually, psoriasis is less pruritic than eczema.

Psoriatic lesions tend to be clearly demarcated from normal surrounding skin, and the scale of psoriasis tends to be thicker and micaceous in appearance. However, psoriasis may at times be clinically indistinguishable from atopic dermatitis.

Tinea Pedis, Corporis, Manuum, and Capitis
- A positive KOH test or fungal culture result will indicate these conditions.

 SEE PATIENT HANDOUT, PAGE 445

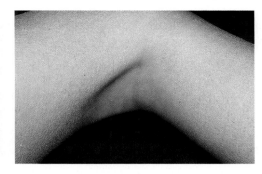

FIGURE 2.21 Ichthyosis vulgaris. This patient has atopic dermatitis and ichthyosis vulgaris lesions that resemble fish scales. Note the characteristic sparing of the popliteal fossa.

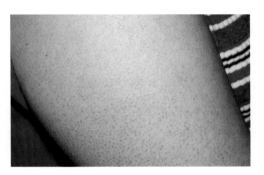

FIGURE 2.22 Keratosis pilaris. This teenager has tiny, rough-textured, red, follicular papules on her lateral upper arms.

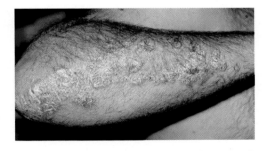

FIGURE 2.23 Psoriasis. Thick "psoriasiform" lesions are on the extensor forearms in this patient.

Topical Steroid Therapy
General Principles

- The application of an appropriately chosen topical steroid will usually bring prompt improvement in a patient with atopic dermatitis.
- Topical steroids should be used only as short-term therapy, if possible, and only against active disease (i.e., with itching and erythema).
- They should not be used for prevention of future lesions or for cosmetic concerns, such as postinflammatory hyperpigmentation.
- "Stronger" is often preferable to "longer" in the use of topical steroids, because long-term application is more often associated with side effects.
- Without question, use of a superpotent topical steroid is preferable to the administration of a systemic steroid, with its potential side effects.
- When the condition is under control, the frequency of application and the potency of the topical steroids are reduced ("downward titration"), or the agents are discontinued.

Face and Body Folds

- For the face and intertriginous regions (the axillae and inguinal creases are areas that are "naturally" occluded), treatment should be initiated with a low-potency cream or ointment, such as over-the-counter hydrocortisone 0.5% or 1%.
- In more severe cases of atopic dermatitis, initial therapy may be with a more potent steroid, followed by a less potent preparation for maintenance ("downward titration"). For example, a higher potency agent, such as hydrocortisone valerate 0.2%, could be used for 2 or 3 days, followed by a lower potency agent, such as desonide 0.05% or over-the-counter 0.5% to 1% hydrocortisone, which is then used for maintenance as needed.

Body

- For nonintertriginous areas of the body, treatment can be initiated with a high-potency cream or ointment, such as triamcinolone acetonide 0.1% or fluocinonide 0.05%. Even a superpotent agent, such as clobetasol 0.05%, may be used for limited periods (no more than 2 to 3 weeks) until control is achieved. Then, therapy may be switched to a lower potency agent, such as hydrocortisone valerate 0.2%. Fluticasone 0.05% cream (Cutivate), has been shown to

be effective as maintenance therapy when it is used twice weekly.

- Ointments are helpful for dry skin conditions. Because of their occlusive properties, they are more lubricating than other formulations; they also tend to be less irritating and less sensitizing. Their popularity increases in colder, dryer weather. For patients with widespread skin involvement, a 1-lb jar of triamcinolone acetonide cream or ointment is quite economical.

Infection

- If necessary, topical steroids can be given concurrently with systemic antibiotics, such as cephalexin, or dicloxacillin. This combination is sometimes helpful if evidence of coexisting staphylococcal or streptococcal infection ("impetiginization") of the skin is present.
- Topical mupirocin (Bactroban) ointment may be applied as an alternative to oral antibiotics.
- During flare-ups, the acute, open, weeping, crusted lesions that develop from infection or scratching may be treated with a drying, antibacterial agent, such as Burow's solution, before the application of topical steroids.

Topical Immunomodulator Therapy

- **Tacrolimus (Protopic) ointment** is a nonsteroidal immunomodulator that has been shown to reduce the symptoms of atopic dermatitis. It is used as an alternative to topical steroids, particularly when the eruption involves the face or intertriginous areas, such as the axillae and groin, where the long-term use of high-potency steroids is limited. It is also a good agent for long-term maintenance.
- It has potential as a topical steroid-sparing agent. It is available as an ointment in 0.1% and 0.03% concentrations. Tacrolimus 0.1% has been approved for the treatment of atopic dermatitis in adults. The lower, 0.03% concentration is designated for short-term and intermittent long-term treatment of atopic dermatitis in children (aged 2 years and older) and in adults. When applied twice daily, tacrolimus may cause transient side effects, such as burning and itching. This burning and itching may result in patients' refusal to continue applying the medication.
- **Elidel (pimecrolimus)**, a 1% cream, is less likely to be irritating, and the cream base is not as greasy as Protopic ointment.

(continued)

MANAGEMENT (*continued*)

Other Therapeutic Measures

- Oral H_1 antihistamines such as diphenhydramine (Benadryl) and hydroxyzine (Atarax) may reduce itching, but they are often effective only when they induce sleep, an unacceptable side effect for many patients.
- Oozing, exudative lesions may be soothed and dried with Burow's solution or by bathing in a tub with antipruritic emollients, such as an Aveeno oatmeal bath preparation.
- Sun exposure, ideally in the early morning and late afternoon—when humidity is lowest—may significantly improve atopic dermatitis.
- When a patient does not have access to natural sunlight, phototherapy with ultraviolet B and, less commonly, ultraviolet A rays is often very effective for widespread skin involvement.
- Tar baths, as well as tar preparations formulated as ointments, pastes, and gels, may be used concurrently with topical steroids or alternated with them. (Before the advent of topical steroids, tar preparations were the mainstay of treatment.) Several coal tar preparations available over the counter are Zetar emulsion, Balnetar, and Doak Tar Oil.
- Emotional stress in patients or in their families may contribute to atopic dermatitis. Measures to reduce stress include support groups and family psychotherapy.
- Systemic steroids, immunosuppressive therapy with systemic agents such as cyclosporine, or short-term hospitalization is sometimes necessary in patients with severe unresponsive generalized atopic dermatitis.
- For patients with secondary herpes simplex infection (Kaposi's varicelliform eruption), oral antiviral therapy and possibly hospitalization may be required.

Unsuccessful Treatments

- Treatments that do not seem to improve atopic dermatitis include vitamins, mineral or dietary supplements, and other nutritional supplements.
- Topical ointments containing diphenhydramine and doxepin are potentially contact allergens and thus are contraindicated.

General Management

Bathing

How often the person who has atopic dermatitis should bathe has been the subject of controversy and misunderstanding. There are many reasons not to restrict frequent bathing:

- Bathing removes crusts, irritants, potential allergens, and infectious agents.

- Bathing provides pleasure and reduces stress.
- Bathing hydrates the skin and allows better delivery of corticosteroids and moisturizers.

Bathing Tips

- Mild, moisturizing soaps such as Dove or nonsoap cleansers such as Cetaphil Lotion should be used.
- Patients should use a nonsoap cleanser, or—on parts of the body that are free of eczema—a mild emollient soap.
- The patient should be cautioned not to use soap on lesional skin (many people are erroneously led to believe that "good soaps" may actually help inflamed skin).
- Excessive bathing that is not followed immediately by application of a moisturizer tends to dry the skin.
- Excessive toweling and scrubbing should be avoided.

Prevention of Atopic Dermatitis

The following measures may help the patient to avoid or reduce exposure to trigger factors such as dry skin, irritants, overheating and sweating, and allergens.

- Dry skin: Moisturizers, particularly in the dry winter months, should be applied immediately after bathing, to "trap" water in the skin. In warm climates or in the summer, however, moisturizers may actually be irritating or may interfere with healing.
  - **Suggested ointments:** Vaseline Petroleum Jelly, Aquaphor
  - **Suggested creams and lotions:** Eucerin, Cetaphil, Lubriderm, Curel, Moisturel
- Irritants: Nonirritating fabrics, such as cotton, should be worn. Wool clothing may induce itching.
- Overheating and sweating: Excess dryness or humidity should be avoided. An air conditioner or humidifier in a child's bedroom may help to avoid the dramatic changes in climate that may trigger outbreaks. (Unfortunately, humidifiers do not seem to help very much.)
- Allergens: Some evidence indicates that the environmental elimination of certain airborne substances, such as house dust mites, may bring some lasting relief. A great deal of controversy surrounds the influence of dietary manipulation and the value of skin testing and hyposensitization on the course of atopic dermatitis. Although some foods may provoke attacks, eliminating them will rarely bring a lasting improvement or cure. Skin tests and allergy shots may actually provoke attacks of atopic dermatitis.

POINTS TO REMEMBER

- Topical steroids should be applied only to active disease (inflamed skin).
- When topical steroids are applied immediately after bathing, their penetration and potency are increased.
- Low-potency topical steroids are recommended for use on the face and in skin folds, such as the perineal area and underarms.

HELPFUL HINTS

- There are primarily two causes of eczema: one comes from the outside (contact dermatitis), and other comes from the inside (atopic dermatitis).
- Patients and their parents, caregivers, and teachers should be educated about the manifestations and management of atopic dermatitis.
- The National Eczema Association can be contacted at: (503) 228-4430 or http://www.eczema-assn.org.

SEE PATIENT HANDOUT, PAGE 445

Numerous common clinical variants of eczema are recognized: nummular eczema, lichen simplex chronicus, prurigo nodularis, asteatotic eczema, neurotic excoriations, hand eczema, and nonspecific eczematous dermatitis. These disorders are usually found in patients with an atopic history. On occasion, however, they manifest in patients without an atopic predisposition; in such instances, a methodic search for an exogenous cause, such as a contact dermatitis, is often necessary. Included here are stasis dermatitis and seborrheic dermatitis, which are also eczematous eruptions that may or may not be related to an atopic history.

NUMMULAR ECZEMA

DESCRIPTION OF LESIONS

The lesions of nummular eczema are coin-shaped, usually itchy, eczematous patches and plaques that often occur in clusters (Figure 2.24). Although this disorder is usually seen in patients who have a history of atopy, it is not uncommon in patients without such a history.

DISTRIBUTION OF LESIONS

Lesions are mainly seen on the legs. Lesions sometimes clear centrally and resemble tinea corporis (ringworm). Healing or resolving lesions often display postinflammatory hyperpigmentation, particularly in dark-skinned patients (Figure 2.25).

DIAGNOSIS

The diagnosis of nummular eczema is based on the clinical appearance and, if necessary, negative results of a KOH examination.

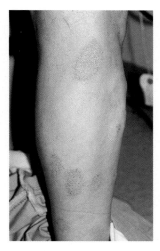

FIGURE 2.24 Nummular eczema. Erythematous, coin-shaped lesions are seen in a typical location.

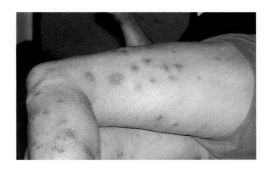

FIGURE 2.25 Nummular eczema. These coin-shaped scaly lesions show evidence of postinflammatory hyperpigmentation.

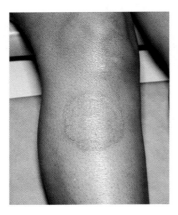

FIGURE 2.26 Tinea corporis (ringworm). Note the annular appearance, central clearing, and "active" scaly border that demonstrate hyphae on potassium hydroxide examination.

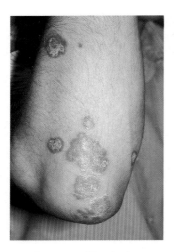

FIGURE 2.27 Psoriasis. These lesions with whitish, micaceous scale are seen in a typical location.

 DIFFERENTIAL DIAGNOSIS

Tinea Corporis (Figure 2.26)
• Lesions of tinea corporis are usually clear in the center (annular).
• In tinea corporis, the KOH examination or fungal culture is positive.

Psoriasis (Figure 2.27)
• Psoriasis is less likely to itch than is nummular eczema.
• Psoriatic lesions frequently occur on elbows and knees and show a whitish or micaceous scale.

Lichen Simplex Chronicus (see later)
• Focal lichenified plaques are noted.
• Often, a positive atopic history is present.

MANAGEMENT

• Nummular eczema can be controlled by an intermediate-strength topical corticosteroid, such as triamcinolone acetonide cream 0.1% applied sparingly two to three times daily.
• If necessary, a high-potency topical corticosteroid, such as clobetasol cream 0.05% once or twice daily, may be used.
• Recalcitrant cases may require occlusion—provided by a polyethylene wrap or Cordran (flurandrenolide) tape—or intralesional corticosteroid injections.
• Long-term treatment can be accomplished with less potent topical corticosteroids.

POINT TO REMEMBER
• Nummular eczema is frequently misdiagnosed as tinea corporis.

LICHEN SIMPLEX CHRONICUS

Also known as *neurodermatitis*, lichen simplex chronicus is a common, chronic, usually solitary, pruritic eczematous eruption caused by repetitive rubbing and scratching. It is seen most commonly in adults, particularly in patients with other atopic manifestations, such as asthma and allergic rhinitis.

CLINICAL MANIFESTATION AND DISTRIBUTION OF LESIONS

Patients with lichen simplex chronicus have a focal lichenified plaque or multiple plaques, most often on the nape of the neck, scalp, external ear canals, wrists, extensor forearms, ankles (Figure 2.28), pretibial areas, or inner thighs. Lichen simplex chronicus may also involve the vulvae, scrotum, and perianal area (pruritus ani). Patients often have only one area of involvement (circumscribed dermatitis). Chronic or paroxysmal pruritus is the primary symptom. Diagnosis is readily apparent and is made on clinical grounds.

 ## DIFFERENTIAL DIAGNOSIS

Tinea Cruris and Candidiasis
- A chronic itchy vulvar or scrotal rash may also suggest a fungal infection such as tinea cruris or candidiasis.

Inverse Psoriasis
Inverse psoriasis (Figure 2.29) should be considered in lesions that involve the inguinal creases and perianal area.

 ### MANAGEMENT
- The most important aspect of therapy is the elimination of scratching and rubbing. Unfortunately, many patients scratch themselves in their sleep.
- Like nummular eczema, lichen simplex chronicus may be treated with an intermediate-strength topical corticosteroid. If necessary, a high-potency topical corticosteroid can be used.
- Occlusion, when required, has the added advantage of preventing patients from scratching or rubbing—or, at least, reminding them not to do so.
- Oral antihistamines may be helpful at bedtime because of their sedative effect.
- Tacrolimus (Protopic) ointment 0.03% may prove beneficial in patients with vulvar or perianal lichen simplex chronicus. (Patients should be warned about the potential for stinging and burning when tacrolimus ointment is applied to these sensitive areas.)
- Alternatively, pimecrolimus (Elidel) cream 1% may be effective. It is less irritating than protopic ointment.

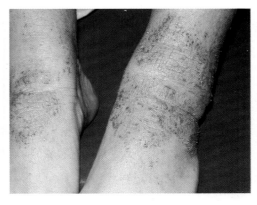

FIGURE 2.28 Lichen simplex chronicus. These focal lichenified plaques involve the distal pretibial area and ankle. This patient not only scratched the lesions, but also she persistently rubbed them with her contralateral heels.

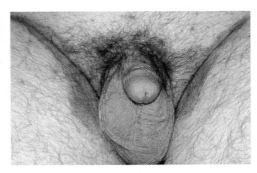

FIGURE 2.29 Inverse psoriasis. This eruption could easily be mistaken for tinea cruris or candidiasis.

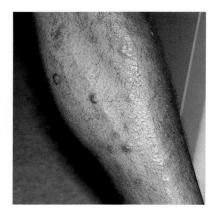

FIGURE 2.30 Prurigo nodularis. These intensely pruritic excoriated papules on the pretibial shafts show marked postinflammatory hyperpigmentation.

PRURIGO NODULARIS

Another chronic, but much less common, variant of atopic dermatitis is prurigo nodularis. It is seen in the same clinical context as lichen simplex chronicus and may be considered a papular or nodular form of it.

DESCRIPTION OF LESIONS

Lesions are reddish, brown, or hyperpigmented dome-shaped papules or nodules (Figure 2.30).

CLINICAL MANIFESTATION AND DISTRIBUTION OF LESIONS

- Lesions are most commonly noted on the pretibial shafts and sometimes on the extensor areas of the arms.
- They are often crusted or excoriated—pruritus may be intense.
- Healing results in significant postinflammatory hyperpigmentation.

MANAGEMENT

- Prurigo nodularis tends to be very resistant to topical corticosteroids.
- Intralesional corticosteroid injections may be helpful.
- Thalidomide (50 to 300 mg per day) has been reported as effective in recalcitrant cases. (Thalidomide should not be used in women who are pregnant. In the United States, only physicians who are part of a special registry are permitted to administer this drug.)

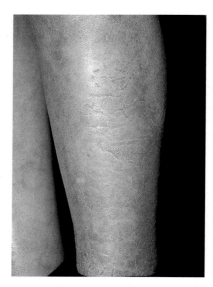

FIGURE 2.31 Asteatotic eczema *(erythema craquelé)*. These scaly patches with superficial fissures resemble a cracked antique china vase or a dry riverbed.

ASTEATOTIC ECZEMA

A common form of dermatitis, asteatotic eczema appears in dry, cold, winter months. It is also referred to as *winter eczema,* and because its lesions consist of scaly patches with superficial fissures that resemble a cracked antique china vase, it is sometimes called, *erythema craquelé.* It occurs only in adults.

CLINICAL MANIFESTATION AND DISTRIBUTION OF LESIONS

- The condition may be pruritic.
- Lesions consist of characteristic scaly patches with very shallow erythematous fissures resembling a cracked, dry riverbed (Figure 2.31).
- They are located most commonly on the shins, arms, hands, and trunk.

DIFFERENTIAL DIAGNOSIS

The differential diagnosis of asteatotic eczema includes **xerosis** (dry skin) and very mild cases of **nummular eczema.**

MANAGEMENT

- Asteatotic eczema is usually managed readily by having the patient bathe less frequently and apply moisturizers regularly.
- A very effective treatment is Lac-Hydrin (12% ammonium lactate cream or lotion), which is available only by prescription, and the similar preparation, AmLactin, which can be obtained without a prescription. These agents are applied immediately after bathing.
- If necessary, pruritic lesions will respond readily to low- to moderate-strength topical corticosteroids.

NEUROTIC EXCORIATIONS

Patients with neurotic excoriations compulsively pick at their skin. Lesions may accompany or exacerbate atopic dermatitis, or they may have been preceded by atopic dermatitis or an insect bite; most often, however, no precipitating cause can be determined.

CLINICAL MANIFESTATION AND DISTRIBUTION OF LESIONS

- Lesions frequently suggest an "outside job," with erosions and grouped linear crusts.
- Postinflammatory hyperpigmentation and whitish hypopigmented lesions indicate chronicity.
- Deep ulcerations with geometric shapes suggest **factitia** (Figures 2.32 and 2.33), a self-induced condition caused by habitual scratching or picking. In factitia, lesions tend to show a wide range of bizarre patterns uncharacteristic of any disease. The presence of factitia may imply that the patient has severe emotional problems.

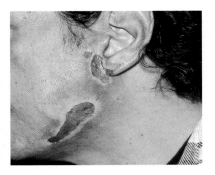

FIGURE 2.32 Factitial ulcerations. These were created by the patient. Note their geometric appearance. The patient has a severe psychiatric disorder.

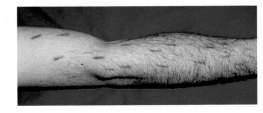

FIGURE 2.33 Factitial purpura. These purpuric lesions were obviously self-induced.

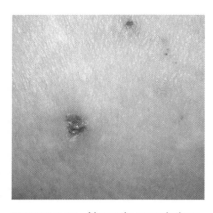

FIGURE 2.34 Neurotic excoriations. Lesions tend to be located on the upper back or ankles, areas that are easily reachable.

- The lesions of neurotic excoriation tend to be located on the upper back or ankles—areas that are easily reachable, especially by the dominant hand (Figure 2.34).
- Factitial lesions may appear anywhere and often have bizarre shapes.
- Many patients with neurotic excoriations or factitia may also show signs and symptoms of a neurosis (e.g., obsessive–compulsive disorder) or delusional psychosis that underlies the repetitive self-destructive behavior.

DIAGNOSIS

- The diagnosis is either given by the patient, who readily admits that the lesions are self-created, or the lesions themselves may be indicative.
- Bizarre lesions and a "belle indifférence" affect on the part of the patient suggest factitial dermatitis as the cause.

MANAGEMENT

- High-potency topical corticosteroids, topical corticosteroids under occlusion, and intralesional corticosteroids are sometimes useful, but these treatments will be ineffective if the underlying psychologic cause is not addressed.
- Bedtime antihistamines are sometimes helpful.
- Psychotherapy or psychopharmacologic drugs should be used, if indicated.

Many people, particularly the elderly, have chronic, recurrent, itchy, eczematous dermatitis without the typical distribution of atopic dermatitis (Figure 2.35). These patients may have no apparent atopic history. Frequently, they complain of dry or sensitive skin that tends to become drier and itchier in winter months. The eruption tends to worsen with aging, as the skin loses some of its barrier function and lubrication (asteatosis). Lesions tend to occur on the arms, legs, and upper back.

DIAGNOSIS AND DIFFERENTIAL DIAGNOSIS

Nonspecific eczematous dermatitis is a diagnosis of exclusion when no underlying cause, such as a contact allergen, scabies, or occult fungal infection (tinea incognito), is found.

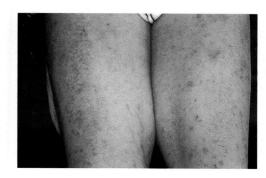

FIGURE 2.35 Nonspecific eczematous dermatitis, with itchy, ill-defined patches of eczema.

MANAGEMENT

- Treatment consists of an intermediate-strength topical corticosteroid.
- If necessary, a higher potency topical corticosteroid may be used. Patients with nonspecific eczematous dermatitis should avoid the use of soap on affected areas. In dry winter months, moisturizers may be beneficial.

ATOPIC HAND ECZEMA (CHRONIC HAND DERMATITIS)

BASICS

When eczema involves the hands and is caused by exposure to an irritant or an allergic contactant, the diagnosis is contact dermatitis (see later).

When there is no suggestive history or documentation of an exogenous cause of hand eczema, the diagnosis is most likely atopic hand eczema (also known as **chronic hand dermatitis**). Most patients with atopic hand eczema report an atopic history, such as a personal or familial atopic diathesis (e.g., asthma, hay fever, sinusitis), or patients may have had a previous episode of atopic dermatitis or a concurrent manifestation elsewhere on the body. Even with these findings, a diligent history must be taken. In addition, patch testing with putative allergens may be performed if an exogenous cause is suspected. Keep in mind that it is also common for both exogenous (contact) and endogenous (atopic) factors to be at work in the same patient.

Whatever the origin, hand eczema is often a cause of social embarrassment and can result in performance problems in the workplace. The onset of atopic hand eczema is uncommon before adolescence. After middle age, the frequency of acute episodes tends to decrease.

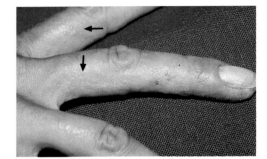

FIGURE 2.36 Atopic hand eczema, dyshidrotic or wet type. The characteristic vesicles *(arrows)* on the sides of the fingers are shown here.

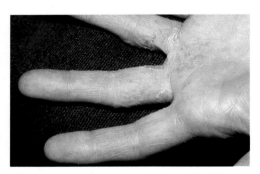

FIGURE 2.37 Atopic hand eczema, dyshidrotic or wet type, subacute. The vesicles are beginning to dry, and the lesions are becoming scaly. Note the older vesicles that are turning golden brown.

DESCRIPTION OF LESIONS, CLINICAL MANIFESTATIONS, AND DISTRIBUTION OF LESIONS

For descriptive purposes, atopic hand eczema may be divided into two clinical types that may overlap in the same patient: a wet type and a dry, scaly type.

Wet Type

Dyshidrotic eczema, the wet type (Figure 2.36), was formerly referred to as *pompholyx* (the Greek word for bubble), which describes the following:

- Itchy, clear vesicles are seen in this condition.
- The vesicles are typically located on the sides of the fingers, but they can also occur on the palms and, less commonly, on the soles of the feet and the lateral aspects of the toes. The term dyshidrotic is a misnomer based on the erroneous assumption that the vesicles were caused by trapped sweat. We now understand that they result from inflammation and foci of intercellular edema ("spongiosis"), which becomes loculated in the thicker stratum corneum of the palms and soles.
- Initially, the very small and clear vesicles resemble little bubbles.
- Later, as they dry and resolve without rupturing, they turn golden brown (Figure 2.37).

Dry, Scaly Type

In nondyshidrotic hand eczema—the dry, scaly type (Figure 2.38)—the following are noted:

- Lesions are scaly and red.
- The skin surface often loses its flexibility and develops painful fissures.
- Scaly, hyperkeratotic, lichenified plaques may arise.
- Fingertips may become dry, wrinkled, red, and fragile, with resultant painful fissures and erosions (Figure 2.39).
- The central palm or palmar aspect of the hands and fingers is also commonly affected in patients with chronic hand eczema. Hyperkeratotic palmar eczema is characterized by highly itchy hyperkeratotic palms.
- Fissures in the folds of the hands and fingers are painful and can limit the use of the hands.
- As with the dyshidrotic type of hand eczema, oozing and secondary bacterial infection ("honey-crusted" skin) can occur.
- With long-standing disease, patients' fingernails may reveal dystrophic changes (e.g., irregular transverse ridging, pitting, thickening, discoloration) when the nail matrix (root) becomes involved (Figure 2.40).

FACTORS THAT MAY TRIGGER RECURRENCES

Many of the triggers that exacerbate eczema are ubiquitous in daily life and in certain work settings. They include the following:

- Emotional stress.
- Environmental conditions (including seasonal changes, hot or cold temperatures, humidity).
- Contact allergens (including nickel, balsams, paraphenylenediamine, chromates) and irritants (including soaps).
- *Staphylococcus aureus.* This microbe is thought to play a role in the exacerbation of eczema because it is virtually omnipresent on the skin of patients with atopic dermatitis. Colonization with *S. aureus* results in the secretion of toxins (superantigens) that promote skin inflammation. The importance of *S. aureus* is supported by the observation that treatment with an anti–*S. aureus* antibiotic (in combination with topical corticosteroids) is effective not only in patients with obvious impetiginized eczema, but also in patients without superinfection.

DIAGNOSIS

The diagnosis of atopic hand eczema is usually made on clinical grounds or when other causes are excluded.

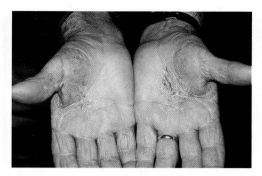

FIGURE 2.38 Atopic hand eczema, dry, scaly, type. Scaly, hyperkeratotic, lichenified plaques and painful fissures are shown here.

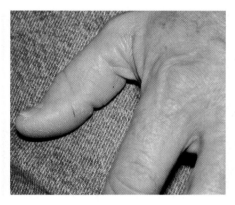

FIGURE 2.39 Atopic hand eczema, dry, scaly type. The fingertips have become dry, and fragile, with a resultant painful fissure on the thumb.

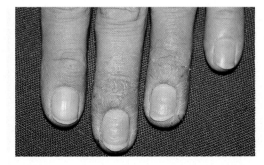

FIGURE 2.40 Atopic hand eczema. This patient's middle fingernails show dystrophic changes, transverse ridging, and cuticle loss solely on those fingers where eczema is present in the proximal nail folds.

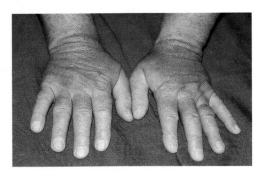

FIGURE 2.41 Contact dermatitis. This eczematous dermatitis on the dorsa of the hands was caused by exposure to lanolin.

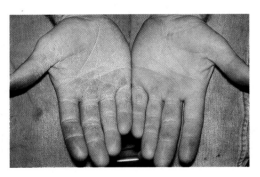

FIGURE 2.42 Tinea manuum. Only one palm shows a well-demarcated plaque. The scale of this palm was positive for fungus.

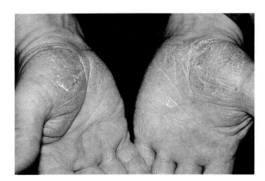

FIGURE 2.43 Psoriasis of the palms. These palmar lesions can easily be mistaken for eczema or tinea.

◀▶◆ **DIFFERENTIAL DIAGNOSIS**

Contact Dermatitis (Figure 2.41)

- This is suspected, particularly if the eruption is on the dorsum of the hands or feet.
- The patient has a history of exposure to a suspected contactant.

Tinea Manuum (Figure 2.42)
- This is suggested by well-demarcated plaques on the palms (usually on one palm only) and soles or a positive KOH examination or fungal culture.

Psoriasis on the Palms (Figure 2.43)
- This may be indistinguishable from hand eczema.
- Pustular psoriasis of the palms may also, at times, be indistinguishable from pustular dyshidrotic hand eczema.
- The patient may have evidence of psoriasis elsewhere on the body or a personal or family history of psoriasis.

Scabies
This diagnosis should be considered if there is an acute pruritic vesicular eruption in the web spaces of the fingers.

MANAGEMENT

Mild Cases
Patients with mild cases of atopic hand eczema are managed as follows:

- Mild cleansers or soap substitutes are recommended.
- Protective cotton-lined gloves are used for washing dishes or other similar tasks.
- Fastidious hand protection is necessary, with emollient barrier creams, protective gloves, and the avoidance of irritants and allergens.
- For oozing and infected lesions, compresses with Burow's solution (10% aluminum acetate) are applied. This treatment promotes drying and has an antibacterial effect. The solution is applied in a 1:40 dilution two or three times daily until bullae resolve (usually, within a few days).
- Topical corticosteroids are the mainstay of treatment. Ointments penetrate skin better than creams do, but patients may prefer to use creams during the day. Most patients require medium-potency corticosteroids (e.g., triamcinolone 0.1%), with or without occlusion. However, higher potency corticosteroids (e.g., fluocinonide 0.05%) can be used on an as-needed basis. Lower strength corticosteroids (e.g., hydrocortisone valerate 0.2%) may sometimes be applied for long-term maintenance.
- Protopic ointment (tacrolimus) 0.1% and Elidel cream (pimecrolimus) 1%, may also be effective.

(continued)

Severe Cases

Severe atopic hand eczema is often very difficult to manage.

- Applying corticosteroids under occlusion is occasionally effective when it is done early in the course of an eruption. However, potent topical corticosteroids applied under plastic or vinyl occlusion and superpotent topical corticosteroids can be used only intermittently and for short periods, because they increase the risk for atrophy.
- Systemic antibiotics should be administered for obvious or suspected secondary infection.
- Short-term use of systemic corticosteroids may be required for very severe flares. They should be given very infrequently, however.
- Treatment of hyperkeratotic palmar eczema is notoriously difficult. Acitretin (Soriatane), an aromatic retinoid, often helps to control hyperkeratosis. Therapy may have to be continued indefinitely.
- Other measures, such as PUVA (oral psoralen plus topical ultraviolet A), oral cyclosporine, azathioprine, and low-dose methotrexate, are used for severe, refractory cases.
- Superficial X-irradiation has been used in some patients who have resistant chronic hand eczema.

 SEE PATIENT HANDOUT, PAGE 449

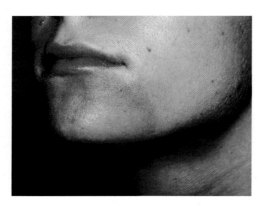

FIGURE 2.44 Irritant contact dermatitis. The localized erythema on this boy's face was due to irritation from benzoyl peroxide.

BASICS

Contact dermatitis is an inflammatory reaction of the skin that is caused by an external agent. The appearance of the eruption and a careful history often give clues to the offending agent. The two types of contact dermatitis are irritant and allergic.

Irritant Contact Dermatitis

Also known as nonallergic contact dermatitis, irritant contact dermatitis (ICD) is an erythematous, scaly, sometimes eczematous eruption that is not caused by allergens (Figure 2.44). It is a direct toxic reaction to rubbing, friction, or maceration, or to exposure to a chemical or thermal agent. Its severity depends on the concentration of the irritant, its thermal energy, its abrasiveness, and the duration of exposure, among other factors. ICD may occur in anyone.

The eruption of ICD is confined to the areas of exposure, as exemplified by diaper rash, "dishpan hands," and reactions that occur under an adhesive dressing or where a topical medication was applied. Examples of irritants include alkalis, acids, solvents, soaps, detergents, and numerous chemicals found in the home and workplace that damage the skin after repeated contact. Patients who have atopic dermatitis are more likely to develop ICD, as a result of their inherent skin sensitivity.

Diagnosis, when not clearly evident, is based on a careful history and the ruling out of allergic contact dermatitis (ACD), which is discussed later. Management is fairly simple. Patients should be told to avoid the offending agent or to minimize contact with it.

DIAPER DERMATITIS (DIAPER RASH)

BASICS

A common example of ICD is diaper dermatitis (diaper rash), referred to as "napkin dermatitis" in the United Kingdom. Diaper dermatitis applies to eruptions that occur in the area covered by a diaper. Irritant diaper dermatitis is by far the most common rash in infancy, but it is not restricted to that age group because it can affect persons of any age group who wear diapers, such as incontinent patients.

Pathogenesis

Diaper dermatitis is essentially the result of overhydration of the skin that is irritated by chafing, by soaps and detergents, and by prolonged contact with urine and feces. The ammonia that is produced as a breakdown product of urea by bacteria in feces is considered an exacerbating factor. Added to this wet, macerated, excrement-laden milieu are the occlusive effect of rubber or plastic diapers and the constant contact of moisture from cloth diapers when they are not changed right away. Diaper dermatitis may also be caused by, or intensified by, the presence of atopic dermatitis, seborrheic dermatitis, or a secondary infection by *Candida albicans*. (*C. albicans* is often isolated from the perineal area in many of these infants; whether it is the cause or effect of the rash is controversial.)

CLINICAL MANIFESTATIONS AND DESCRIPTION OF LESIONS

- Erythema, scale, and possibly papules and plaques are present; occasionally, vesicles and bullae occur.
- With neglect, lesions may erode and ulcerate.
- Beefy redness and satellite pustules suggest a primary or secondary infection of diaper dermatitis with *Candida*.

DISTRIBUTION OF LESIONS

- Lesions typically **spare the creases** (genitocrural folds) (Figure 2.45).
- The eruption may conform to, and be limited to, the diaper area, or it may affect the lower abdomen, genitalia, perineum, and buttocks.
- Primary candidal diaper dermatitis should be considered in an immunocompromised patient, particularly if the creases are involved. This diagnosis can be confirmed by KOH examination.

 DIFFERENTIAL DIAGNOSIS

Atopic Dermatitis of the Diaper Area
- In general, patients with atopic dermatitis are more likely to experience ICD; nonetheless, the diaper area is often remarkably spared (Figure 2.46).
- Other evidence of atopic dermatitis is present; the patient has a family history of atopy.

Seborrheic Dermatitis (Intertriginous Seborrheic Dermatitis) (see Seborrheic Dermatitis later)
- The creases are involved, and the patient may have lesions elsewhere such as the axillae or scalp *(cradle cap)*.

Other less common conditions to consider in the differential diagnosis are tinea cruris, impetigo, child abuse, Kawasaki's disease, and psoriasis, particularly if there is a positive family history or other evidence of psoriasis. In addition, other rare diseases such as Letterer–Siwe disease (a form of histiocytosis X) and acrodermatitis enteropathica (from zinc deficiency) should be considered in recalcitrant cases. Leiner's disease is a very rare eruption resembling seborrheic dermatitis that is associated with diarrhea and a failure to thrive.

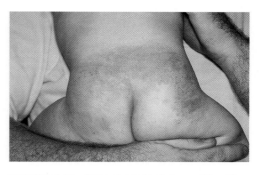

FIGURE 2.45 Irritant contact dermatitis. The patient has a diaper rash with an eruption conforming to the shape of a diaper.

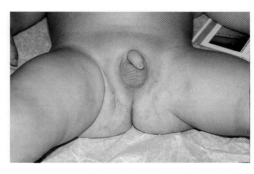

FIGURE 2.46 Atopic dermatitis. Note the involvement of the inguinal creases.

MANAGEMENT

General preventive measures to minimize friction, absorb moisture, and protect the skin from urine and feces include the following:

- The use of disposable or superabsorbent diapers holds moisture in and keeps it away from the skin.
- Frequent diaper changes should be done promptly after voiding or soiling.
- Rubber and plastic pants should be avoided.
- Soap-free cleansers such as Cetaphil Lotion are recommended.
- Absorbent baby powders such as Desitin cornstarch powder, Zeasorb powder, and Johnson's Baby Powder are useful.
- Aquaphor ointment and pure white petrolatum ointment (Vaseline Petroleum Jelly) act by trapping water beneath the epidermis.

Specific Measures of Treatment
- The first-line therapy is zinc oxide ointment. There are many inexpensive over-the-counter products that contain zinc oxide such as Balmex, Desitin, and A and D ointment.
- Petrolatum, zinc oxide, aluminum acetate solution (1-2-3 Paste) is a "tried and true" combination product that both protects skin and has a drying effect. It should be applied after each diaper change.
- Low-potency over-the-counter hydrocortisone 1% or 1/2% cream or ointment is often all that is necessary for uncomplicated diaper dermatitis.
- Stronger topical steroids such as desonide 0.05% or hydrocortisone valerate 0.02% cream or ointment may be used for short periods, if necessary.
- Potent topical steroids, particularly fluorinated preparations such as contained in Lotrisone, are to be avoided in the diaper area.
- If the presence of *C. albicans* is suspected, particularly if there is no improvement after several days, a topical antifungal preparation such as the over-the-counter miconazole (Micatin) or ketoconazole should be applied. Consider adding nonabsorbable oral nystatin in recalcitrant cases.

 POINTS TO REMEMBER

- Avoid the use of potent topical steroids in the diaper area.
- Educate parents and caregivers to change diapers frequently, to wash the patient's genitalia with warm water and mild soap, and to use superabsorbent disposable diapers.
- Consider referral to a dermatologist, particularly in persistent, unresponsive cases.

Allergic Contact Dermatitis

BASICS

A true allergic reaction that precipitates eczematous dermatitis, ACD is caused by an allergen (antigen) that produces a delayed (type IV) hypersensitivity reaction. It occurs only in sensitized persons. ACD is not dose dependent, and it may spread extensively beyond the site of original contact. ACD is seen less commonly in young children, the elderly, and African-Americans.

Examples of allergic contact sensitizers include jewelry, metal (Figure 2.47), cosmetics, topical medications, rubber compounds, plants, and the countless chemicals that are found in the home and work environments. The best-known example of ACD is caused by poison ivy and poison oak (rhus dermatitis).

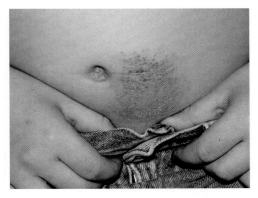

FIGURE 2.47 Allergic contact dermatitis. This boy developed an eczematous eruption at the site where the nickel snap on his blue jeans contacted his skin.

RHUS DERMATITIS

In the United States, poison ivy and poison oak are the principal causes of rhus dermatitis. Poison ivy is found throughout the country. Poison oak is more commonly found in the western United States. Poison sumac, another cause of rhus dermatitis, is found only in woody, swampy areas.

The three plants belong to the same genus, *Toxicodendron*, which is the "poisonous" branch of the genus *Rhus*. Each of the three plants contains penta- and heptadecylcatechol, the sensitizing allergens, in their resinous oils (urushiol). The plants' invisible oils may reach the skin not only through direct contact but also through garden tools, pet fur, golf clubs, or the smoke of a burning plant. Identical or related antigens are found in the resin of the Japanese lacquer tree, ginkgo trees, cashew nut shells, the dye of the India marking nut (used as a clothing dye in India), and the skin of mangoes. All cause similar skin rashes in sensitized people.

In the eastern United States, rhus dermatitis occurs mainly in the spring and summer. In the western and southeastern United States, where outdoor activity is common all year, rhus dermatitis may occur in any season. Approximately 85% of the population will develop a reaction on exposure to one of the plants.

DESCRIPTION OF LESIONS

The characteristic eruption, which consists of intensely pruritic linear streaks of erythematous papules, "juicy" vesicles, and blisters, appears to be factitious (i.e., caused by an "outside job") (Figure 2.48). The rash typically occurs 2 days after contact with the plant, but initial reactions have been noted within 12 hours of contact and as long as 1 week later.

Generally, exposed areas of the body are affected first. The rash may later involve covered areas that have come into contact with the plant oil. For example, the external vulva or perianal areas may be affected after women with rhus dermatitis use toilet paper that has been contaminated by plant oil from their hands. In men, involvement of the penis is sometimes a diagnostic sign.

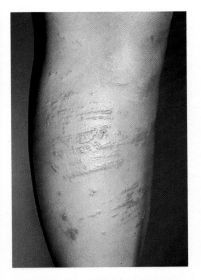

FIGURE 2.48 Allergic contact dermatitis. Poison ivy caused this eruption. Note the "outside job" appearance of the linear streaks of papules and vesicles.

DIAGNOSIS

- The diagnosis of rhus dermatitis is based on history of exposure to an antigen and the characteristic distribution of the lesions. Contrary to common belief, the fluid in blisters does not contain the resinous oil, and it cannot transfer the rash to others or cause the rash to spread on the affected person. Further dissemination, or autoeczematization, is believed to occur through hematogenous spread and subsequent immune-complex deposition in the skin. This spread may occur within 5 to 7 days after the initial office exposure, and the resulting rash may last for 3 weeks or more.

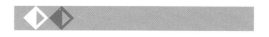

◁◆ DIFFERENTIAL DIAGNOSIS

Conditions to be included in the differential diagnosis are as follows:

Other Forms of Contact Dermatitis
Plants
- Plants such as meadow grass may cause a reaction that resembles rhus dermatitis.

Insect Bites (Figure 2.49)
- Bites, particularly those from bedbugs, often cause a linear eruption that may occasionally be confused with rhus dermatitis.

Scabies
- In scabietic infestations, other family members may report itching. Scabies has its own characteristic distribution of lesions: in the finger webs, wrists, genitals, and axillae.

Herpes Zoster (Figure 2.50)
- Nonpainful herpes zoster, with its linear series of blisters, can cause diagnostic confusion.

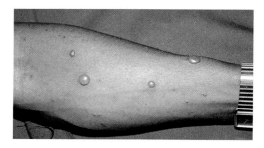

FIGURE 2.49 Vesicobullous insect bite reaction. This could easily be mistaken for poison ivy.

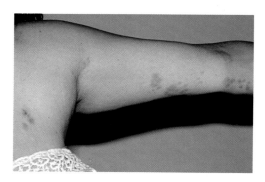

FIGURE 2.50 Herpes zoster. This linear eruption could also be mistaken for poison ivy.

MANAGEMENT

A limited eruption and mild itching may be relieved by the following:

- Cool showers and application of frozen vegetable packages such as frozen peas may help.
- Cool baths with colloidal oatmeal agents such as Aveeno are recommended.
- Cool compresses of Burow's solution help to dry vesicles and bullae.
- Calamine lotion is useful.
- Potent or superpotent topical corticosteroids, such as clobetasol cream 0.05% two or three times daily, can be prescribed.
- Oral antihistamines are helpful, particularly at bedtime. In severe cases with widespread eruption and marked pruritus, topical therapy may need to be supplemented with the following:
  - Systemic corticosteroids. Prednisone is usually used, in a tapering dosage schedule that often starts at 1 mg/kg and decreases by 5 mg every 2 days for at least 2 weeks and for as long as 3 weeks. The dosage may be increased again if flares occur during the tapering regimen. Prednisone tablets should be taken with meals, and the entire daily dose may be taken all at once, rather than in divided doses throughout the day. (Possible side effects of short-term systemic corticosteroids include gastrointestinal upset, sleep disturbances, and mood changes. Hyperactivity, anxiety, depression, and even paranoia have been reported.)
  - Intramuscular corticosteroids. Triamcinolone diacetate or hexacetonide may be used if the patient has gastrointestinal intolerance to oral corticosteroids.

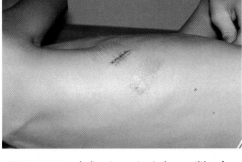

FIGURE 2.51 Irritant contact dermatitis. A Band-Aid caused a focal irritant reaction in this patient.

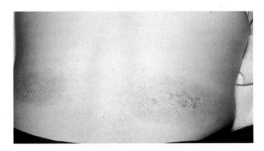

FIGURE 2.52 Allergic contact dermatitis. This patient reacted to the rubber in the elastic waistband of her underpants. Note sparing at the sites where the garment did not come into constant contact with the skin.

SEE PATIENT HANDOUT, PAGE 451

OTHER FORMS OF ALLERGIC CONTACT DERMATITIS

Other than the *Toxicodendron* species, the most common contact allergens are nickel, thimerosal (a mercurial preservative), neomycin (a topical antibiotic), formaldehyde (found in shampoo and cosmetics), *para*-phenylenediamine (found in certain hair dyes), and quaternium-15 (a preservative often found in cosmetics) (Figures 2.51 to 2.54). Patterns of distribution and shapes of the rash may be clues to the specific allergen, as in, for example, dermatitis from rubber in underpants, neomycin in eardrops, or nickel in earrings.

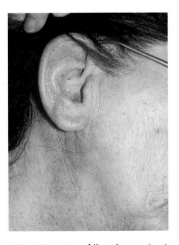

FIGURE 2.53 Allergic contact dermatitis. This contact dermatitis is secondary to neomycin in ear drops.

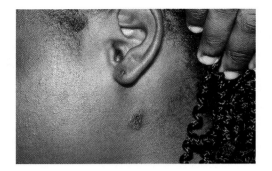

FIGURE 2.54 Allergic contact dermatitis. Nickel in earrings caused this dermatitis on the ear lobe and neck.

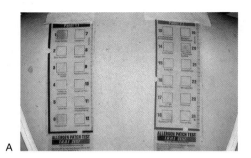

A

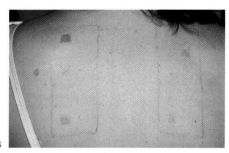

B

FIGURE 2.55 Test patches. *A:* These test patches will be removed after 48 hours. *B:* The final reading at 96 hours shows positive reactions to various allergens.

DIAGNOSIS

Patients should be questioned regarding their daily habits and occupational exposures, so any possible contactants can be revealed. Patch testing is used as an aid to identify specific allergens in patients with histories suggestive of ACD (Figure 2.55). The allergens most commonly responsible for ACD are standardized and are available commercially. The allergens, which are fixed in dehydrated gel layers, are taped against the skin of the patient's back for 48 hours and are then removed. A final reading is performed at 96 hours. The area is examined for evidence of contact dermatitis. The presence of erythema, papules, or vesicles (i.e., an acute eczematous reaction) is strongly positive. A bullous reaction is extremely positive. Interpretation of patch test results and correlation with clinical findings require experience and are generally performed by dermatologists.

 DIFFERENTIAL DIAGNOSIS

Conditions to include in the differential diagnosis are the following:

- ICD
- Other types of acute and chronic eczematous dermatitis
- Systemic drug reactions

 MANAGEMENT

Patients with ACD may be managed with the following:

- Identification and removal of the inciting agent
- Advice on how to avoid the inciting agent
- Treatment with topical or systemic corticosteroids, if necessary

 POINTS TO REMEMBER

- In patients with severe rhus dermatitis, it is important to continue prednisone for 2 to 3 weeks because a shorter course may allow a rebound of the condition.
- Patch testing may be the only way to differentiate ACD from ICD.

HELPFUL HINTS

- Methylprednisolone Dosepaks usually do not provide enough days of treatment for most patients who have rhus dermatitis.
- During the tapering prednisone regimen for treatment of severe rhus dermatitis, patients may experience a rebound of the eruption and itching. When this rebound occurs, it may be suggested that patients increase the dosage back to the one that worked the day before and then titrate downward thereafter.
- There are advantages to prescribing doses consistently in increments of 5 mg. It is easier for the patient and health care provider to keep track of the dosage schedule, and tablets usually do not have to be broken in half to decrease the dose.

Prevention

To prevent rhus dermatitis, patients can learn to recognize its plants:

- "Leaves of three, let it be." If work or hobbies involve frequent exposure to poisonous plants, a barrier cream may be applied before exposure.
- When people come into contact with the plant or its oil, they should wash with soap and cold water as soon as possible. All exposed clothing should be laundered.
- Vaccines against poison ivy and other immunizations given orally or as injections may be result in serious negative side effects and often fail.

SEBORRHEIC DERMATITIS

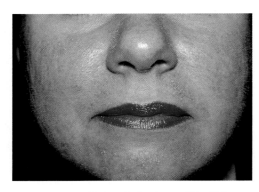

FIGURE 2.56 Seborrheic dermatitis. This patient has extensive scaling and erythema on her face.

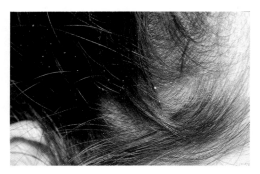

FIGURE 2.57 Dandruff. This patient shows scale without erythema.

BASICS

Seborrheic dermatitis is a very common, chronic inflammatory dermatitis. Its characteristic distribution involves areas that have the greatest concentration of sebaceous glands: scalp, face (Figure 2.56), presternal region, interscapular area, umbilicus, and body folds (intertriginous areas).

Many people experience some degree of dandruff—a whitish scaling of the scalp that is sometimes itchy and is fairly easily controlled with dandruff shampoos (Figure 2.57). When dandruff is accompanied by erythema, a sign of inflammation, it is referred to as seborrheic dermatitis. When seborrheic dermatitis occurs in the body folds, it is called intertrigo, or intertriginous seborrheic dermatitis.

Seborrheic dermatitis is seen more commonly in male patients and often begins after puberty. There appears to be a hereditary predisposition to its development. When it presents in patients who are infected with the human immunodeficiency virus (HIV), seborrheic dermatitis may serve as an early marker of the acquired immunodeficiency syndrome. Seborrheic dermatitis is also seen commonly in patients with Parkinson's disease, and in patients taking phenothiazines.

Seborrheic dermatitis has many features in common with chronic eczema and psoriasis: Typical lesions of seborrheic dermatitis often appear in patients with psoriasis, and the histologic features of the lesions of seborrheic dermatitis resemble those of both eczema and psoriasis. In fact, some dermatologists do not consider seborrheic dermatitis a distinct nosologic entity, but instead assign it to various forms of eczema or psoriasis. In the latter case, the term "seborrhiasis" has been used. In the United Kingdom, seborrheic dermatitis is referred to as "seborrhoeic eczema."

Pathogenesis

Traditionally, seborrheic dermatitis has been described as idiopathic. Some evidence, however, indicates that *Pityrosporon ovale,* a small yeast, may play a part in its pathogenesis because seborrheic dermatitis occasionally responds to antifungal medications, such as ketoconazole. Because seborrheic dermatitis occurs only where the sebaceous glands are found, sebum has also been thought to play a role, although no link has been shown.

DESCRIPTION OF LESIONS

The appearance of the lesions of seborrheic dermatitis varies depending on their location. On the face, lesions are red, with or without an overlying whitish scale, or they may appear as orange-yellow greasy patches. On the scalp, seborrheic dermatitis may range from a mild erythema and scaling to thick, armorlike plaques that are indistinguishable from psoriasis ("sebopsoriasis").

When lesions occur in body folds, they often consist of sharply defined, bright red plaques that may develop fissures.

DISTRIBUTION OF LESIONS

The eruption of seborrheic dermatitis tends to be bilaterally symmetric in its distribution:

- **Scalp, face.** Lesions appear on the forehead, eyebrows, eyelashes, cheeks, beard, and nasolabial folds (Figures 2.58 and 2.59).
- **Ears.** Lesions occur behind the ears and in the external ear canal (Figure 2.60).

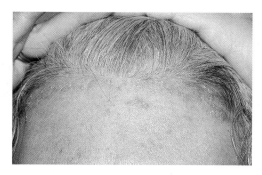

FIGURE 2.58 Seborrheic dermatitis. Scale and erythema are evident along the frontal hairline.

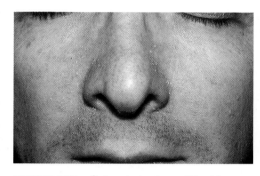

FIGURE 2.59 Seborrheic dermatitis. Here we see typical involvement of the cheeks and nasolabial folds.

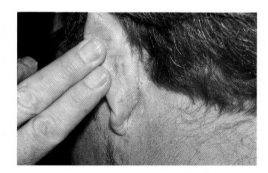

FIGURE 2.60 Seborrheic dermatitis. This patient has involvement of retroauricular area.

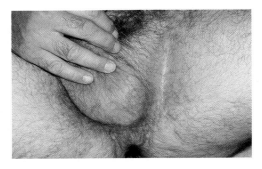

FIGURE 2.61 Intertrigo (intertriginous seborrheic dermatitis). This patient has an itchy erythematous rash in his inguinal creases. This condition is frequently confused with tinea cruris and cutaneous candidiasis.

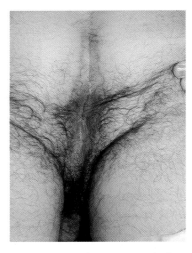

FIGURE 2.62 Inverse psoriasis. This intergluteal erythematous plaque is often indistinguishable from intertrigo.

- **Body folds.** Body folds and anogenital areas are affected—inframammary areas, axillae, inguinal creases (Figure 2.61), and intragluteal crease and perianal area (Figure 2.62).

CLINICAL MANIFESTATIONS

- On the scalp, there may be itching and scale with resultant dandruff that, embarrassingly, often falls on clothing.
- Facial seborrheic dermatitis usually flares in the winter and improves in the summer. Many patients, however, report provocation of the condition after sun exposure.
- When fissures develop in the body folds and umbilicus, symptoms consist of burning, itching, oozing, and pain.

CLINICAL VARIANTS

- Nonspecific vulvitis and balanitis and the interscapular "itchy back syndrome" are considered variants of seborrheic dermatitis by some dermatologists.
- Seborrheic dermatitis in infants (see earlier) is generally self-limiting and usually disappears by 8 months of age. It presents as either *cradle cap*, a buildup of a scaly, greasy adherent plaque on the vertex of the scalp, or as erythematous lesions in body folds. Both these presentations probably represent different conditions than adult seborrheic dermatitis.

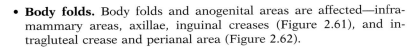 **DIFFERENTIAL DIAGNOSIS**

The differential diagnosis of seborrheic dermatitis varies depending on the age, sex, and ethnic background of the patient and, particularly, on the location of lesions. Clinical and laboratory features also help to distinguish seborrheic dermatitis from its look-alikes:

Scalp
Psoriasis
- Psoriatic lesions elsewhere on body
- Family history of psoriasis

Eczematous Dermatitis
- Eczematous lesions elsewhere on body
- Atopic history
- Onset often before adolescence

Tinea Capitis
- Focal areas of alopecia
- Positive KOH examination or positive fungal culture
- Prevalent in urban African-American toddlers

Face
Prerosacea, Rosacea
- Telangiectasias
- Acnelike papules and pustules (rosacea)
- Absence of scale

"Butterfly" Rash of Systemic Lupus Erythematosus (Figure 2.63)
- Positive antinuclear antibody test
- Other features of lupus

Tinea Faciale
- Lesions generally annular (ring-shaped) with an asymmetric distribution
- Positive KOH examination or positive fungal culture

Body Folds and Genitalia
Inverse Psoriasis (Figure 2.62)
- Possibly indistinguishable from seborrheic dermatitis (see Chapter 3, "Psoriasis")
- Negative KOH examination
- No growth on fungal culture

Tinea Cruris
- Arcuate shape with advancing "active border" with central clearing
- Positive KOH examination or fungal culture

Candidiasis
- "Beefy" red plaques, "satellite pustules"
- Positive KOH examination
- Fungal culture positive for *Candida* species
- Most common in patients with diabetes

Eczematous Dermatitis, such as Atopic Dermatitis
- Ezcematous lesions elsewhere on the body
- Atopic history
- Marked pruritus

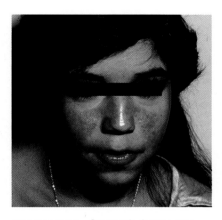

FIGURE 2.63 Systemic lupus erythematosus. This young girl has the classic "butterfly" rash of lupus.

MANAGEMENT

Treatment options for seborrheic dermatitis vary according to the site of the lesions.

Scalp
Mild scalp seborrheic dermatitis generally responds to the numerous commercially available antidandruff, antiseborrheic shampoos that contain one or more of the following ingredients: zinc pyrithione, coal tar, salicylic acid, selenium sulfide, ketoconazole, and sulfur.

- The shampoos should be left on for at least 5 minutes after lathering.
- For itching and inflammation, a medium-strength topical steroid in a gel or solution formulation may be used only if necessary.

Severe scalp seborrheic dermatitis ("sebopsoriasis") is often managed in the same manner as psoriasis of the scalp. Potent topical steroids are frequently preceded by keratolytic agents to remove thick scale, to allow the medications to penetrate the scalp.

- Scale may be removed as often as necessary, usually two to three times per week at the beginning and then whenever it builds up again.

(continued)

Body Fold Areas
- Other areas of the body, including body folds and genital areas, are similarly treated with low-potency topical steroids.

Face
- Seborrheic dermatitis of the face quickly responds to topical steroids, but this treatment requires long-term maintenance and vigilance to avoid atrophy, telangiectasias, and rosacealike side effects.
- To minimize these unwanted reactions, low-potency topical steroids may be alternated with ketoconazole cream 2%; occasionally, ketoconazole cream alone affords control.
- Very low-potency topical steroids are used, with caution, when treating seborrheic dermatitis of the eyelid.

Intertriginous Areas
- Other areas of the body, including body folds and genital areas, are similarly treated with low-potency topical steroids.

"Cradle Cap"
- Minor amounts of scale can be removed with mild antiseborrheic shampoos that contain sulfur and salicylic acid, such as Sebulex.
- Stronger keratolytic agents such as 2% to 6% salicylic acid in petrolatum are used for thick, dense, adherent scale. Mineral oil or olive oil also help to remove scale.
- Very mild topical steroids may be applied to reduce inflammation and itching.

 POINTS TO REMEMBER

- Seborrheic dermatitis is often confused with psoriasis, rosacea, and fungal infections.
- Ketoconazole cream is often used in conjunction with topical steroids.
- As with all steroid-responsive dermatoses, topical steroids should be *used only for brief periods.*

 HELPFUL HINTS

- Seborrheic dermatitis of the scalp is not seen in preadolescent children; therefore, excessive use of shampoos should not be encouraged in this age group. The child may have atopic dermatitis, which will only be aggravated by frequent shampooing.
- Protopic ointment (tacrolimus) 0.1% and Elidel cream (pimecrolimus) 1%, may also be effective in the treatment of facial and intertriginous seborrheic dermatitis.

SEBORRHEIC DERMATITIS FORMULARY

SCALP
Shampoos/gels/lotions

Antiseborrheics   Pyrithione zinc (Head & Shoulders*) shampoo
Coal tar (Neutrogena T/Gel*) shampoo
Coal tar (Zetar*) shampoo and emulsion
1% selenium sulfide (Selsun Blue*) shampoo
2.5% selenium sulfide shampoo
1% ketoconazole shampoo (Nizoral*)

Antifungals   2% ketoconazole shampoo (Nizoral)

Keratolytics (agents that remove excessive scale)   Sulfur 2%, salicylic acid 2% (Sebulex*) shampoo
Tar plus salicylic acid (Neutrogena T/Sal*) shampoo

Topical corticosteroids

Medium potency   Betamethasone valerate foam 0.1% (Valisone)
Desoximetasone (Topicort) gel 0.05%
Fluocinolone acetonide (Capex†) shampoo 0.01%

High potency   Fluocinonide (Lidex) gel or solution 0.05%

Superpotency   Clobetasol gel or scalp application 0.05%

FACE AND INTERTRIGINOUS AREAS
Topical steroids

Very low potency   Hydrocortisone cream or ointment 0.5% to 1%*

Low potency   Desonide (DesOwen) cream, lotion 0.05%

Medium potency   Hydrocortisone valerate (Westcort) cream, ointment 0.2%

Topical creams/ ointments

Antifungals   Ketoconazole (Nizoral*) 1% cream
Ketoconazole (Nizoral) 2% cream

Immunomodulators   Tacrolimus 0.03% and 0.1% (Protopic) ointment
Pimecrolimus 1% (Elidel) cream

---

*Available over the counter.
†This shampoo contains a mid-potent topical steroid. It is used two or three times weekly, as needed.

STASIS DERMATITIS

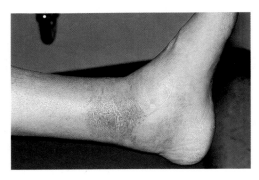

FIGURE 2.64 Acute stasis dermatitis. This patient has the earliest signs of stasis dermatitis—pruritus, erythema, scale (eczematous dermatitis), and slight distal hyperpigmentation.

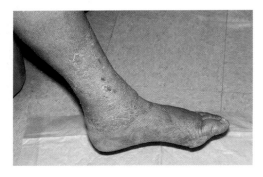

FIGURE 2.65 Subacute stasis dermatitis. This patient shows symptoms of more advanced stasis dermatitis—increased scale, peripheral edema, erosions, crusts, and secondary bacterial infection.

BASICS

Stasis dermatitis (or **gravitational dermatitis**) is an eczematous eruption most commonly located on the lower legs. It often appears on the medial ankles of middle-aged and elderly patients. It is a consequence of chronic venous insufficiency ("leaky valves") and is seen more often in women, particularly those with a genetic predisposition to develop varicosities. Stasis dermatitis may also occur in patients with acquired venous insufficiency resulting from surgery (e.g., vein stripping or harvesting of saphenous veins for coronary bypass), deep venous thrombosis, or other types of traumatic injury to the lower venous system.

Pathogenesis

Traditionally, the following sequence of events has been proposed to explain the pathogenesis of stasis dermatitis: Varicose veins → reversed flow through incompetent valves → diminished venous return → increased hydrostatic capillary pressure → peripheral edema and relative tissue hypoxia. The preceding schema may account for the pruritic, eczematous eruption seen in the early stages of stasis dermatitis; however, several other theories besides this one offer explanations for the exact mechanism at the tissue level, and the issue is still cause for debate.

PROGRESSION OF LESIONS

Lesions begin with erythema and scale (eczematous dermatitis) (Figure 2.64). Later, the rash may become subacute, with more intense erythema, edema, erosions, crusts, and secondary bacterial infection (Figure 2.65). The rash may progressively lead to the chronic stages of stasis dermatitis, in which pigmentary changes occur. After an initial redness (from extravasated red blood cells), affected areas turn reddish brown (from iron left from the breakdown of red blood cells). Postinflammatory hyperpigmentation (from melanin) also occurs. These colors may overlie a cyanotic background. Ultimately, the skin thickens and becomes less supple and nonpitting, and it feels permanently bound down and fibrotic ("woody") on palpation.

DISTRIBUTION OF LESIONS

Most cases of stasis dermatitis and associated ulcers are located on the medial malleolus.

- When symptoms progress, lesions may spread to the foot or calf.

CLINICAL MANIFESTATIONS

- Large venous varicosities may be evident proximal to the eruption, and superficial varicosities may surround the affected area (Figure 2.66).
- Pruritus may occur.
- Ankle edema that is initially pitting later becomes fibrotic and non-pitting.
- Even during the inactive periods of the eruption, the skin remains thickened and permanently pigmented.

Possible complications of stasis dermatitis include the following:

- **Venous stasis ulcers** can occur as a result of trauma (e.g., scratching), bacterial infection, or improper care of the rash (Figure 2.67). Ulcers sometimes produce a dull pain that is relieved by elevation.
- Induration may progress to **lipodermatosclerosis,** which has a classic "inverted water bottle" appearance.
- **Autoeczematization (id reaction),** is a widespread, often explosive, acute eczematous eruption that is presumably triggered by secondary bacterial infection (impetiginization) of eczema, with resultant circulating immune complexes released from the site of the stasis dermatitis lesions (Figure 2.68). It is hypothesized that patients become sensitized to their own tissue breakdown products.

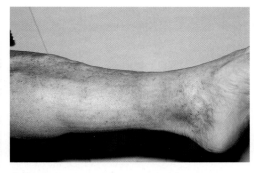

FIGURE 2.66 Chronic stasis dermatitis. Large venous varicosities are evident proximal to the eruption, and superficial varicosities surround the affected area. The eruption is inactive, but the skin remains thickened and permanently pigmented.

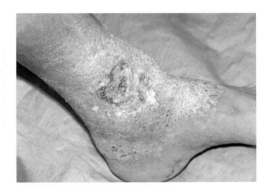

FIGURE 2.67 Stasis dermatitis with venous stasis ulcer. Note the eczematous eruption, the nonpitting edema ("woody" fibrosis) surrounding the ulcer.

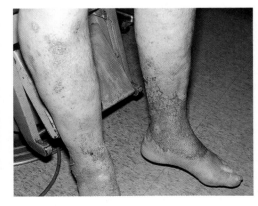

FIGURE 2.68 Stasis dermatitis with secondary autoeczematization. This patient's ankle eruption has become widespread, as a result of impetiginization of the eczema on her legs.

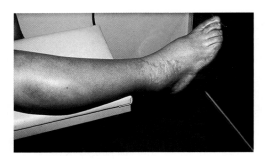

FIGURE 2.69 Cellulitis. This patient has a painful, tender, pretibial plaque.

 DIFFERENTIAL DIAGNOSIS

Typical stasis dermatitis is generally an obvious diagnosis, but it is often confused with the following:

- **Cellulitis** (Figure 2.69) often resembles stasis dermatitis.

Other Diagnoses
- The presence of ulceration should point to other possible conditions, such as arterial disease, skin cancer, and pyoderma gangrenosum.

 MANAGEMENT

Stasis Dermatitis
Diminished Venous Return
Venous return can be increased by engaging in regular exercise, such as brisk walking and bicycling.

- The leg should be elevated above the level of the heart. (Sitting with the affected leg elevated by a stool is inadequate.) At night, leg elevation can be accomplished by propping up the foot end of the bed on blocks that are 15 to 20 cm high.

Edema
Significant edema may be managed with compressive therapy, the mainstay of therapy for venous insufficiency.

- Support hose helps to decrease the stretching of blood vessels. Elastic bandages and specialized compression (Jobst-type) stockings that deliver a controlled gradient of pressure are strongly recommended.
- The patient's peripheral arterial circulation should be assessed (clinically or with a Doppler study) before compression is recommended.

Rash
The eczematous rash (stasis dermatitis) should be carefully managed with topical therapy.

- Burow's solution soaks to help dry oozing or infected areas.
- A mild- to moderate-strength topical corticosteroid ointment (such as desonide 0.05%, hydrocortisone valerate 0.2%, or, if necessary, triamcinolone 0.1%) applied twice daily is usually sufficient to treat the eczematous rash and to alleviate any itching.
- Patients should be advised not to apply topical corticosteroid preparations directly to stasis ulcers because the preparations may interfere with healing. Long-term use of potent topical corticosteroids may promote the development of atrophy and should be avoided.
- Also to be avoided are over-the-counter preparations that contain benzocaine, lanolin, or neomycin. (Patients with stasis dermatitis tend to develop contact dermatitis quite easily.)

(continued)

Infection

Obvious superficial infections (impetiginization) should be treated with systemic antibiotics that have activity against *S. aureus* and *Streptococcus species* (e.g., dicloxacillin, cephalexin, or cefadroxil).

- A widespread autoeczematized eruption may require treatment with both systemic corticosteroids and oral antibiotics.

Stasis Ulcers

Stasis ulcers are managed by treating the underlying eczematous dermatitis, controlling weight, preventing infection, and using compression dressings and Unna's boots.

- Unna's boot is a commercially available bandage (Dome-Paste bandage, Gelocast bandage) that is impregnated with zinc oxide paste. It is best applied in the morning before edema progresses. After application, the bandage hardens into a cast. The boot decreases edema, promotes healing, and serves as a barrier from trauma (e.g., from scratching). It should be changed weekly until the ulcer heals.
- If feasible, corrective surgery, such as skin grafts or vascular procedures, may be another option.
- Venous ulcers can also be treated with moist wound healing methods, high-compression therapy, fibrinolytic agents, and newer modalities, such as growth factors, matrix materials, and biologically engineered tissue. (These methods are beyond the scope of this chapter.)

POINTS TO REMEMBER

- Stasis dermatitis is often misdiagnosed as cellulitis.
- Infected stasis dermatitis should be considered in patients who develop a sudden onset of extensive generalized eczematous dermatitis (autoeczematization).
- Contact dermatitis or autoeczematization should be considered in patients who become clinically worse despite appropriate topical treatment.
- Compression is the mainstay of therapy for venous insufficiency and venous leg ulceration. It is the standard of care, even though it is not preferred by patients (it is cosmetically objectionable and uncomfortable) and it is not easy for health care providers to apply (it is labor-intensive).

HELPFUL HINT

- Sitting in a reclining chair while reading or watching television can help to promote venous return.

Psoriasis

Overview

Psoriasis is a red and scaly chronic skin condition of unknown cause. A patient's main concern is the unsightly appearance of lesions. The visibility and persistence of psoriasis often lead patients to feel self-conscious and unclean. The emotional toll and the personal struggle to come to terms with it are expressed in an autobiographic short story, "At War with my Skin," by John Updike, who has severe psoriasis. After undergoing an operation for a broken leg, Updike reflects, "I chiefly remember amid my pain and helplessness being pleased that my shins, at that time, were clear and I would not offend the surgeon."

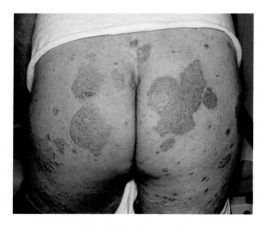

FIGURE 3.1 Psoriasis. Large plaques.

About 30% of patients with psoriasis have a family history of the disease. It affects 1% to 2% of the world's population. However, psoriasis is much less common in West Africans, African-Americans, Native Americans, and Asiatic people than it is in whites. It is found equally in men and women.

Psoriasis most frequently begins in the second or third decade of life, but it can first present in infants or in the elderly. Ten percent of patients with psoriasis also develop psoriatic arthritis, which may precede or follow the onset of skin lesions. A person who has psoriasis often spends an excessive amount of time treating skin lesions and trying to hide them, as well as searching for external causes and possible cures.

Psoriasis is often a major blow to the ego that stifles social activities, sexual spontaneity, job opportunities, participation in sports, and use of public swimming pools, for example. Because psoriasis is a visible disease, it may arouse a fear of contagion, as well as repugnance and avoidance from persons who are not used to seeing it.

The young child with psoriasis has the additional burden of embarrassment caused by the undisguised scrutiny and thoughtless remarks of other children. The parent may have to cope with guilt for having genetically passed psoriasis on to the child.

Pathophysiology

Psoriatic lesions result from an increase in epidermal cell turnover. The cell's transit time from the basal layer of the epidermis to the stratum corneum is decreased from the normal 28 days to 3 or 4 days. This "turned-on" epidermis, with its rapid accumulation of cells, accounts for the *characteristic lesion of psoriasis: a red papule or plaque surmounted by a white or silvery (micaceous) scale* (Figures 3.1 through 3.3). The scale can be accounted for by the great increase in cellular kinetics that does not allow time for shedding. Psoriasis is now considered an immunologic disease, and most current therapies—including corticosteroids, phototherapy, photochemotherapy, methotrexate, and cyclosporine—are directed at the suppression of responsible T cells.

Histopathology (Illustration 3.1)

The histopathologic findings demonstrate the altered cell kinetics of psoriasis:

- Increased mitosis of keratinocytes, fibroblasts, and endothelial cells. Skin biopsies typically show:
  - Marked thickening (acanthosis) and also thinning of the epidermis with resultant elongation of the rete ridges
  - Parakeratosis (nuclei retained in the stratum corneum)
- And the inflammatory process:
  - Dermal inflammation (lymphocytes and monocytes)
  - Epidermal inflammation (polymorphonuclear cells) in the stratum corneum that may form microabscesses of Munro

DISTRIBUTION OF LESIONS

The distribution of thickened, reddened, silvery or whitish scaly plaques can range from only a few small asymptomatic lesions, to larger plaques that cover extensive areas of the body, to generalized exfoliative erythroderma.

Psoriasis tends to be remarkably symmetric. It usually spares the face. Lesions are most commonly located as follows:

- The large extensor joints (elbows, knees, and knuckles) are commonly involved.
- The anogenital region (perineal and perianal areas, glans penis) is often affected.
- The palms and soles are frequently involved.
- When lesions occur primarily in the intertriginous areas (axillae, inframammary, perineal, and perianal areas, and inguinal creases), this manifestation is referred to as **inverse psoriasis.**
- Trunk lesions may be small, guttate (teardrop-shaped) plaques or large plaques.
- When psoriasis involves only the scalp and retroauricular areas, it is sometimes referred to as "*sebopsoriasis*" or "*seborrhiasis*") (see Chapter 2, "Eczema").
- When the entire body is involved, generalized, disseminated plaques or **exfoliative dermatitis** may be evident.
- Psoriasis commonly is a cause of **nail deformity.**
- **Psoriatic arthritis** occurs in 5% to 10% of patients who are diagnosed with psoriasis.

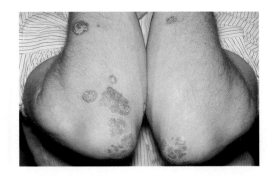

FIGURE 3.2 Psoriasis. The characteristic primary lesion of psoriasis is the well-circumscribed, red papule or plaque surmounted by a silvery (micaceous) or whitish scale.

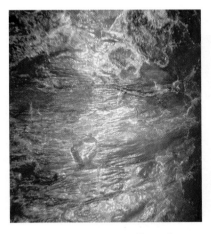

FIGURE 3.3 Psoriasis. The silvery, shiny luster of the micaceous scale is noted.

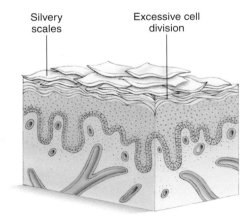

Silvery scales   Excessive cell division

Psoriasis

Illustration 3.1 Psoriasis: Silvery scales and excessive cell division.

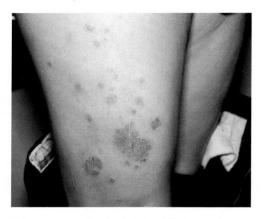

FIGURE 3.4 Psoriasis. The *Köebner phenomenon* is evident in this diabetic patient, who developed psoriatic plaques at the sites of insulin injections.

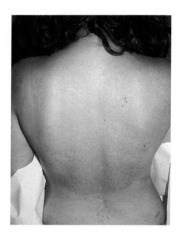

FIGURE 3.5 Psoriasis. The *Köebner phenomenon* is localized to the area of sunburn. The region that had been covered by the patient's bathing suit is almost free of lesions.

CLINICAL MANIFESTATIONS

Pruritus

Psoriasis generally is asymptomatic, but it can become quite pruritic and uncomfortable, particularly during acute flare-ups or when it involves the scalp or intertriginous (skin folds) regions. It also can cause pain, functional impairment, and embarrassment when it involves the palms or soles.

The Köebner Phenomenon or Isomorphic Response

Psoriatic lesions can appear to spread to, or crop up in, apparently normal areas of the skin that are traumatized by noxious stimuli, such as needle injections (Figure 3.4), a sunburn (Figure 3.5), or scratching and rubbing (see Chapter 4, "Lichen Planus").

Psychosocial Problems

Emotional stress has been implicated in the acute exacerbations and progression of psoriasis. In a vicious cycle, the poor self-image that may be incited by lesions can create more stress. The health care provider should recognize the psychological ramifications of psoriasis—anxiety, social isolation, alcoholism, depression, suicidal ideation—as possible associations and outcomes of this benign skin disease.

Drugs that Adversely Influence Psoriasis

- **Alcohol.** Alcohol overindulgence has been reputed to exacerbate psoriasis.
- **Drugs.** Antimalarials, beta-blockers, systemic interferon, and lithium carbonate have been reported to worsen psoriasis; however, preexisting psoriasis is not necessarily a contraindication to their use.
- **Systemic corticosteroids.** These agents are no longer advocated as a treatment for psoriasis. They have been known, albeit rarely, to trigger severe acute, potentially fatal pustular psoriasis that occurs after withdrawal of the steroid.

Course

- Psoriasis is an erratic condition with an unpredictable, waxing-and-waning course. It has no known cure.
- During episodes of physical illness or pregnancy, psoriasis may worsen or may suddenly clear.
- Many patients tend to improve during the summer and worsen in the colder times of the year. This fluctuation is presumably the result of the positive influence of sunlight on psoriasis.
- There have been anecdotal reports of patients with psoriasis who were "cured," and some patients claim that they "grew out of it." This situation may be explained by either a misdiagnosis of the original skin problem or by cases of acute guttate psoriasis that resolved without recurrence.

DIAGNOSIS

- The diagnosis of psoriasis is made on clinical grounds. However, a skin biopsy or fungal studies may be performed to rule in or rule out other possible diagnoses.

CLINICAL VARIANTS

The clinical presentations of psoriasis listed here create a somewhat artificial classification, which is based on the characteristics or morphology of the predominant type of lesion and its distribution. There may be composites of these different types in a given patient. Because each type is managed somewhat differently and has its own differential diagnosis, each is discussed separately.

- Localized plaque psoriasis
- Generalized plaque psoriasis
- Acute guttate psoriasis
- Erythrodermic psoriasis (exfoliative dermatitis secondary to psoriasis)
- Psoriasis in children
- Human immunodeficiency virus (HIV)–induced psoriasis
- Inverse psoriasis (on the groin, penis, perianal, axillae, and inframammary regions)
- Psoriasis of the palms and soles
- Scalp psoriasis
- Psoriatic nails
- Psoriatic arthritis
- Other rare clinical variants: localized pustular psoriasis (Hallopeau) and the rare generalized pustular psoriasis of Von Zumbusch

HELPFUL HINTS

- If there is one word to choose to describe psoriasis, "capricious" is the one that would be used to express its unpredictable course.
- **The National Psoriasis Foundation** provides information about psoriasis to educate patients, the public, and health care providers. National Psoriasis Foundation, 6600 S.W. 92nd, Suite 300, Portland, OR 97223; 800-723-9166. www.psoriasis.org.

SEE PATIENT HANDOUT, PAGE 453

Differential Diagnosis
The differential diagnosis of psoriasis varies, depending on the type and location of lesions. In general, psoriasis most often must be differentiated from the following:

- Eczematous dermatitis
- Superficial fungal infections
- Seborrheic dermatitis
- Parapsoriasis and cutaneous T-cell lymphoma (mycosis fungoides)

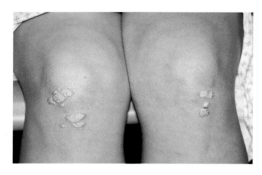

FIGURE 3.6 Psoriasis. Here the scale is white. Note the symmetry of the lesions.

BASICS

In its mildest manifestation, psoriasis is an incidental finding. It may consist of nail pitting or mildly erythematous, scaly patches on the elbows or knees. The patient is frequently unaware of or not troubled by psoriasis in this form. Localized plaque psoriasis, the most common presentation of psoriasis, may remain limited and localized (Figure 3.6), or it may become unstable and widespread.

DIAGNOSIS

- If the typical well-demarcated whitish or silvery plaque is present in the usual locations, the diagnosis of psoriasis is quite evident.
- Other helpful diagnostic features include a family history of psoriasis and nail findings.
- If necessary, other tests, such as a skin biopsy and fungal examinations, can be performed to rule out other conditions.

 DIFFERENTIAL DIAGNOSIS

Eczematous Dermatitis (Lichen Simplex Chronicus)/Atopic Dermatitis
- The patient or a close relative has a **history of atopy** (Figure 3.7).
- Flexural distribution is noted.
- **Lichenification** (exaggeration of normal skin markings is the hallmark lesion) is present.
- Lesions are **poorly demarcated;** they blend gradually into normal surrounding skin.
- Usually, lesions **itch,** and crusts and excoriations may be seen.

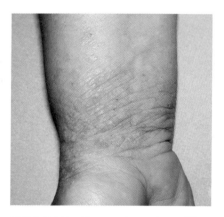

FIGURE 3.7 Eczematous dermatitis (lichen simplex chronicus). Note the flexural distribution, lichenification, and poor demarcation of this lesion (it blends gradually into normal surrounding skin).

Nummular Eczema (Figure 3.8)

- An atopic history may or may not be present.
- An extensor or flexural distribution is noted, most often on the legs.
- "Coin-shaped" patches and plaques are present.
- Usually, lesions itch, with possible crusts and excoriations.

Tinea Corporis (Figure 3.9)

- Patients have a possible history of exposure to fungus.
- Lesions usually are annular ("ringlike"), round and clear in the center.
- The potassium hydroxide (KOH) examination or fungal culture is positive.
- Lesions usually itch.

Parapsoriasis

- Idiopathic multiple, barely elevated patches are usually found on the trunk and arms (similar to pityriasis rosea).
- There are small and large plaque variants.

Mycosis Fungoides (Cutaneous T-Cell Lymphoma) (Figure 3.10)

- "Smudgy" patches and plaques or tumors are noted, usually on the buttocks and trunk.
- Lesions are often pruritic.
- A biopsy may show cutaneous T-cell lymphoma.

Bowen's Disease (Squamous Cell Carcinoma *In Situ*)

- Patients have a solitary lesion.
- The lesion may resemble a typical psoriatic plaque.
- It is unresponsive to topical steroids.

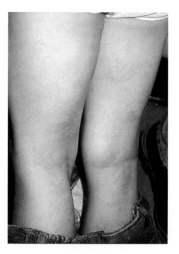

FIGURE 3.8 Nummular eczema. "Coin-shaped" patches and plaques are located on the legs.

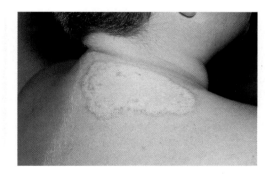

FIGURE 3.9 Tinea corporis. The lesion is annular (clear in the center).

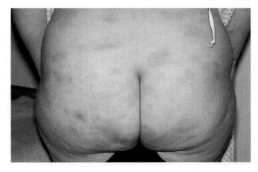

FIGURE 3.10 Mycosis fungoides (cutaneous T-cell lymphoma). Lesions have characteristic "smudgy," poorly-defined patches and plaques in a typical location.

MANAGEMENT

Principles

Treatment of psoriasis is aimed at decreasing size and thickness of plaques, relieving pruritus, and improving emotional well being. Ultimately, the measure of successful treatment includes both objective and subjective determinations.

The types of treatment selected are determined by some of the following factors:

- The age of patient. Many oral agents that are used to treat severe psoriasis, such as methotrexate and oral retinoids, are less likely to be used in a child. Very young children, particularly infants, are not able to cooperate with phototherapy treatment.
- The type of psoriasis.
- The site and extent of involvement.
- The health care provider's experience in managing psoriasis. (Management of mild to relatively moderate psoriasis can be performed by primary care clinicians. Moderate to severe psoriasis is best treated by dermatologists.)
- The availability of facilities, such as a phototherapy unit.
- The presence of psychosocial problems, such as anxiety, depression, alcoholism, and substance abuse.

Topical Corticosteroids

The use of a potent topical steroid for a limited period, followed by a less potent topical steroid for maintenance, has become a popular method for treating psoriasis and many inflammatory dermatoses (see Introduction, "Topical Therapy and Topical Steroids").

Advantage
- Rapid onset in decreasing erythema, inflammation, and itching

Disadvantages
- Tachyphylaxis is common
- Expensive, especially when large areas are treated
- Steroid rosacea, local atrophy, hypothalamic-pituitary-adrenal suppression possible if these agents are used incorrectly

Additional Suggestions
- Consider rotational dosing, for example, agents used for 2 weeks and then not used for 1 week; or agents used on weekends and a moisturizer or topical calcipotriene used during the week.

Topical Vitamin D

Calcipotriene 0.005% (Dovonex ointment, cream, and solution), a topical vitamin D_3 preparation, is indicated for mild to moderate plaque psoriasis.

Advantages
- Potency equivalent to betamethasone valerate
- Effective in reducing scale
- No tachyphylaxis reported

Disadvantages
- Expensive
- Slower onset of action than topical steroids; good for long-term maintenance therapy
- Occasionally irritating, especially intertriginous areas and face

Additional Suggestions
- Use in rotational therapy with topical steroids.

Topical Retinoids

Tazarotene 0.05% or 0.1% (Tazorac cream and gel) is a topical retinoid derivative that is applied once daily. This agent has delayed onset of action; however, psoriasis that is cleared with tazarotene appears to remain in remission longer than psoriasis treated with topical steroids alone. It is generally used in conjunction with medium-potency topical steroids to increase therapeutic efficacy and to decrease the irritation that commonly occurs when it is used alone. Tazarotene should not be applied to nonpsoriatic skin.

Advantages
- Remissions are possibly longer than with topical steroids alone
- No tachyphylaxis reported

Disadvantages
- Expensive
- Slower onset of action than topical steroids
- Often irritating

Additional Suggestions
- Use in conjunction with topical steroids to minimize irritation (e.g., tazarotene at bedtime and a topical steroid in the morning).

Topical Tar Preparations

Before the advent of topical steroids, tar preparations were the mainstay of therapy for most inflammatory dermatoses. Currently, they are used less often.

(continued)

MANAGEMENT (*continued*)

Additional Suggestions

- Agents such as liquor carbonis detergens, Balnetar, Doak Tar Oil, Estar gel, PsoriGel, and T-Derm tar oil are currently used.

Topical Anthralin

Anthralin, a topical anthracene preparation, has been used to treat psoriasis since the 19th century. Anthralin is a coal tar derivative that evolved as an answer to many of the side effects of crude coal tar. It may be used for shorter periods, such as for half an hour. This is referred to as short-contact anthralin therapy (SCAT). This treatment has gained popularity in Europe. Its major drawbacks are that skin irritation may occur, and there is generally a reversible brownish purple staining of the skin.

Occlusion of Topical Steroids

Generally a medium-potency agent is applied and is then covered with a polyethylene wrap such as Saran Wrap for several hours or overnight, if tolerated. Cordran tape is similarly effective.

Advantage

- Increases the potency of topical steroids

Disadvantage

- Occlusion has same disadvantages of not occluding, but side effects are more common

Additional Suggestions

- A plastic shower cap can be used during treatment of the scalp with topical steroids; the resultant occlusion increases efficacy.

Intralesional Steroids

Intralesional triamcinolone acetonide (Kenalog, 2.5 to 5 mg/mL) is delivered intradermally with a 30-gauge needle. The plaque is infiltrated until it blanches. This procedure may be repeated at 4- to 6-week intervals.

Advantages

- Useful with limited number of lesions
- Rapid acting
- Longer duration of remission

Disadvantages

- Painful
- Possible local atrophy and telangiectasias
- Requires office visits to administer injections

Innovative Management Strategies

Rotational Therapy

An innovative approach in the management of psoriasis consists of cycling or rotating different treatment modalities (see earlier). This strategy presumably decreases cumulative side effects and drug tolerance (tachyphylaxis), and it often allows for lower dosages and shorter durations of therapy for each agent.

As an example, the use of a superpotent topical steroid, such as clobetasol, may be applied for 2 weeks, discontinued for 1 or 2 weeks, and then restarted. Alternatively, clobetasol may be used on weekends only.

The use of agents such as UVB, PUVA, and methotrexate, which are reserved for more severe, extensive psoriasis, can also be rotated, whereby treatment may be used from 12 to 24 months and then changed to another modality. On clearing of the condition, treatment is stopped until the psoriasis recurs, at which point another agent is used.

Combination Therapy (see later)

With RePUVA, which combines an oral retinoid (Re) with the photochemotherapy of PUVA, it is possible to lower the dosage of both treatment modalities and to achieve better clinical responses in many patients.

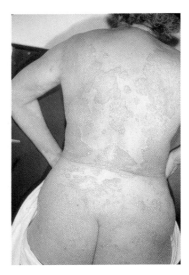

FIGURE 3.11 Psoriasis. Extensive, large plaques are evident on this patient.

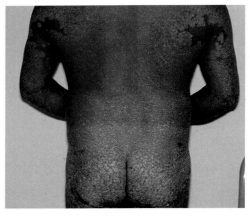

FIGURE 3.12 Psoriasis. Exfoliative dermatitis.

BASICS

Psoriasis can flare very quickly and unexpectedly to cover 20% to 80% of the body. Therapy for widespread psoriasis differs from that for more localized disease. In such cases, topical therapy alone becomes less effective, more expensive, time consuming, and labor intensive when it is administered to larger regions (Figures 3.11 and 3.12).

MANAGEMENT

UV light treatment (phototherapy) and systemic medications may be necessary to treat widespread psoriasis.

Phototherapy
- It is well known that most cases of psoriasis improve with sunlight exposure. This observation has led to the development of various methods to deliver UV light artificially.
- The two forms of UV light that are used clinically are UVB and UVA.
- UVB is usually administered in a dermatologist's office or a psoriasis daycare center. Treatment is given two to three times per week.
- The administration of topical tar preparations before light exposure is known as Goeckerman therapy.
- UVB is tried first because it has fewer side effects than does UVA.
- UVA is given with oral psoralen (PUVA). The drug psoralen is activated by the skin's exposure to UV light. PUVA is also administered in a dermatologist's office or a psoriasis day care center.
- Studies have indicated a link between PUVA therapy and the development of squamous cell and basal cell carcinomas and possibly malignant melanoma.

Systemic Therapy
Options include methotrexate, retinoids, and cyclosporine.

- Oral methotrexate is reserved for patients with psoriasis that is difficult to treat. Because of its hepatotoxicity, this drug should be used only with extreme care. Methotrexate has been associated with hepatic fibrosis and bone marrow suppression.
- Oral acitretin (Soriatane) is an oral retinoid drug. The retinoid family of drugs is related to vitamin A. These agents are potent teratogens; therefore, they are not given to women capable of having children. Cheilitis is a symptom seen in virtually all patients taking retinoids. Retinoids can cause lipid elevation, muscle weakness, myalgias, hair loss, nail changes, skin fragility, premature epiphyseal closure or calcification, and ossification of ligaments and tendons.
- Oral cyclosporine (Neoral). The use of cyclosporine requires careful monitoring, to avoid significant risks to kidney function and blood pressure.

BASICS

Rarely, a patient may develop a sudden or subacute appearance of generalized scaling and erythema (Figures 3.13 and 3.14), often with accompanying fever and chills. This condition, exfoliative dermatitis, can be the presenting symptom of psoriasis or a subsequent complication of limited psoriatic disease (see Chapter 25, "Cutaneous Manifestations of Systemic Disease").

Some of the trigger factors that may lead to exfoliative dermatitis in patients with psoriasis are as follows:

- After administration of systemic or superpotent topical corticosteroids in patients with preexisting psoriasis.
- Topical therapy that is irritating or produces severe contact dermatitis can trigger the condition.
- High levels of emotional stress have been implicated.
- Medical procedures (e.g., surgery) or certain conditions (e.g., infections) can precipitate the problem.

Alternatively, psoriasis may initially present as exfoliative dermatitis.

MANAGEMENT

Treatment of exfoliative dermatitis secondary to psoriasis may involve some of the measures used for generalized plaque psoriasis (e.g., UV light therapy, oral agents) in addition to the following:

- Bed rest
- Cool compresses
- Lubrication with emollients
- Antipruritic therapy with oral antihistamines
- Low- to moderate-strength topical corticosteroids
- Hospitalization, in extreme cases

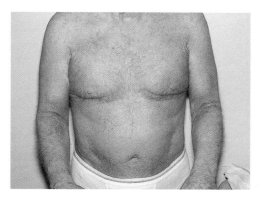

FIGURE 3.13 Psoriasis. Exfoliative dermatitis. Frontal view of patient in Figure 3.12.

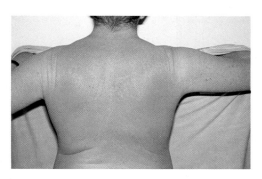

FIGURE 3.14 Psoriasis. Erythrodermic variant.

PSORIASIS IN CHILDREN

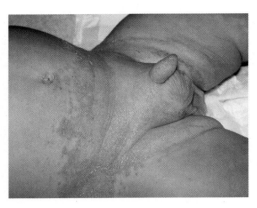

FIGURE 3.15 Psoriasis. These plaques could easily be confused with a diaper rash or atopic dermatitis.

BASICS

In approximately 10% of patients, psoriasis begins before the age of 10 years (Figure 3.15). An early onset portends more severe disease, and there is often an associated family history of the disease.

In some infants, psoriasis begins as a diaper rash, which may be difficult to distinguish from an irritant dermatitis, atopic dermatitis, or cutaneous candidiasis. The rash may clear; however, the child later may develop psoriasis. Conversely, psoriasis may present with typical plaques, such as those seen in adults.

Infantile or childhood psoriasis deserves particular attention. It requires intensive educational guidance and counseling of the patient and family.

MANAGEMENT

Many of the treatments that are used in adults, such as superpotent topical steroids, phototherapy, methotrexate, and retinoids, are generally avoided in children. Low- to medium-potency topical steroids, SCAT, and natural sunlight, if available, are also used in children. All of these treatments should be administered with caution.

BASICS

This type of psoriasis refers to the sudden onset of multiple guttate (teardrop-shaped) lesions (Figures 3.16 and 3.17). It is often the initial presentation of psoriasis in children or young adults.

Acute guttate psoriasis is occasionally preceded by a group A beta-hemolytic streptococcal pharyngitis (positive throat culture or serologic evidence of antistreptolysin O). These patients should be treated promptly with appropriate antibiotic therapy, because it has been reported that some of these patients have self-limited cases of psoriasis. Long-term follow-up has indicated that many of these patients with "one-time" cases of psoriasis eventually proved to have recurrences suggesting typical psoriasis.

  DIFFERENTIAL DIAGNOSIS

- Pityriasis rosea
- Drug eruption
- Secondary syphilis

MANAGEMENT

- UVB phototherapy or natural sunlight exposure
- Appropriate antibiotic therapy, such as penicillin or erythromycin for group A beta-hemolytic streptococcus

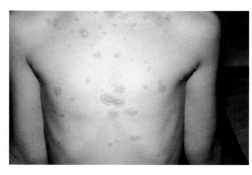

FIGURE 3.16 Psoriasis (acute guttate). This 11-year-old child had recent group A beta-hemolytic streptococcal pharyngitis.

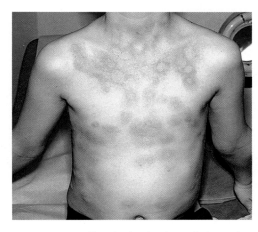

FIGURE 3.17 Psoriasis. Acute guttate variant. This is the same patient as in Figure 3.16 after 4 weeks treatment with penicillin and topical anthralin (brown stains are due to the anthralin).

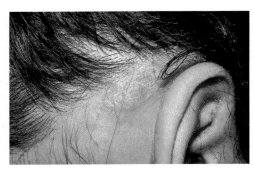

FIGURE 3.18 Psoriasis of the scalp. This discrete, scaly plaque is one of many this patient has on her scalp.

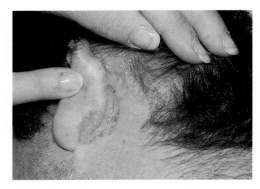

FIGURE 3.19 Psoriasis of the scalp and ears. Note the lesions behind this patient's ear and along the hairline.

BASICS

Psoriasis may involve the scalp alone, or the scalp may be affected along with other areas. In scalp psoriasis, the plaques are often thick and well demarcated with a whitish scale (Figure 3.18). The plaques are frequently hidden in the scalp or behind the ears, but most often they extend beyond the hairline. They become more obvious when the hair is held back and when the retroauricular area is examined (Figure 3.19). Occasionally, the external ears and ear canals are involved.

Features of Scalp Psoriasis

- Pruritus and scratching may exacerbate the condition (Köebner phenomenon).
- Lesions range from flaky dandruff to thick, extensive, armorlike plaques.
- Scalp psoriasis does not cause hair loss.
- When severe, it is particularly difficult to treat because hair blocks UV light and topical applications of medications.

 DIFFERENTIAL DIAGNOSIS

Adults
Seborrheic dermatitis
- Seborrheic dermatitis may be indistinguishable from mild scalp psoriasis.

Children
Eczematous dermatitis of scalp
- Eczematous lesions may be present elsewhere on the body.
- An atopic history is usually present.

Tinea capitis
- A positive KOH test and/or fungal culture result.

MANAGEMENT

Mild Cases

Patients with minimal scaling and thin plaques (similar to what is seen in seborrheic dermatitis) can often be managed with anti-dandruff shampoos and a topical steroid used as needed for itching and for thicker scales. Over-the-counter options include shampoos that contain tar (Zetar, T/Gel), selenium sulfide (Selsun Blue, Head and Shoulders), or salicylic acid (T/Sal).

A shampoo containing ketoconazole 2% (Nizoral) is available by prescription. Medium-potency topical steroid in a solution (e.g., Fluonid) or gel (e.g., Topicort) can be applied one to two times daily as needed. Gel or lotion preparations reach the scalp more readily than do ointments or creams.

Severe Cases

In patients with thick scales and plaques, the scale must be removed before the plaques can be treated. Scale removal is accomplished by applying a 2% to 6% salicylic acid preparation (e.g., Keralyt Gel) one to three times per week. This regimen may be sufficient to keep scale under control, thus allowing penetration of a topical steroid.

After the scale is removed, a medium-potency topical steroid is used. A fluocinonide solution or gel or desoximetasone (Topicort) gel can be applied once or twice daily as needed, under shower cap occlusion overnight, or for 3 to 4 hours during the day. If necessary, a superpotent topical steroid such as clobetasol propionate lotion or gel can be used without occlusion. In recalcitrant situations, a superpotent topical steroid can be applied under occlusion once or twice per week.

Injections of intralesional triamcinolone (3 to 5 mg/mL) in a limited amount (using 1 to 2 mL or less per treatment) every 4 to 8 weeks are used to target particularly itchy areas and may bring longer remissions. Calcipotriene (Dovonex) lotion can be used as maintenance or rotational therapy.

 POINTS TO REMEMBER

- Scalp psoriasis is often inaccessible to UV; therefore, treatment is limited to intensive topical measures.
- Use rotational or pulse treatment to avoid tachyphylaxis (tolerance).
- For maintenance treatment after control, use topical steroids in the lowest strength possible in a pulse-dosing or rotating manor with agents such as calcipotriene (Dovonex) lotion.

 SEE PATIENT HANDOUT, PAGE 457

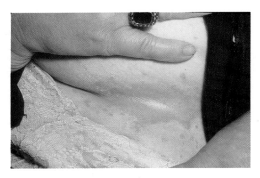

FIGURE 3.20 Inverse psoriasis. Inframammary involvement, shown here, is often misdiagnosed as cutaneous candidiasis.

BASICS

Psoriasis seen in intertriginous areas such as the axillae, inframammary folds (Figure 3.20), perineal and perianal areas, scrotum, glans penis, and inguinal creases is referred to as inverse psoriasis (Figures 3.21 and 3.22).

Typically, lesions are red, glistening, well-demarcated plaques that lack scale. This manifestation is seen when two apposing surfaces of skin rub together, such as under the breasts. The constant rubbing does not allow scale to build up. Fissures may occur in the groin and gluteal creases (Figure 3.23).

Inverse psoriasis is commonly misdiagnosed by nondermatologists as tinea or candidiasis. Accordingly, it is often treated with topical antifungal agents.

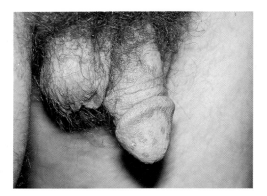

FIGURE 3.21 Inverse psoriasis. Involvement of the penis is not unusual.

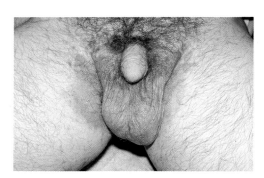

FIGURE 3.22 Inverse psoriasis. Note involvement of the scrotum. This is often misdiagnosed as cutaneous candidiasis or tinea cruris.

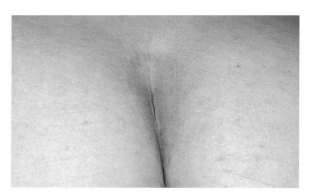

FIGURE 3.23 Inverse psoriasis. Intragluteal involvement is not unusual. Note the painful fissure.

DIFFERENTIAL DIAGNOSIS

Tinea Cruris
- This has a scalloped, active border (Figure 3.24).
- It generally spares the scrotum and penis.
- The KOH examination and fungal cultures are positive for dermatophytes.

Cutaneous Candidiasis
- Lesions have a "beefy red" color.
- Satellite pustules are seen beyond the border of the plaques (Figure 3.25).
- The KOH examination is positive for budding yeast.
- Culture for *Candida* species is positive.

Atopic Dermatitis
- Eczematous lesions may be seen elsewhere on the body.
- The patient has an atopic history.

Seborrheic Dermatitis
- It may be indistinguishable from psoriasis (*intertriginous seborrheic dermatitis*).

Irritant Intertrigo and Contact Dermatitis
- May occur secondary to obesity or maceration
- May be caused by contactants such as antiperspirants.

When lesions are present on the glans penis, nonspecific balanitis (more commonly seen in elderly men) and balanitis from candidal species should be considered in the differential diagnosis. Pruritus ani also may be confused with inverse psoriasis.

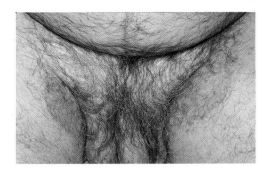

FIGURE 3.24 Tinea cruris. Note the scalloped border. The potassium hydroxide examination is positive. The scrotum is spared in this patient.

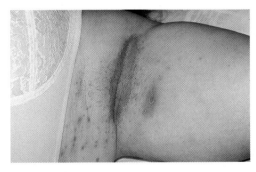

FIGURE 3.25 Cutaneous candidiasis. Note the "satellite pustules" in this diabetic patient.

MANAGEMENT

The lowest-potency nonfluorinated topical steroids are used to avoid atrophy and striae. Treatment should be monitored regularly (multiple prescription refills should be avoided). To achieve rapid improvement, treatment may be initiated with a higher-potency steroid that is used for several days before it is changed to a lower-potency agent.

Face and Intertriginous Areas (Inverse Psoriasis)

Less potent topical steroids such as hydrocortisone cream 0.5% to 1% (Cortaid, an over-the-counter preparation) or desonide 0.05% or hydrocortisone valerate 0.2% (Westcort) may be applied once or twice daily.

- **Calcipotriene (Dovonex) cream or ointment** may be used primarily (if it is not irritating) or in rotation with a mild topical steroid.
- Tacrolimus (Protopic) ointment 0.03% or 0.1% once or twice daily.
- Pimecrolimus (Elidel) cream 1% once or twice daily.

POINTS TO REMEMBER

- Inverse psoriasis, by virtue of its location, cannot benefit from UV light therapy.
- Intertriginous areas are moist and occluded; therefore, the penetration and efficacy of topical agents are increased in these regions.
- Topical steroids are more likely to produce striae (linear atrophy) in these areas.

BASICS

Psoriasis that manifests on the palms and soles presents a difficult therapeutic challenge. The palms or soles alone may be affected, or these areas may be a part of more extensive psoriasis on the body. There are two variants:

- **Hyperkeratotic type.** Like its counterparts elsewhere, this form of psoriasis is characterized by well-demarcated scaly plaques (Figures 3.26 and 3.27). The location of these lesions presents additional problems to patients such as pain, impairment of function, fissuring, bleeding, and embarrassment.
- **Pustular type.** This rare form of psoriasis has historically has many clinical descriptions and eponyms. It is most commonly seen in adults, and lesions tend to be symmetric and well defined. It favors the insteps of the feet, the heels, and the thenar and hypothenar eminences. Less commonly, it appears on the palms (Figure 3.28).

 DIFFERENTIAL DIAGNOSIS

Contact Dermatitis
- This is suspected, particularly if the eruption is on the dorsum of the hands or feet.
- The patient has a history of exposure to a suspected contactant.

Hand Eczema or Dyshidrotic Eczema (see Chapter 2, "Eczema")
- "Sago-grain" vesicles are visible.
- Pruritus is present.
- Hand eczema may be indistinguishable from psoriasis.
- The patient has evidence of eczema elsewhere on the body or a personal or family history of atopy.

Tinea Manuum and Pedis
- A "two-feet, one-hand" presentation is noted (see Chapter 7, "Superficial Fungal Infections").
- The KOH examination or fungal culture is positive.

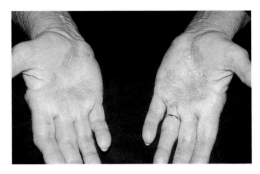

FIGURE 3.26 Psoriasis. This patient's lesions are symmetric. She also has similar plaques on her feet.

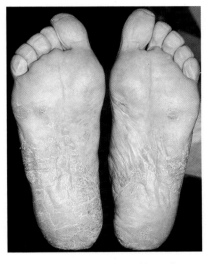

FIGURE 3.27 Psoriasis. Note the clear demarcation between involved and uninvolved skin.

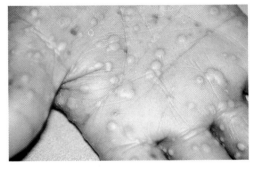

FIGURE 3.28 Psoriasis. This is the pustular variant of psoriasis.

MANAGEMENT

Topical treatment is the first line of therapy. Because the palms and soles present the greatest barrier to cutaneous penetration, the most potent topical steroids are used, often under occlusion. Treatment options include the following:

- Superpotent topical steroids, such as clobetasol propionate, are first tried without occlusion, but occlusion (under vinyl or rubber gloves) may be used if necessary.
- Anthralin, overnight or as SCAT, is useful.
- Salicylic acid preparations may be used to remove scale, if necessary.
- Emollients are helpful.
- Calcipotriene (Dovonex) ointment or cream is used. Vinyl or rubber gloves may be worn over calcipotriene.

When a patient is not responding to topical therapies, treatment options can include phototherapy and systemic measures such as the following:

- UVB is administered.
- PUVA: **UVA** therapy involves the ingestion of a photoactivating drug that is followed in 90 minutes to 2 hours by exposure to UV light given in the UVA spectrum. As with UVB, treatment is given two to three times per week until clearing, followed by a maintenance regimen.
- Oral retinoids, such as etretinate, are prescribed.
- RePUVA (low-dose etretinate combined with PUVA) is useful.
- Oral methotrexate may be given.
- Oral cyclosporine may be administered.
- Neoral, a cyclosporine that is easily absorbed, is used.

POINT TO REMEMBER

- Palmoplantar psoriasis is a difficult therapeutic challenge.

BASICS

Involvement of nails is very common in patients with psoriasis (see Chapter 13, "Diseases and Abnormalities of Nails"). Psoriatic nail dystrophy is a chronic, primarily cosmetic condition. However, in some instances, thickened psoriatic toenails can become painful, and psoriatic fingernail deformities may interfere with function. Psoriatic nail dystrophy is more common in patients with psoriatic arthritis.

Typical Nail Changes

- **Pitting** is the most characteristic nail finding in psoriasis. (It may also be seen in alopecia areata, eczematous dermatitis, and as a normal finding in some nails.) It is produced by tiny punctate lesions that arise from the nail matrix (nail root) and appear on the nail plate as it grows (Figure 3.29).
- **Onycholysis** represents a separation of the nail plate from the underlying pink nail bed. The separated portion is white or yellow-white and opaque, in contrast to the pink translucence of the attached portion (Figure 3.30).
- **"Oil spots,"** or **"drops,"** are orange-brown colorations appearing under the nail plate. They are presumably the result of psoriasis of the nail bed (Figure 3.31).
- Thickening, or **subungual hyperkeratosis,** is a buildup of scale beneath the nail plate. It resembles onychomycosis, with which it is often confused and may coexist, particularly in toenails (Figure 3.32).

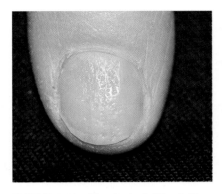

FIGURE 3.29 Psoriasis (pitting). The result of tiny punctate lesions that arise from the nail matrix, pitting appears on the nail plate as it grows.

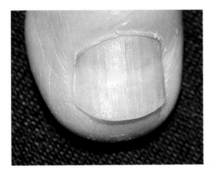

FIGURE 3.30 Psoriasis (onycholysis). The nail plate has separated from the underlying pink nail bed. The separated portion is white or yellow white and opaque, in contrast to the pink translucence of the attached portion.

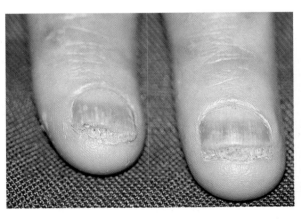

FIGURE 3.32 Psoriasis (subungual hyperkeratosis). A buildup of scale beneath the nail plate resembles onychomycosis. Also note in this figure "oil spots" and onycholysis.

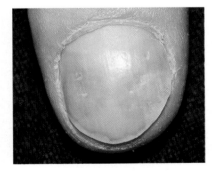

FIGURE 3.31 Psoriasis ("oil spots" or "drops"). Orange-brown coloration appears under the nail plate, presumably the result of psoriasis of the nail bed.

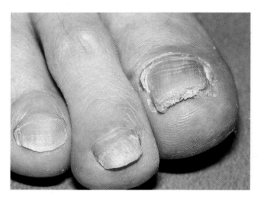

FIGURE 3.33 Onychomycosis. The subungual hyperkeratosis is similar to psoriasis; however, a fungal culture grew a dermatophyte.

- In onychomycosis, the KOH examination or fungal culture is positive. This disorder may be indistinguishable from psoriatic nails; in fact, both conditions can coexist in the same nail (Figure 3.33).
- Eczematous dermatitis with secondary nail dystrophy lacks subungual hyperkeratosis. Eczema is noted in the area of the proximal nail fold.

MANAGEMENT

Treatment is generally unrewarding, but some measures can be helpful:

- Careful trimming and paring of the nails are recommended.
- The application of potent topical steroids is followed by covering of the nail with plastic wrap or a plastic glove.
- Steroid can be injected into the nail matrix. (The injection is quite painful.)

POINT TO REMEMBER

- Nail dystrophy is more common in patients with psoriatic arthritis.

HELPFUL HINT

- Tazarotene (Tazorac) gel 0.01%, applied to the proximal nail fold nightly, has been shown to reduce onycholysis and pitting of psoriatic nails. (It has no effect on thickening and severe dystrophy.)

BASICS

Although psoriatic arthritis can be seen at any age, it most often begins between the ages of 35 and 45 years. It develops before or, more often, after the outbreak of skin manifestations of psoriasis. An earlier onset of psoriatic arthritis in adulthood can portend a worse prognosis that may include destructive arthropathy. Psoriatic arthritis has the following clinical features:

- A test for the rheumatoid factor is usually negative.
- It is seen in 5% to 10% of patients with psoriasis.
- Psoriatic arthritis is more likely seen in patients with severe cutaneous disease.
- Nail involvement is more frequently noted in patients with psoriatic arthritis.
- Peripheral psoriatic arthritis may be indistinguishable from Reiter's syndrome.

Types

There are five clinical patterns of psoriatic arthritis:

- Asymmetric involvement of one or several small or medium-sized joints is the most common initial presentation of psoriatic arthritis; if a finger joint is affected initially, the result is sometimes referred to as a "sausage finger deformity" (Figure 3.34).
- Mild involvement of the distal interphalangeal joints is considered the classic form of psoriatic arthritis. It is often accompanied by nail disease.
- Symmetric joint involvement resembles rheumatoid arthritis. (A test for the rheumatoid factor is negative, however.)
- Involvement of the joints in the axial skeleton that resembles, and may overlap with, ankylosing spondylitis.
- Mutilating, grossly deforming, arthritis mutilans may occur (Figure 3.35).

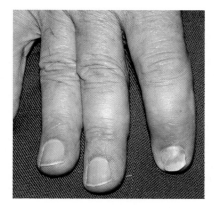

FIGURE 3.34 Psoriatic arthritis. "Sausage finger deformity" of the distal interphalangeal joint. Note onycholysis.

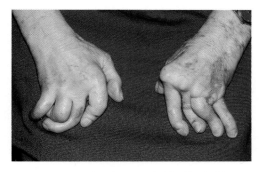

FIGURE 3.35 Psoriatic arthritis ("arthritis mutilans"). This patient has severe psoriatic arthritis with marked deformities and subluxations of the small bones of the hands. Note also the characteristic onycholysis on the nails.

MANAGEMENT

Treatment consists of analgesics, primarily nonsteroidal anti-inflammatory drugs, and methotrexate. Etanercept (Enbrel) has been approved by the United States Food and Drug Administration for the treatment of psoriatic arthritis. Etanercept is self-administered subcutaneously twice weekly. Evidence suggests that this drug, a tumor necrosis factor inhibitor, will prove to be valuable in the treatment of severe psoriasis, even in patients who do not have psoriatic arthritis. Etanercept can also be used in combination with methotrexate in patients who do not respond adequately to methotrexate alone.

FORMULARY FOR THE TOPICAL TREATMENT OF PSORIASIS

NOTE: *The formulary that follows is not comprehensive. It lists proprietary names and attempts to designate generic equivalents whenever possible. It is intended to provide more than enough treatment options; it contains more agents than most dermatologists tend to use on a regular basis.*

GENERIC NAMES	BRAND NAMES

KERATOLYTIC AGENTS

Salicylic acid 6%	Keralyt Gel*
Salicylic acid 5%	Hydrisalic Gel*

TOPICAL STEROIDS
Listed in order of decreasing potency

Superpotent

Clobetasol propionate cream/ointment/gel 0.05%	Temovate, Cormax
Clobetasol propionate lotion, foam	Temovate, Cormax scalp application, Olux
Diflorasone diacetate ointment 0.05%	Psorcon
Halobetasol propionate cream/ointment 0.05%	Ultravate
Flurandrenolide (24- and 80-inch rolls)	Cordran tape 4 μ g/cm^2

Very strong

Desoximetasone cream/ointment 0.25%/gel 0.05%	Topicort
Fluocinonide cream/ointment/solution/gel 0.05%	Lidex

Strong

Triamcinolone acetate ointment 0.1%/cream 0.5%	Aristocort A
Betamethasone valerate 0.1% foam	Luxiq

Medium-strong

Hydrocortisone valerate ointment 0.2%, NF	Westcort

Mild-medium

Hydrocortisone valerate cream 0.2%, NF	Westcort
Alclometasone dipropionate cream/ointment 0.05%, NF	Aclovate
Desonide cream/ointment/lotion 0.05%, NF	DesOwen

Mild

Hydrocortisone cream/ointment/lotion 0.5%, 1.0%, 2.5%, NF	Cortaid, Cortizone-5*

TOPICAL VITAMIN D$_3$

Calcipotriene 0.005% solution	Dovonex cream/ointment, scalp

TOPICAL RETINOIDS

Tazarotene 0.05%, 0.1%, cream/gel	Tazorac cream/gel

TOPICAL IMMUNOMODULATORS

Tacrolimus ointment 0.03%, 0.1%	Protopic ointment
Pimecrolimus 1% cream	Elidel

ANTHRALIN PREPARATIONS

Anthralin 0.1%, 0.25%, 0.5%	Drithocreme
Anthralin 0.25%, 0.5%	Dritho-Scalp
Anthralin 1% cream	Psoriatec

TAR PREPARATIONS

	Estar*
	PsoriGel*
	Balnetar*
	Doak tar oil*

NEWER APPROACHES TO PSORIASIS THERAPY:
The following "biologic" agents are the latest systemic agents that are currently being evaluated for the treatment of psoriasis and psoriatic arthritis:

Alefacept (Amevive): monoclonal antibody
Efalizumab (Xanelim): monoclonal antibody
Etanercept (Enbrel)
Infliximab (Remicade)

NF, non fluorinated.
*Available over-the-counter.

CHAPTER 4

Inflammatory Eruptions of Unknown Cause

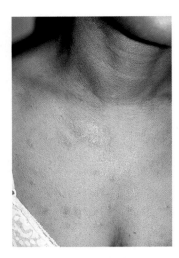

FIGURE 4.1 Pityriasis rosea. This patient has a herald patch on her chest. Other, smaller lesions can be seen.

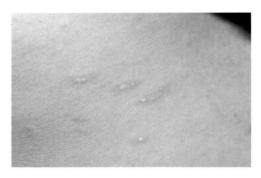

FIGURE 4.2 Pityriasis rosea. Multiple lesions with fine scale. Note the elliptic ("football") shape of lesions.

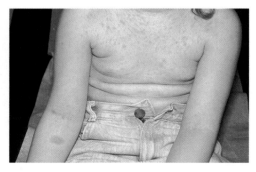

FIGURE 4.3 Pityriasis rosea. The herald patch is on the flexor forearm.

BASICS

Pityriasis rosea, which means "fine pink scale," is an acute, benign, self-limiting eruption with a characteristic clinical course. Pityriasis rosea tends to occur in the spring and fall, and although it may occur at any age, it is seen mostly in young adults and older children. The cause is unknown; however, the occasional clustering of cases and seasonal appearances suggest an infectious, transmissible origin.

Pathogenesis

Reports have suggested a role for human herpesvirus 7, but this has not been confirmed. Despite the prevailing opinion that pityriasis rosea is caused by an infectious agent, it does not appear to be very contagious; household contacts and schoolmates usually do not develop the eruption.

DESCRIPTION OF LESIONS

* The typical course of pityriasis rosea often begins with the larger *herald patch* (Figure 4.1), a 2- to 5-cm, scaly lesion that may exhibit central clearing and therefore may mimic tinea corporis.
* The herald patch is followed in several days to 2 weeks by multiple characteristic oval or elliptic erythematous patches with fine, thin scale on their surface (Figure 4.2).

DISTRIBUTION OF LESIONS

* The initial lesion, the herald patch, is most commonly observed on the trunk, neck, or extremities (Figure 4.3).
* Subsequent lesions appear on the trunk, neck, arms, and legs in an "old-fashioned bathing suit" distribution.

- The long axis of the lesions runs parallel to skin tension lines. This gives a "Christmas tree" pattern on the trunk (Figure 4.4).

CLINICAL MANIFESTATIONS

- Itching is usually absent or mild but may be severe.
- Pityriasis rosea is a self-limiting benign disorder; it usually lasts for 6 to 8 weeks.
- On resolution, postinflammatory pigment changes (hyperpigmentation) can occur, particularly in dark-skinned people.
- Recurrences are rare.

CLINICAL VARIANTS

- Pityriasis rosea can occur with less typical presentations such as those in which the herald patch is not noted by the patient or clinician. Moreover, in dark-skinned patients, the lesions may be vesicular and uncharacteristically pruritic.

The eruption may be limited in its distribution, or it may present in an inverse fashion involving the groin, axillae, or distal extremities *(inverse pityriasis rosea)* (Figure 4.5).

- Eruptions resembling those of pityriasis rosea also can occur in association with many drugs. These include barbiturates, bismuth, captopril, clonidine, diptheria toxoid, gold, isotretinoin, ketotifen, levamisole, metronidazole, and D-penicillamine.

DIAGNOSIS

The diagnosis is made clinically in most cases. In general, laboratory tests are not necessary or helpful, with the following exceptions:

- A potassium hydroxide (KOH) examination may be helpful when only the herald patch is present, to help rule in or rule out tinea corporis; similarly, a KOH examination may be used to distinguish tinea versicolor from pityriasis rosea.
- If the eruption includes lesions on the hand and feet, or if the patient is sexually active, then a rapid plasma reagin (RPR) or venereal disease research laboratory (VDRL) test should be performed to rule out secondary syphilis.
- A skin biopsy can be done when the eruption is atypical, the diagnosis is uncertain, or the disease has not resolved after 3 to 4 months.

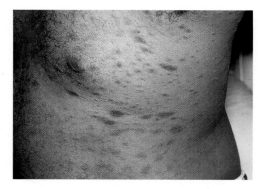

FIGURE 4.4 Pityriasis rosea. Here the "Christmas tree" pattern is evident.

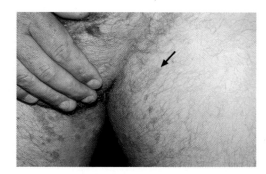

FIGURE 4.5 Atypical (inverse) pityriasis rosea in an inguinal distribution. The herald patch is present in the left inguinal area.

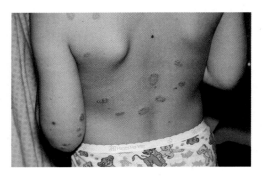

FIGURE 4.6 Guttate psoriasis. Thicker scale—actually plaques—than seen in pityriasis rosea is noted.

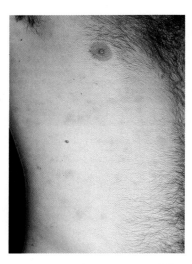

FIGURE 4.7 Secondary syphilis. Papulosquamous lesions appear on the trunk, similar to pityriasis rosea.

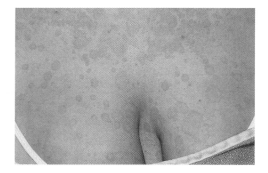

FIGURE 4.8 Tinea versicolor. The oval, tan patches are positive on potassium hydroxide examination.

 DIFFERENTIAL DIAGNOSIS

Guttate psoriasis (Figure 4.6)
- The abrupt onset is easily confused with pityriasis rosea.
- Scale is silvery and thicker than that of pityriasis rosea.

Secondary Syphilis
- Lesions are often seen on the palms, soles, and face, as well as the trunk (Figure 4.7).
- The RPR or VDRL test is positive.

Tinea Versicolor
- Round or oval macules or patches are present.
- Pigmentation is varied ("versicolor").
- The KOH examination is positive (Figure 4.8).

Drug Eruption or Viral Exanthem
- Lesions are redder, less scaly, and tend to be itchier than in pityriasis rosea.
- There may be other symptoms (e.g., fever).

Nummular Eczema
- "Coin-shaped" patches and plaques are present.
- Lesions tend to be on the legs.
- This condition generally itches.

Parapsoriasis
- Lesions may be similar to those of pityriasis rosea.
- This diagnosis should be considered in "pityriasis rosea" that persists for longer than 8 weeks.

MANAGEMENT

- Treatment is often unnecessary in most cases, because pityriasis rosea is usually a self-limiting, asymptomatic condition with no sequelae.
- All that is usually necessary is to advise the patient about the usual course of the rash and its noncontagious nature.
- Sunlight exposure may speed resolution of the eruption.
- Follow-up or referral to a dermatologist should be made if the rash persists beyond the typical 8 to 12 weeks.
- In cases of severe pruritus, oral antihistamines or topical steroids may help to alleviate the itching. The sedative effect of the antihistamines may help the patient to sleep better at night. On occasion, systemic steroids (prednisone 0.5 to 1 mg/kg per day for 7 days) can be used in patients with severe pruritus.

POINTS TO REMEMBER

- Lesions characteristically appear "from the neck to the knees."
- Pityriasis rosea is observed in otherwise healthy people, most frequently in children and young adults.
- Patients should be told that pityriasis rosea is a benign condition that will resolve over the next 6 to 12 weeks without treatment.
- Secondary syphilis should be considered in the differential diagnosis, especially when lesions are present on the palms and soles.

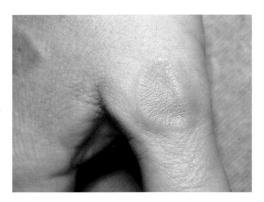

FIGURE 4.9 Granuloma annulare. This lesion is a typical annular plaque with central clearing.

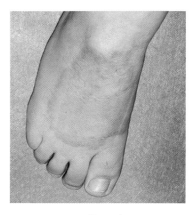

FIGURE 4.10 Granuloma annulare. This child has a typical annular plaque. The center of the lesion demonstrates hyperpigmentation.

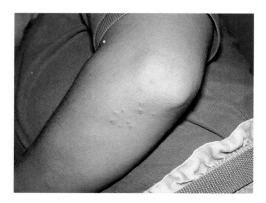

FIGURE 4.11 Granuloma annulare. Papules of granuloma annulare are located below the elbows in a middle-aged woman.

BASICS

Granuloma annulare is an idiopathic, generally asymptomatic, ring-shaped grouping of dermal papules. The papules are composed of focal granulomas that coalesce to form curious circles or semicircular plaques, which are often misdiagnosed as "ringworm." The condition is seen most frequently in very young children, in whom it is usually self-limiting.

Granuloma annulare is also seen in women by a 2.5:1 female-to-male ratio. In adults, granuloma annulare tends to be more chronic. There is also an adult form of disseminated granuloma annulare, which may be associated with diabetes.

Pathophysiology

Proposed pathogenic mechanisms include cell-mediated immunity (type IV), immune complex vasculitis, and an abnormality of tissue monocytes. None of these theories has convincing supporting evidence.

DESCRIPTION OF LESIONS

- Lesions are skin-colored or red firm papules, with no epidermal change (scale).
- The lesions may be individual, isolated papules, or they may be joined in annular or semiannular (arciform) plaques with central clearing (Figure 4.9). The centers of the lesions may be slightly hyperpigmented and depressed relative to their borders.
- Occasionally, granuloma annulare may present as subcutaneous nodules that are similar to rheumatoid nodules.

DISTRIBUTION OF LESIONS

- The dorsal surfaces of the feet, the hands and fingers, and the extensor aspects of the arms and legs are the most common sites of presentation.
- Although any part of the cutaneous surface may be involved, lesions are most often symmetrically distributed on dorsal surfaces of hands, fingers, and feet (acral areas) (Figure 4.10).
- In adults, lesions may also be found around the elbows (Figure 4.11) and on the trunk.
- Subcutaneous nodules may be seen on the arms and legs.

CLINICAL MANIFESTATIONS

- Granuloma annulare is generally asymptomatic and is usually only a cosmetic problem.

DIAGNOSIS

- The diagnosis is most often made on clinical grounds.
- Granuloma annulare has a characteristic histopathologic appearance. It consists of foci of altered collagen and mucin surrounded by granulomatous inflammation of histiocytic and lymphocytic cells. The degenerative collagen is referred to as *necrobiosis*.

  DIFFERENTIAL DIAGNOSIS

Tinea Corporis ("Ringworm")
- Scale is present at the "active border" (Figure 4.12).
- Lesions are annular "ringlike" (clear in the center).
- An asymmetric distribution of lesions is noted.
- The KOH examination or fungal culture is positive.
- Lesions generally are pruritic.

Erythema Migrans Rash of Lyme Disease
- Lesions of erythema migrans are larger than those associated with granuloma annulare (Figure 4.13).
- The rash is self-limited.
- Lesions are not as firm to palpation as noted in granuloma annulare.

Cutaneous Sarcoidosis
- This is seen most commonly in adult blacks and Scandinavians.
- Lesions often appear periorificially or develop in scars.
- Other diagnostic features of sarcoidosis are usually present.
- Annular sarcoidosis may be indistinguishable from granuloma annulare.

Rheumatoid Nodules
- These may be indistinguishable from subcutaneous nodules of granuloma annulare.

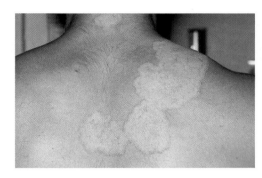

FIGURE 4.12 Tinea corporis. Scale is present at the "active border." Note the asymmetric distribution of lesions.

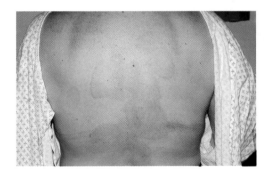

FIGURE 4.13 Erythema migrans rash of Lyme disease. Lesions are larger than those associated with granuloma annulare.

MANAGEMENT

- The patient should be reassured of the benign nature of this condition.
- Localized lesions in children are best left untreated.
- Potent topical steroids, if desired, may be used alone or under polyethylene occlusion (see Introduction, "Topical Therapy and Topical Steroids").

Intralesional triamcinolone acetonide (Kenalog), in a dose of 2 to 4 mg/mL, is injected directly into the elevated border of the lesions with a 30-gauge needle. The plaque is infiltrated until it blanches. This may be repeated at 4- to 6-week intervals.

- Cryotherapy with liquid nitrogen is used, but it frequently results in hypopigmentation or hyperpigmentation.

 POINTS TO REMEMBER

- Diabetes mellitus may be associated with the generalized form of granuloma annulare.
- Generalized forms of granuloma annulare are more difficult to treat and are less likely to resolve spontaneously.

BASICS

Lichen planus is a pruritic, idiopathic eruption with characteristic shiny, flat-topped (Latin: *planus*, "flat") papules on the skin, often accompanied by mucous membrane lesions. The papules are characterized by their violaceous color, polygonal shape, and, sometimes, fine scale. Lichen planus is most commonly found on the extremities, genitalia, and mucous membranes. Lesions can also involve the hair and nails.

Lichen planus is relatively uncommon; it is seen predominantly in adults and occurs in women more often than men. More than two-thirds of patients are between 30 and 60 years old; however, the condition can occur at any age.

Pathophysiology
Lichen planus is a cell-mediated immune response of unknown origin. An association is noted between lichen planus and hepatitis C infection, chronic active hepatitis, and primary biliary cirrhosis.

DESCRIPTION OF LESIONS

The "Seven Ps" (Figure 4.14)

1. Lesions are often **pruritic,** but they may be asymptomatic.
2. Lesions are often **purple** (actually, violaceous).
3. Lesions tend to be **planar** (flat-topped).
4. Lesions form **papules** or **plaques.**
5. Lesions may be **polygonal.**
6. Lesions may be **pleomorphic** in shape and configuration, that is, oval, annular, linear, confluent (plaquelike), large, and small, even on the same person.
7. Lesions tend to heal with residual **postinflammatory hyperpigmentation.**

Other Clinical Findings Associated with Lichen Planus
- The Köebner phenomenon (isomorphic response) (Figure 4.15) is seen as a reaction to trauma such as scratching (see Chapter 3, "Psoriasis").

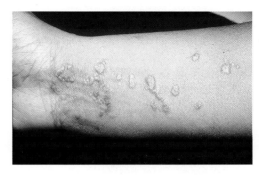

FIGURE 4.14 Lichen planus. Flat-topped, violaceous, polygonal papules on the flexor wrists are present. There are active and resolving lesions. Note the postinflammatory hyperpigmentation.

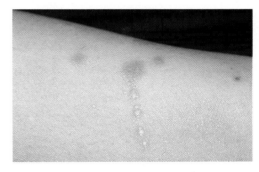

FIGURE 4.15 Lichen planus. The Köebner phenomenon (isomorphic response) results from scratching.

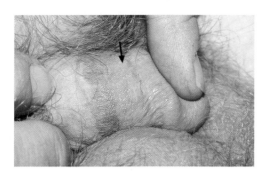

FIGURE 4.16 Lichen planus. Wickham's striae are white streaks *(arrow)* on the surface of lesion on glans penis after mineral oil is applied.

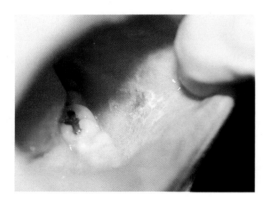

FIGURE 4.17 Lichen planus. Oral lesions, with a white, lacy pattern and erythematous erosion on the buccal mucosa.

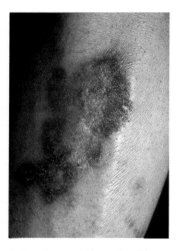

FIGURE 4.18 Hypertrophic lichen planus. Darkly pigmented hypertrophic lesions are present on the pretibial shaft.

- Wickham's striae are characteristic white streaks that are best visualized on the surface of lesions after mineral oil is applied (Figure 4.16).
- Mucous membrane lesions are characterized by white lacy streaks in a netlike pattern or by atrophic erosions or ulcers (Figure 4.17) (see Chapter 12, "Disorders of the Mouth, Lips, and Tongue").
- Nail lesions may exhibit a mild dystrophy to a total loss of the nails.
- Scalp lesions result in scarring follicular alopecia *(lichen planopilaris)*.

DISTRIBUTION OF LESIONS

- The flexor areas such as the wrists, pretibial shafts, scalp, trunk, and glans penis are most often affected.
- Mucous membrane involvement is common and may be found without skin involvement. Lesions are most commonly found on the tongue and buccal mucosa; they are characterized by white or gray streaks forming a linear or reticular pattern.
- Genital involvement is common in men with cutaneous disease. Typically, an annular configuration of papules is seen on the glans penis. Less commonly, linear white streaks (Wickham's striae) can be seen on male genitalia. Vulvar involvement can range from reticulate papules to severe erosions.

CLINICAL MANIFESTATIONS

- Pruritus and the cosmetic appearance of lesions are the major concerns to patients.
- Lichen planus is a self-limited disease that usually resolves within 8 to 12 months; however, lesions may persist for months and then spontaneously disappear.
- In some instances, the condition can last for years, or even a lifetime.
- Oral lesions may become ulcerative and painful; rare malignant transformation to squamous cell carcinoma has been documented.
- Hypertrophic lesions tend to be extremely pruritic.
- Vulvar lesions can result in dyspareunia, burning, and pruritis.

CLINICAL VARIANTS

Variations in lichen planus include the following:

- **Hypertrophic:** These extremely pruritic lesions are most often found on the extensor surfaces of the lower extremities (Figure 4.18), especially around the ankles. Hypertrophic lesions are often chronic; residual pigmentation and scarring can occur when the lesions eventually clear.

- **Atrophic:** Atrophic lichen planus is characterized by a few lesions, which often develop into hypertrophic lesions.
- **Erosive:** These lesions are found on the mucosal surfaces and evolve from sites of previous lichen planus involvement.
- **Follicular:** Lichen planopilaris is characterized by keratotic papules that may coalesce into plaques. Scarring alopecia may result.

Other eruptions resembling lichen planus are seen in the following conditions:

- Drug-induced lichen planus associated with gold, thiazides, captopril, and antimalarials
- Lichenoid reactions associated with graft-versus-host disease
- Lichen planus associated with hepatitis C

DIAGNOSIS

- Lichen planus is often very easy to diagnose by its appearance, despite its range of clinical presentations.
- The presence of Wickham's striae is diagnostic.
- Characteristic oral lesions are helpful in making the diagnosis.
- Skin biopsy is performed, if necessary.

 DIFFERENTIAL DIAGNOSIS

Lichen Simplex Chronicus (Figure 4.19; see Chapter 2, "Eczema")

- Lichenification is present.

Lichenoid (Lichen Planus–Like) Eruptions
- Skin lesions are indistinguishable from those of classic lichen planus.
- Oral lesions are lacking.
- Patients have a history of drug ingestion or bone marrow transplantation, for example.

Other Diagnoses
- Pityriasis rosea
- Guttate psoriasis
- Tinea corporis

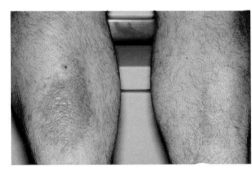

FIGURE 4.19 Lichen simplex chronicus. This patient has itchy pretibial hypertropic plaques.

MANAGEMENT

Mild cases can be treated symptomatically with antihistamines and fluorinated topical steroids. Patients with more severe cases, especially those with scalp, nail, and mucous membrane involvement, may require systemic therapy.

- The first-line treatments of cutaneous lichen planus are potent topical steroids.
- Systemic steroids in short tapering courses may be necessary for symptom control and possibly more rapid resolution.
- Oral acitretin (Soriatane) has been tried with some success.
- Many other treatments are of uncertain efficacy because of the lack of randomized controlled trials.
- For lichen planus of the oral mucosa, topical steroids are usually tried first. Topical tacrolimus (Protopic) ointment 0.03% and 0.1% has been tried with some success.

POINT TO REMEMBER

- Lichen planus is seen frequently enough and has a sufficiently unusual array of features to be recognizable to the nondermatologist.

Superficial Bacterial Infections, Folliculitis, and Hidradenitis Suppurativa

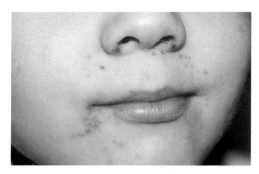

FIGURE 5.1 Impetigo. Dried stuck-on appearing "honey-crusted" lesions in a typical location.

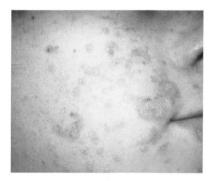

FIGURE 5.2 Impetigo. This child has a mixture of intact bullae and drying crusts.

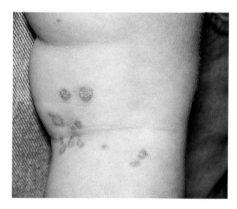

FIGURE 5.3 Impetigo. Here intact blisters are not present; only the flaccid remains (scaly collarettes) of bullae are seen.

BASICS

Impetigo is a primary superficial bacterial infection of the skin. It is a common, highly contagious finding in preschoolers. The two forms of the disease—bullous and nonbullous (crusted) impetigo—are caused by *Staphylococcus aureus* and group A beta-hemolytic streptococci, respectively. Impetigo traditionally has been divided into these two varieties, but because they are clinically more or less indistinguishable, it is probably less confusing to use the term impetigo to describe both of them. In fact, both organisms can be present at the same time.

Children younger than 6 years have a higher incidence of impetigo than do adults; however, the condition may occur in persons of all ages. Impetigo rarely progresses to systemic infection, although poststreptococcal glomerulonephritis is a rare complication. When impetigo presents as a secondary infection of preexisting skin disease or traumatized skin, it is referred to as **impetiginization** or secondary impetiginization.

S. aureus may colonize preexisting dermatoses, with resulting secondary impetiginization. Examples include the following:

- Impetiginized eczema
- Impetiginized stasis dermatitis
- Impetiginized herpes simplex and varicella infections
- Impetiginized scabies and insect bites
- Impetiginized lacerations and burns

DESCRIPTION OF LESIONS

- Impetigo begins as a thin-roofed vesicle or bulla that ruptures and often leaves a peripheral collarette of scale or a darker, hemorrhagic crusted border.
- Oozing serum dries and gives rise to the classic golden-yellow, "honey-crusted" lesion. Lesions appear to be stuck on (Figure 5.1 and 5.2).
- In time, a varnishlike crust develops centrally that, if removed, reveals a moist red base.
- Intact bullae usually are not present; they often demonstrate a collarette of scale or the flaccid remains of bullae (Figure 5.3).

DISTRIBUTION OF LESIONS

- The face is commonly involved, particularly in and around the nose and mouth, in children.
- However, lesions may occur anywhere on the body.

CLINICAL MANIFESTATIONS

- Spread of lesions is by autoinoculation.
- Lesions are usually asymptomatic, but they may itch.
- The infection is self-limiting—even without treatment—and generally spontaneously resolves after a few weeks.
- Healing takes place without scarring, but it may cause temporary postinflammatory hyperpigmentation in dark-skinned persons.
- Recurrent or persistent impetigo may indicate a carrier state in the patient or the patient's family.

DIAGNOSIS

- Diagnosis is usually made on clinical grounds.
- Bacterial culture and sensitivity testing are recommended if standard topical or oral treatment does not result in improvement.
- A bacterial culture of the nares may be obtained to determine whether a patient is a carrier of *S. aureus*.
- Urinalysis is necessary to evaluate for acute poststreptococcal glomerulonephritis if the patient develops edema or hypertension. Hematuria, proteinuria, and cylindruria are indicators of renal involvement.

 ## DIFFERENTIAL DIAGNOSIS

Tinea Corporis (Figure 5.4)
- The potassium hydroxide examination or fungal culture is positive.
- Central clearing of lesions is noted.

Much less commonly considered in the differential diagnosis are primary bullous diseases such as bullous dermatosis of childhood and bullous pemphigoid.

 ### MANAGEMENT

- Antibacterial soaps such as povidone-iodine (Betadine) or chlorhexidine (Hibiclens) are used twice daily.
- Gentle débridement of lesional crusts is done with a washcloth and antibacterial soap.
- Mupirocin 2% (Bactroban) ointment or cream applied three times daily may be used alone to treat very limited cases of impetigo. It is used until all lesions are cleared. This ointment applied topically has been shown to be as effective as oral antibiotics.
- For widespread involvement, an oral staphylocidal penicillinase-resistant antibiotic, such as cephalosporin, dicloxacillin, or erythromycin, may be used alone or in conjunction with topical antibiotics.
- For patients with recurrent impetigo or for *S. aureus* nasal carriers, mupirocin 2% (Bactroban) cream or ointment can be applied inside the nostrils three times daily for 5 days each month, to reduce bacterial colonization in the nose.
- Patients who are chronic nasal carriers also can be treated with rifampin.

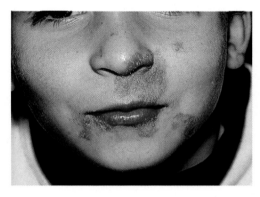

FIGURE 5.4 Tinea corporis (faciale). This young boy was initially treated with topical antibiotics for presumptive impetigo.

 ### POINTS TO REMEMBER

- Rarely, poststreptococcal glomerulonephritis (but not rheumatic fever) has been reported to follow impetigo caused by certain strains of streptococci.
- Family members should be evaluated as potential nasal carriers of *S. aureus* and treated, if necessary.

 ### HELPFUL HINT

- Chronic or recurrent impetigo should alert the clinician to the possibility of an impaired immune status.

PERIANAL STREPTOCOCCAL DERMATITIS (PERIANAL CELLULITIS)

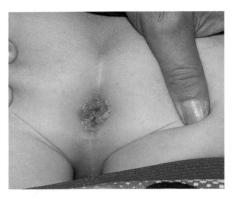

FIGURE 5.5 Perianal streptococcal dermatitis. Erythematous plaque with a collarette of scale on the anus of this 4-year-old boy.

BASICS

This fairly common condition that occurs in children 3 to 4 years of age is probably recognized more frequently by pediatricians than by dermatologists. It is caused by group A beta-hemolytic streptococci.

CLINICAL MANIFESTATIONS

- Most commonly, the eruption presents as a bright pink to red erythema that extends 2 to 3 cm from the anus (Figure 5.5).
- Infrequently, fissuring, pain, and a mucoid discharge may be present.
- Generally, this lesion is asymptomatic and is discovered on inspection by parents.
- On occasion, itching may be a complaint, and if cellulitis develops, there may be pain on defecation.

DIAGNOSIS

- This is most often a clinical diagnosis, confirmed by isolation of group A beta-hemolytic streptococci from lesional skin.

 DIFFERENTIAL DIAGNOSIS

- Pinworm infestation
- Psoriasis
- Atopic dermatitis
- Candidiasis
- Inflammatory bowel disease
- Most important: Sexual abuse

 MANAGEMENT

- The treatment of choice is penicillin V, 50 mg/kg per day in four divided doses. This is combined with topical mupirocin (Bactroban) ointment or cream twice a day.
- Penicillin-allergic patients may be given a cephalosporin or erythromycin.

 HELPFUL HINT

- Flares of guttate psoriasis have been associated with this condition.

Overview

Folliculitis, in its broadest sense, may be defined as a superficial or deep infection or inflammation of the hair follicles. It has multiple causes: various infections, physical or chemical irritation, occlusive dressings or clothing, and the use of topical or systemic steroids. Hereditary forms of folliculitis such as follicular eczema are generally classified as atopic dermatitis (see Chapter 2, "Eczema"). The deeper forms of inflammatory folliculitis that involve the entire follicular structure, such as **folliculitis decalvans,** occur most commonly in black men and women (see Chapter 10, "Hair and Scalp Disorders Resulting in Hair Loss").

Folliculitis may also be seen as a secondary infection in conditions such as eczema, scabies, and excoriated insect bites. It is more commonly found in patients who are diabetic, obese, or immunocompromised. Viral folliculitis may be seen in patients with herpes simplex infections, particularly in patients with human immunodeficiency virus (HIV) infection.

STAPHYLOCOCCAL FOLLICULITIS

BASICS

Bacterial folliculitis is more commonly found in patients who are diabetic, obese, or immunocompromised. Coagulase-positive *S. aureus* is the responsible pathogenic bacterium in most cases of infectious folliculitis.

CAUSES AND PRECIPITATING FACTORS

As in cases of inflammatory folliculitis (see Chapter 2, "Eczema"), bacterial folliculitis may be seen after the following:

- Repeated trauma (such as waxing, plucking, and shaving)
- Wearing of restrictive clothing, such as tight jeans
- Excessive sweating

DESCRIPTION OF LESIONS

- **A pustule or papule with a central hair** is the primary lesion in folliculitis. The central hair shaft may not always be visible (Figure 5.6).
- Follicular lesions tend to manifest a **gridlike pattern** on hair-bearing areas of the body (Figure 5.7).
- Lesions are often polymorphic, displaying a mixture of papules and pustules, or they may be monomorphic and consist solely of papules.
- In darkly pigmented patients, primary lesions may consist of obvious papules or pustules; alternatively, only secondary, hyperpigmented lesions arranged in a follicular pattern may be all that is clinically visible.

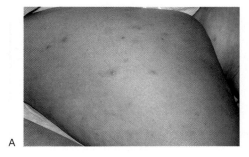

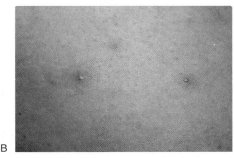

FIGURE 5.6 *A:* Staphylococcal folliculitis. Pustules and papules can be seen on this woman's thigh. *B:* Staphylococcal folliculitis. This is a close-up view of *A.*

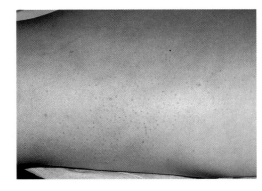

FIGURE 5.7 Irritant folliculitis. This woman developed small erythematous papules after shaving her legs. Note the gridlike (follicular) pattern.

DISTRIBUTION OF LESIONS

- Lesions occur primarily on hair bearing areas—the face, scalp, thighs, and body folds.
- The axillae, groin, and legs are particularly prone to folliculitis when they are regularly shaved.

CLINICAL MANIFESTATIONS

- Lesions of folliculitis elicit mild discomfort and cosmetic concern.

CLINICAL VARIANTS

- Tender, painful, folliculitis involving an eyelash is called a hordeolum, or "sty" (Figure 5.8).
- Similarly, folliculitis may affect a single nasal hair follicle and may produce a tender erythematous papule or pustule in, or on, the distal nose or near the tip of the nose.

DIAGNOSIS

This is generally diagnosed by clinical findings. In cases resistant to treatment, the following procedures may be performed:

- **Gram stain and bacterial culture.** In typical cases, a Gram stain shows gram-positive cocci, and culture grows *S. aureus*.
- **Nasal culture.** The patient and, if necessary, the patient's family members may require a nasal culture to look for *S. aureus*.

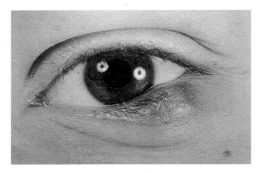

FIGURE 5.8 Hordeolum (sty). This is a painful localized infection or inflammation of the eyelid margin involving hair follicles of the eye lashes.

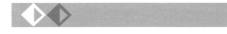 **DIFFERENTIAL DIAGNOSIS**

Acne Vulgaris and Other Acnelike Conditions
- **Keratosis pilaris** is frequently confused with acne and folliculitis (see Chapter 2, "Eczema").
- Because keratosis pilaris involves the hair follicles, it manifests in a gridlike pattern, similar to that of folliculitis.
- Lesions have a rough texture and are persistent.

Insect Bite Reactions
- Lesions are grouped in a nonfollicular pattern (Figure 5.9).

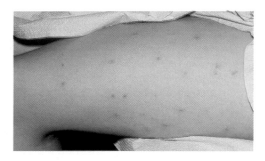

FIGURE 5.9 Insect bites. These flea bites are grouped in a characteristic nonfollicular ("breakfast, lunch, and dinner") pattern.

MANAGEMENT

Mild Cases
- Mild cases of bacterial folliculitis can sometimes be prevented or controlled with antibacterial soaps.
- In addition, topical antibiotics, such as erythromycin 2% topical solution or clindamycin (Cleocin) 1% solution, may be applied once or twice a day to the affected areas.

Chronic and Recurrent Cases
Chronic and recurrent cases of bacterial folliculitis present a difficult therapeutic problem:

- If staphylococcal colonization is present, mupirocin 2% (Bactroban) ointment should be applied to the nasal vestibule twice a day for 5 days to eliminate the *S. aureus* carrier state.
- Family members may be treated similarly, if necessary. Rifampin (600 mg per day for 10 to 14 days) may also eliminate the carrier state.
- Even in cases of negative bacterial cultures, a systemic antibiotic is often needed for coverage of *S. aureus* because it is the most common pathogen. This organism is often resistant to penicillin, and thus dicloxacillin (250 to 500 mg four times a day) or a cephalosporin, such as cephalexin (1 to 4 g per day in two doses) is generally the first choice. Minocycline (50 to 100 mg twice a day) is sometimes used for methicillin-resistant *S. aureus*.

 POINTS TO REMEMBER

- Bacterial cultures should be considered in cases resistant to therapy.
- Consider culturing and treating family members in cases of chronic bacterial folliculitis.

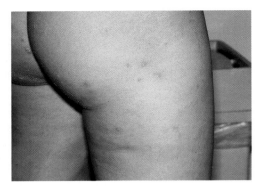

FIGURE 5.10   Hot tub folliculitis ("hot tub buns"). Multiple pruritic follicular papules and pustules occurred on the buttocks and trunk of this woman 3 days after she had bathed in a hot tub. Bacterial culture grew *Pseudomonas aeruginosa.*

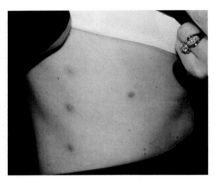

FIGURE 5.11   Hot tub folliculitis. This woman developed very itchy erythematous papules after bathing in a Jacuzzi.

PSEUDOMONAS (HOT TUB) FOLLICULITIS

Pseudomonas folliculitis, which may be acquired from communal hot tubs, is caused by *P. aeruginosa* infection. Although they have increased the incidence of folliculitis, hot tubs are often overlooked as a cause. Jacuzzis, therapeutic whirlpools ("whirlpool folliculitis"), public swimming pools, and the use of loofah sponges may also be a source of *Pseudomonas* infection. *Pseudomonas* folliculitis has been found to occur under diving suits and after wax depilation.

DESCRIPTION OF LESIONS

Lesions of hot tub folliculitis consist of intensely pruritic or tender follicular papules or pustules that are most often found on the trunk (the area covered by a bathing suit) (Figures 5.10 and 5.11).

CLINICAL MANIFESTATIONS

- Pruritic lesions occur 1 to 3 days after bathing in a hot tub, whirlpool, or public swimming pool.

DIAGNOSIS

- The diagnosis is based on a history of exposure.
- *Pseudomonas* organisms can be isolated in patients with this condition.

MANAGEMENT

- Hot tub folliculitis usually resolves spontaneously, but it may not if it is very extensive or symptomatic.
- If necessary, it may be treated with oral ciprofloxacin (500 mg twice a day for 5 days).

FOLLICULITIS: OTHER TYPES

Irritant, Frictional, or Chemical Folliculitis
Nonbacterial, or sterile, folliculitis can arise from physical or chemical irritation. Such irritants include leg waxing, leg shaving, axillary shaving, and hair plucking. Chemical depilatories, electrolysis, occlusive dressings, and excessive sweating can also contribute to this problem, as well as wearing tight jeans. Nonbacterial folliculitis may also be related to working conditions, such as the use of greases or oils, and to the application of various cosmetics. Bacteria such as *S. aureus* are not infrequent secondary invaders.

Steroid-Induced Acne and Rosacea
Topical or systemic steroid treatment may lead to steroid-induced acne, which is actually a form of folliculitis. Diagnosis of these conditions is aided by a history of potent topical or systemic steroid use (Figure 5.12).

Eosinophilic Pustular Folliculitis
Eosinophilic pustular folliculitis, another form of sterile folliculitis, has intensely pruritic lesions that resemble urticaria papules. It is seen in patients with acquired immunodeficiency syndrome (see Chapter 24, "Cutaneous Manifestations of HIV Infection").

Folliculitis from Fungi
Pityrosporum Folliculitis
This acnelike eruption, seen on the trunk, is caused by yeast forms of *Pityrosporum ovale* and *P. orbicularis*. Lesions are chronic, erythematous, pruritic papules and pustules that usually appear on the back and chest in a follicular pattern (Figure 5.13). This condition is seen more frequently in the summer. *Pityrosporum* folliculitis should be considered as a diagnosis when folliculitis resists antibiotics. It looks like acne, but it does not respond to acne therapy.

Majocchi's Granuloma
Tinea corporis of the lower legs may produce tinea folliculitis in women who shave their legs. The organism is introduced into the hair follicle by shaving. The condition is known as *Majocchi's granuloma*.

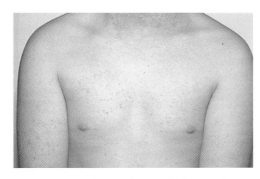

FIGURE 5.12 Systemic steroid-induced folliculitis. This patient is taking systemic steroids for severe asthma.

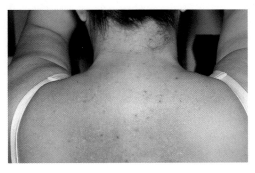

FIGURE 5.13 *Pityrosporum* folliculitis. This pruritic, acnelike eruption was resistant to antibiotics. It looks like acne, but it did not respond to acne therapy.

 POINTS TO REMEMBER

- Bacterial, fungal, or viral cultures should be considered in cases resistant to therapy.
- In HIV-positive patients, a skin biopsy should be performed for suspected cases of eosinophilic pustular folliculitis.

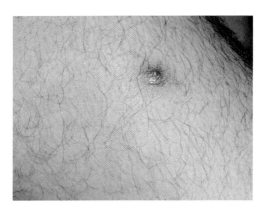

FIGURE 5.14 Furuncle. This patient has a painful, "pointing" furuncular nodule on his thigh.

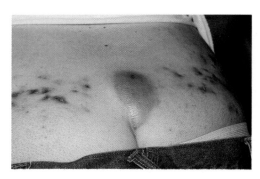

FIGURE 5.15 Abscess. This patient has the follicular occlusion triad, which consists of hidradenitis suppurativa, acne conglobata, and dissecting cellulitis of the scalp. This walled-off lesion began as folliculitis that later became a furuncle and then an abscess. Note the older violaceous scars from previous furuncles and cystic acne lesions.

BASICS

Folliculitis may evolve into a furuncle ("boil"), which is a deeper infection; the term carbuncle refers to an aggregation of furuncles. *S. aureus* is the customary responsible pathogenic bacterium. Furuncles are painful nodules or abscesses (walled-off collections of pus) in an infected hair follicle; they are more common in boys and young adults.

Chronic or recurrent furunculosis is a difficult therapeutic problem that is often the result of nasal carriage of *S. aureus*. Like folliculitis, furunculosis is more common in diabetic patients and in obese persons.

DESCRIPTION OF LESIONS

- It is a tender, painful nodule with overlying erythema (Figure 5.14).
- As the lesion evolves, a fluctuant abscess may form (Figure 5.15).
- If untreated, it may rupture and drain spontaneously.

DISTRIBUTION OF LESIONS

- Hair-bearing areas are commonly involved, with body folds the preferred sites.
- The scalp, face, buttocks, thighs, axillae, and inguinal areas are affected.
- Furuncles are often seen in the axillae, groin, posterior neck, thighs, and buttocks. When they occur in a contiguous cluster on the occipital scalp, they are referred to as carbuncles.

CLINICAL MANIFESTATIONS

- Furuncles can cause throbbing pain and can be quite tender.

DIAGNOSIS

- This is based on the clinical presentation.
- Gram stain generally reveals gram-positive cocci; culture often grows *S. aureus*.

 DIFFERENTIAL DIAGNOSIS

Hidradenitis Suppurativa (see later)
- Chronic, scarring inflammatory disease of apocrine glands is present.
- Abscesses resembling furuncles are noted.
- One often sees comedones and sinus tracts.
- Bacteria are secondary invaders.
- The condition is more common in women.
- It may be indistinguishable from furunculosis in its early stages.

MANAGEMENT
- Furuncles come to a "head" with warm compresses, or they may be incised and drained.
- Systemic staphylocidal antibiotics such as dicloxacillin, erythromycin, or cephalosporin may be added. Minocycline is sometimes used for methicillin-resistant *S. aureus*.

BASICS

- Hidradenitis suppurativa should not be classified as an infection; rather, it is a chronic, recurrent, scarring, inflammatory disease that affects the regions of the skin-bearing apocrine sweat glands: the axillae, inguinal folds, suprapubic area, anogenital area, buttocks, areola, and inframammary area. Bacterial involvement is not a primary pathogenic event.
- Hidradenitis suppurativa is seen mostly in women and only rarely before puberty.
- When hidradenitis suppurativa occurs in African-American women, it tends to be more severe.

Pathophysiology

The exact cause of hidradenitis suppurativa is unknown. Traditionally, it had been considered a primary inflammatory disorder of the apocrine glands (and was sometimes referred to as *apocrinitis* or *apocrine acne*). The current hypothesis suggests that poral occlusion of the hair follicle leads to retention of the secretory products and subsequent inflammation. This hypothesis is supported by the finding that in most biopsy specimens, the apocrine glands are intact and unaffected, and follicular occlusion is constant. Inflammation of the apocrine glands is thus considered to be secondary or incidental. Bacterial involvement is also considered a secondary pathogenic event.

Hormones appear to affect the course of hidradenitis suppurativa. Symptoms often improve during the estrogen-elevation phases of the menstrual cycle. Moreover, the condition often improves during pregnancy, only to flare during the postpartum period.

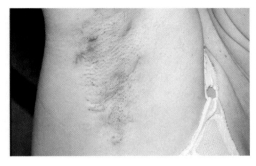

FIGURE 5.16 Chronic hidradenitis suppurativa. This patient has involvement of the axilla with bandlike hypertrophic scars. Note the characteristic paired open comedones and the single furunclelike lesion.

DESCRIPTION OF LESIONS AND CLINICAL MANIFESTATIONS

- Initially, hidradenitis suppurativa presents with nodules and abscesses that may be indistinguishable from furunculosis or common "boils."
- Lesions are painful and tender, and they often become infected secondarily and exude a serosanguineous or foul-smelling purulent material that may stain clothing.
- Hidradenitis suppurativa is often a cause of embarrassment and, possibly, social isolation.
- Lesions recur, new lesions crop up, and old lesions scar in a frustrating, unrelenting process.
- Chronic hidradenitis suppurativa is indicated by the appearance of sinus tract and fistula formation, ulcerations and, eventually, hypertrophic linear bands of scars.
- Characteristic multiple open comedones ("blackheads") develop in long-standing cases.

DISTRIBUTION OF LESIONS

- The most common area of involvement is the axillary area (Figure 5.16); the groin is also frequently involved (Figure 5.17). However, lesions may also be seen on the perineum, the buttocks, and, rarely, the neck and scalp.

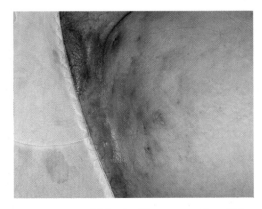

FIGURE 5.17 Hidradenitis suppurativa. This patient has involvement of the inguinal areas, labia majora, and mesial thighs. Her undergarment was stained by the oozing lesions.

DIAGNOSIS

- The multiple lesions of hidradenitis suppurativa that scar and form sinus tracts should be easily distinguishable from other conditions.

 DIFFERENTIAL DIAGNOSIS

In its early stages, hidradenitis suppurativa is most often confused with the following:

- **Recurrent furunculosis** (Figure 5.18). Solitary lesions resemble a furuncle, lymphadenitis, or an infected epidermoid cyst.
- In the vaginal area, an infected **Bartholin's cyst** may resemble a solitary lesion of hidradenitis suppurativa.

Other conditions appear to be related to hidradenitis suppurativa and may coexist in the same patient. The so-called follicular occlusion triad, which consists of hidradenitis suppurativa, acne conglobata, and dissecting cellulitis of the scalp, has been well documented. Pilonidal sinus was later added to the triad, making it a tetrad (Figure 5.15).

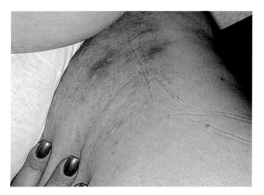

FIGURE 5.18 Furunculosis. This woman has recurrent draining "boils" in the inguinal area.

 MANAGEMENT

- Hidradenitis suppurativa is a difficult, frustrating condition to control.

Preventive Measures during Remissions

The risk for developing hidradenitis suppurativa can be decreased by wearing loose cotton undergarments, to minimize friction and moisture. Other preventive measures include the following:

- The use of absorbent powders
- Weight reduction
- The use of bacteriostatic soaps

Topical Therapy

- Limited and very early disease may be helped somewhat by the daily use of topical antibiotics, such as clindamycin or erythromycin.
- Intralesional corticosteroid injections inserted directly into painful lesions are used to treat limited acute exacerbations.

Systemic Therapy

Prednisone can be used in short courses, particularly if inflammation is severe. A short course of prednisone, 40 to 60 daily, to be tapered over 2 to 3 weeks is often quite effective.

Prednisone may be given alone or, most often, in combination with oral antibiotics, such as minocycline, erythromycin, ciprofloxacin, cephalosporins, or semisynthetic penicillin, given in the usual doses used for soft tissue infections. For example, minocycline, in doses ranging from 50 to 100 mg twice a day, may be used on an episodic basis for weeks or, if necessary, months at a time and then tapered to the lowest dosage that

(continued)

relieves symptoms. Long-term administration of an antibiotic, such as minocycline, can also be used to prevent episodic flares. The efficacy of minocycline seems to be attributable to its anti-inflammatory action, not to its antibiotic effect.

Alternative antibiotics that can be helpful include erythromycin (250 to 500 mg three or four times a day), ciprofloxacin (500 mg twice a day), cephalexin (250 to 500 mg four times a day), and dicloxacillin (250 to 500 mg twice a day).

Systemic retinoids, such as oral isotretinoin (Accutane), have been used with limited benefit in early disease that has not yet produced significant scarring. The systemic retinoids are not as effective in treating hidradenitis suppurativa as they are in treating severe nodular acne; moreover, relapses are very common after seemingly effective treatment is stopped.

Certain oral contraceptives, such as cyproterone acetate (which is not available in the United States), have been reported to be helpful in some cases. Cyclosporine has also been reported to be of some value.

Surgical Measures
- Incision and drainage are performed only on fluctuant lesions. This approach affords short-term relief of troublesome, painful abscesses. Repeated incision and drainage may lead to more scarring and sinus tract formation.
- Severe refractory hidradenitis suppurativa is best treated with wide, complete surgical excision of the involved area, which may produce a definitive cure.
- A narrow excision of inflamed areas may help temporarily, but this method has a high recurrence rate.
- Ablation techniques using a carbon dioxide laser that spares normal tissue have been tried successfully. These techniques may become the standard of surgical treatment.

Prognosis
The course of hidradenitis suppurativa varies.

- Some patients have very mild disease that may be indistinguishable from chronic furunculosis.
- Remissions may occur more frequently as the patient ages or as more scar tissue develops; however, total spontaneous resolution is rare. More commonly reported is a decline in severity at, or after, menopause.

 POINTS TO REMEMBER
- Recurrent tender, furuncles or sterile abscesses in the axillae or groin, on the buttocks, or below the breasts suggest the diagnosis of hidradenitis suppurativa.
- Chronic disease is indicated by the presence of old scars, sinus tracts, and open comedones.

CHAPTER 6

Superficial Viral Infections

BASICS

Warts are extremely common, particularly in the pediatric age group (Figure 6.1), and they are generally easy to diagnose. An estimated 20% of school-age children will at some time have at least one wart. In children, warts tend to regress spontaneously. In many adults and in immunocompromised patients, however, warts often prove difficult to eradicate.

All warts are caused by the human papillomavirus (HPV); to date, more than 150 different subtypes have been identified. The virus infects epidermal keratinocytes, which stimulates cell proliferation. Transmission is primarily through skin-to-skin contact. HPV types 16, 18, and 31, which are noted mainly in the anogenital region, have been associated with potential oncogenicity.

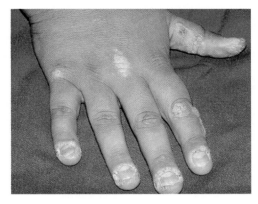

FIGURE 6.1 Verruca vulgaris. This young boy has multiple common warts.

Factors that Predispose to Human Papillomavirus Infection
- Being infected with the human immunodeficiency virus (HIV) is a predisposing factor.
- Taking drugs that decrease cell-mediated immunity (e.g., prednisone, cyclosporine) is another predisposing factor. Transplant recipients who, by necessity, use such medications on a long-term basis have warts that can be very resistant to treatment.
- Taking chemotherapeutic agents also may allow the virus to proliferate.
- During pregnancy, warts may proliferate and then regress post partum.
- Handling raw meat, fish, or other types of animal matter in one's occupation (for example, butchers), is a predisposing factor.

DESCRIPTION OF LESIONS

- A typical wart is a papillomatous, corrugated, hyperkeratotic growth that is confined to the epidermis. Despite a common misconception, warts have no "roots," and there is no "mother wart."
- Warts often vary widely in shape, size, and appearance. The different names for warts generally reflect their clinical appearance, location, or both.
- For example, filiform warts are threadlike, planar warts are flat, and plantar warts are located on the plantar surface of the feet.
- Genital warts, or condyloma acuminatum, may be large and cauliflowerlike, or they may consist of small papules.

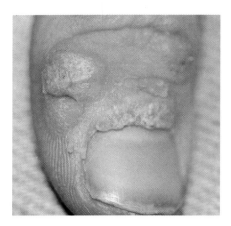

FIGURE 6.2 Common warts. Periungual warts.

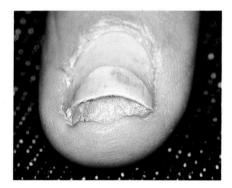

FIGURE 6.3 Common wart. This subungual lesion could easily be mistaken for onychomycosis.

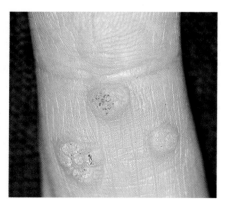

FIGURE 6.4 Common warts. Lesions demonstrate loss of normal skin markings. "Black dots," or thrombosed capillaries, are pathognomonic.

DISTRIBUTION OF LESIONS

- Warts may develop anywhere on the body, but they are most often found at sites subject to frequent trauma, such as the hands and feet.

Viral protein and infectious particles have been detected in the absence of visible skin surface lesions using electron microscopy, polymerase chain reaction, and DNA hybridization techniques. Thus, it is well documented that HPV can exist in a subclinical or latent state. This latency explains the not infrequent recurrence of warts at the same site or at an adjacent site, even when they had been apparently "cured" many years before.

CLINICAL VARIANTS

Common Warts

- Verrucae vulgaris, or common warts, occur most often on the hands and fingers and in the nail area—both periungually and subungually (Figures 6.2 and 6.3). They are frequently seen on the knees and elbows, especially in children.
- Their distribution is generally asymmetric, and lesions are often clustered.

DESCRIPTION OF LESIONS

Common warts generally have a verrucose, or vegetative, appearance.

- Lesions show loss of normal skin markings (e.g., fingerprints and handprints).
- "Black dots," or thrombosed capillaries, are pathognomonic (Figure 6.4).

Seborrheic Keratosis (Benign) (Figure 6.5)
- These lesions occurs in middle aged and older people.
- They are most often seen along the frontal hairline, face, and trunk.
- They have a "stuck-on" appearance.
- They may be indistinguishable from warts.

Solar Keratosis (Actinic Keratosis; Premalignant)
- These lesions occur in elderly, fair-complexioned persons, and they are sometimes associated with a cutaneous horn.
- They are rough-textured papules that appear in sun-exposed areas (see Chapter 21, "Benign Skin Neoplasms")
- Biopsy may be necessary to distinguish these lesions from squamous cell carcinoma.

Other Diagnoses
- **Squamous cell carcinoma under the nail**
  - Biopsy is necessary.
  - This lesion can easily be misdiagnosed as a subungual wart.
- **Onychomycosis**
  - The potassium hydroxide examination or fungal culture is positive.

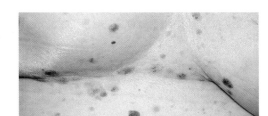

FIGURE 6.5 Seborrheic keratoses. These "stuck-on" appearing lesions, which resemble warts, are often seen in middle-aged and elderly people.

FILIFORM WARTS

Tan, fingerlike projections that emanate from the skin, filiform warts are most commonly seen on the face—usually around the ala nasi (Figure 6.6), mouth, and eyelids—and on the neck.

PLANTAR WARTS

These warts are seen on the plantar surface of the feet in children and young adults. They usually appear on the metatarsal area, heels, and toes in an asymmetric distribution (Figure 6.7).

DESCRIPTION OF LESIONS

- Plantar warts may be painful when they are under pressure, such as during walking.
- Lesions may be solitary or multiple, or they may appear in clusters *(mosaic warts)* (Figure 6.8).

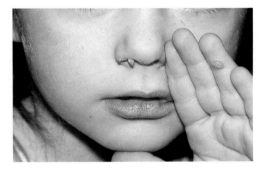

FIGURE 6.6 Filiform and common warts. This child has filiform warts on her nose and a common wart on her finger.

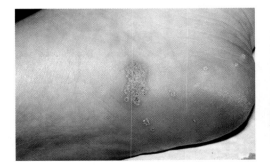

FIGURE 6.8 Mosaic plantar warts. Characteristic "black dots" are seen in this cluster of plantar warts.

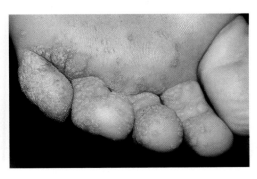

FIGURE 6.7 Mosaic plantar warts. Note the clustering, "kissing lesions" on this patient's toes.

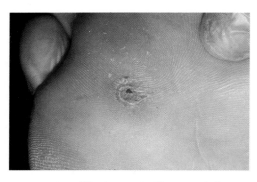

FIGURE 6.9 Plantar wart. Characteristic punctate bleeding is present after paring. Note the loss of skin markings.

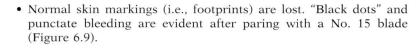

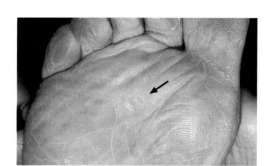

FIGURE 6.10 Corn (clavus). The circular central translucent core resembles a kernel of corn.

- Normal skin markings (i.e., footprints) are lost. "Black dots" and punctate bleeding are evident after paring with a No. 15 blade (Figure 6.9).

DIFFERENTIAL DIAGNOSIS

- **Corns** (clavi) are sometimes difficult to distinguish from warts. Like calluses, corns are thickened areas of the skin that form in response to excessive pressure and friction.
- They are usually hard and circular, with a polished or central translucent core, like the kernel of corn from which they take their name (Figure 6.10).
- Corns most commonly develop at sites subjected to repeated friction and pressure, such as the tops and the tips of toes and along the sides of the feet.
- Corns do not have "black dots," and skin markings are retained, except for the area of the central core.
- Wearing high-heeled shoes, particularly shoes that shift the body weight into a narrow, tapering toe box, can cause corns.
- Lesions are also typically seen between the fourth and fifth toes and are known as "kissing corns."

FLAT WARTS

Verruca plana, or flat warts, are commonly found on the face (Figure 6.11). In men, flat warts are spread by shaving. In women, they often occur on the shins, where lesions are spread by leg shaving. Lesions are also seen on the arms (Figure 6.12) and on the dorsa of the hands. Flat warts tend to resolve spontaneously, sometimes after a sudden increase in number, size, and inflammation.

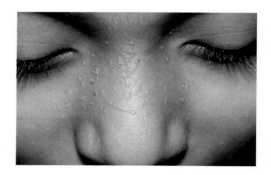

FIGURE 6.11 Flat warts. Lesions are slightly elevated papules the color of the patient's skin. Note the linear configuration resulting from autoinoculation of lesions on the bridge of this child's nose.

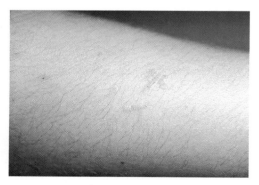

FIGURE 6.12 Flat warts. Lesions are slightly elevated papules the color of the patient's skin. Again, linear autoinoculation is apparent.

DESCRIPTION OF LESIONS

- These small, papular warts resemble a plateau; they are slightly elevated and well defined.
- Papules range in color from flesh-colored to brown. They range in size from 1 to 5 mm. Side lighting may be necessary to see them.
- Sometimes, flat warts show a linear configuration caused by autoinoculation.

 ### DIFFERENTIAL DIAGNOSIS

- Flat warts may resemble molluscum contagiosum (see later), which manifests as shiny, waxy, dome-shaped papules with a central white core.

 ### MANAGEMENT

General Principles

The method of treatment depends on the following:

- The age of the patient
- The patient's pain threshold
- The type of wart
- The location of the lesion

The abundance of treatment modalities (see later) is a reflection of the finding that no treatment is uniformly effective. Social factors are also important. For example, a 2-year-old child with a filiform wart located near the ala nasi, or with multiple hand warts, should warrant less aggressive treatment than a 6-year-old child with similar lesions who may suffer from the teasing of other children.

In adults, warts are typically stubborn and can be a frustrating problem to overcome. It is necessary to explain to patients that there is no way actually to kill HPV, and in many patients, when warts regress it is not because they have been "cured" but because the infection has become latent. Treatment of individual warts does not necessarily affect the field of viral particles that are likely to surround each lesion.

Patients may also be reminded that so far there are no cures for acquired immunodeficiency syndrome (AIDS) or the common cold—both of which are caused by viruses—so it is not surprising that the virus that causes warts is difficult to eradicate. Treatment often takes numerous sessions, and, on occasion, warts fail to resolve.

In short, the immune system apparently plays the most significant role in the expression of HPV. Treatment merely prompts or stimulates the immune system into dealing more effectively with the virus.

Wart Heroes

The hero of successful wart treatment is usually the last person to treat the wart, or the last person to recommend a treatment, before the wart regresses. The "wart hero" may have been a wart charmer, a dermatologist, a hypnotist, or a person who recommended a folk medicine remedy, such as the application of garlic or aloe vera. More often than not, warts tend to "cure" themselves over time, especially in immunocompetent patients. This outcome should be borne in mind and explained to patients early in the course of therapy.

Painful, aggressive therapy should be avoided initially, unless there is a pressing need to eliminate the wart. The following suggestions are given in a stepwise fashion, beginning with the least painful methods. *(Note: The use of many of the following topical chemical approaches may be contraindicated during pregnancy or in women who are likely to become pregnant during the treatment period.)*

Topical Salicylic Acid

A keratolytic (peeling) agent, primarily containing salicylic acid, is available in numerous over-the-counter preparations that can be self-administered. These preparations provide the best treatment for small children, in whom warts are usually self-limiting.

Technique

Plantar warts may be treated by applying 17% salicylic acid solution or a 40% salicylic acid plaster cut to the size of the wart. The solution is left on overnight; the plaster may be left on for 5 to 6 days. For best results with any of these keratolytic agents, the affected area should be hydrated first by soaking it in warm water for 5 minutes before application of the agent.

Advantages

- Usable on periungual warts
- Nonscarring
- Painless to apply
- Relatively inexpensive
- Does not require office visits

(continued)

MANAGEMENT (*continued*)

Disadvantages
- Slow response
- Time-consuming, often daily, application

Cryotherapy with Liquid Nitrogen

Liquid nitrogen (LN_2) may be applied with a cotton swab or with a cryotherapy gun (Cryogun) (see Chapter 26, "Basic Dermatologic Procedures"). The goals are a rapid freeze and a slow thaw. Repeated freeze—thaw cycles increase cell damage. Cryotherapy is best for warts on hands.

Technique

Regardless of whether LN_2 is applied with a saturated cotton swab or with a cryotherapy gun, one should aim to create a 2- to 3-mm zone of freeze around the lesion for a total of 4 to 5 seconds. The time of application varies, depending on the thickness of the lesion.

If possible, an attempt should be made to freeze lesions at a right angle; this approach may lessen the patient's pain and may minimize collateral damage to normal surrounding skin. Repeat the procedure as tolerated or based on previous treatment results, degree of pain, and posttreatment morbidity.

Advantages
- Treatment is fast.
- Many lesions can be treated during one visit.

Disadvantages
- This approach necessitates the availability of an LN_2 unit and holding tank.
- Treatment is painful and must be used cautiously on fingertips and on periungual lesions.
- Overaggressive treatment may cause scarring.
- Treatment often requires multiple office visits.

Light Electrocautery and Blunt Dissection

These methods are best for warts on the knees, elbows, and dorsa of hands. They are also good for filiform warts.

Advantage
- Treatment is tolerable in most adults.

Disadvantages
- Local anesthesia is required. Treatment sometimes necessitates a digital block, which can be very painful, especially on the fingers and soles of feet.
- Treatment may cause scarring.

Laser Ablation

This method is expensive and requires local anesthesia. One study concluded that laser ablation is no more effective in eradicating recalcitrant warts than are the less costly conventional methods described here.

Treatments for Specific Warts

Plantar Warts
- In patients with plantar warts, paring with a No. 15 blade parallel to the skin surface often immediately relieves pain on walking.
- Self-application of salicylic acid preparations or sanding with an emery board or pumice stone often keeps the wart flat and thus painless.
- Large plantar mosaic warts may be helped by 40% salicylic acid plaster. LN_2, blunt dissection, electrodesiccation, and curettage are reserved for more recalcitrant warts or when patients insist on aggressive therapy.

Periungual Warts

Topical cantharidin, a vesicant (potent blistering agent) may be used on periungual warts if salicylic acid or LN_2 fails or is not tolerated.

Flat Warts

Cautious application of LN_2 therapy or light electrocautery can treat flat warts. These destructive measures may be used in combination with the daily application of imiquimod cream (Aldara cream; see later), which reportedly speeds resolution of lesions.

Filiform Warts
- An almost painless method is to dip nontoothed forceps into LN_2 for 10 seconds and then grasp the wart for about 10 seconds. The frozen wart is generally shed in 7 to 10 days (see also Chapter 21, Figure 21.22A and B).
- Alternatively, electrocautery may be used after local anesthesia has been administered.

Other Treatments

Some additional methods of treating recalcitrant warts have met with varying degrees of success. The following treatments often require multiple office visits and may be expensive; some have potential side effects.

- Chemical applications, such as bichloroacetic and trichloroacetic acids and formalin can be used.
- Intralesional bleomycin may be tried.
- Immunotherapy with topical sensitizing agents is an option.
- Results, using oral immunomodulating techniques, such as high-dose oral cimetidine (Tagamet), have been disappointing in most placebo-controlled studies.

POINTS TO REMEMBER

- Freezing and other destructive treatment modalities do not kill the virus but merely destroy the cells that harbor HPV. In other words, when you treat a wart, only the "host" is destroyed, not the virus itself.
- Because HPV persists after therapy, some degree of infectivity and the potential for recurrence may remain, even in the absence of clinical lesions.
- Patients always ask, "How do you know when the warts are gone?" Answer: "When they don't recur."
- How to avoid getting warts? *Never shake hands. Never kiss anyone. Never walk barefoot. Never share towels. Live in a bubble, . . . and . . . there's still a good chance you'll get one.*

HELPFUL HINTS

- Imiquimod (Aldara), a local inducer of interferon, may be applied at home by the patient. It is a 5% cream that is effective for genital warts (condyloma acuminatum). There have been numerous anecdotal reports of the successful use of Aldara cream on flat warts, common warts, and plantar warts.
- Duct tape may be an effective painless alternative to liquid nitrogen. Patients should be instructed to apply duct tape over their warts for 6 weeks. The tape is then removed and the affected area is soaked in water and filed down with an emery board. The tape is reapplied the next morning. Treatment should be continued for a maximum of 2 months or until the wart disappears.

SEE PATIENT HANDOUT, PAGE 465

WART MEDICATIONS FORMULARY

AGENT	APPLICATION	FORMS	COMMENTS
TOPICAL AGENTS: OVER-THE-COUNTER			
DuoFilm solution	Apply daily under occlusion	17% salicylic acid	First hydrate the affected area
DuoFilm patch	Apply daily	40% salicylic acid in rubber-based vehicle	First hydrate the affected area
Dr. Scholl's Callus Removers	Apply daily	40% salicylic acid in rubber-based vehicle	First hydrate the affected area
Occlusal-HP solution	Apply daily	17% salicylic acid in polyacrylic solution	First hydrate the affected area
Compound W gel	Apply daily	17% salicylic acid in flexible collodion	First hydrate the affected area
TOPICAL AGENTS: PRESCRIPTION			
Aldara	Nightly as tolerated	5% imiquimod cream; 12 packets in a box	May be irritating; use occlusion, except for face and skin folds

MOLLUSCUM CONTAGIOSUM

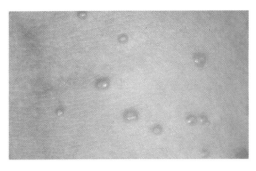

FIGURE 6.13 Molluscum contagiosum. Characteristic dome-shaped, shiny, waxy papules have a central white core.

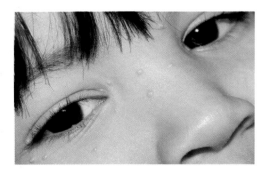

FIGURE 6.14 Molluscum contagiosum. This is a typical distribution of lesions on a child's face. Note the eyelid lesions.

BASICS

Molluscum contagiosum is a common superficial viral infection of the epidermis. It is spread by skin-to-skin contact and is caused by a large DNA-containing poxvirus. It is seen most often in three clinical contexts:

- It occurs in young, healthy children (infants and preschoolers), in whom the incidence decreases after the age of 6 or 7 years.
- It occurs in HIV-positive patients.
- It occurs in young adults who are sexually active and not HIV seropositive.

DESCRIPTION OF LESIONS

- The lesions are dome-shaped, waxy or pearly papules with a central white core (Figure 6.13). Less frequently, the papules are the color of the patient's skin.
- Lesions are generally 1 mm to 3 mm in diameter, but they may coalesce and become **giant mollusca.**
- Frequently, the lesions are grouped.
- The number of lesions varies from 1 to 20 up to hundreds.

DISTRIBUTION OF LESIONS

- Lesions of molluscum contagiosum most often appear on the face and eyelids (Figure 6.14), the trunk, the axilla, and the extremities.
- Usually, lesions are asymmetric in distribution, depending on the sites of initial inoculation.
- They are spread by autoinoculation from picking and rubbing (Figure 6.15).
- Lesions can appear in areas of the skin that are traumatized or inflamed, as seen in the flexural creases in children who have underlying atopic dermatitis at these sites (Figure 6.16).

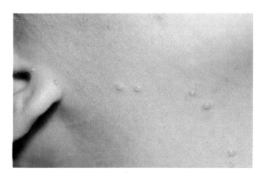

FIGURE 6.15 Molluscum contagiosum. Note the configuration of lesions resulting from autoinoculation.

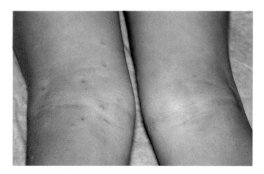

FIGURE 6.16 Molluscum contagiosum. Lesions are present on a background of atopic dermatitis of the flexural creases.

- Lesions may be seen on the external genitalia (Figure 6.17), on the lower abdominal wall, on the inner thighs, and on the pubic area.

CLINICAL MANIFESTATIONS

- Generally asymptomatic, molluscum contagiosum may itch slightly, may be scratched, and may become secondarily infected.
- The course is self-limiting, and recurrences are rare in immune-competent persons.
- Molluscum contagiosum in HIV-positive patients is common (see Chapter 24, "Cutaneous Manifestations of HIV Infection").
  – More than 100 lesions may be seen.
  – They appear most commonly on the face and are spread by shaving (Figure 6.18).
  – The giant molluscum or coalescent double or triple lesions are frequently seen in these patients.
  – The lesions are often chronic and are difficult to eradicate.

DIAGNOSIS

- Typical papules are easily recognized.
- Inspection with a handheld magnifier often reveals the central core.
- A short application of cryotherapy with LN$_2$ accentuates the central core (Figures 6.19).
- A direct microscopic smear of a lesion (crush preparation) demonstrates characteristic "molluscum bodies" (Figure 6.20).
- A shave biopsy is performed, if necessary. Identification of characteristic intracytoplasmic inclusion bodies in histologic or cytologic preparations is made by hematoxylin and eosin staining of biopsy sections.

 DIFFERENTIAL DIAGNOSIS

Warts (Nongenital), Especially Small Flat Warts
Distinguishing features (Figures 6.11 and 6.12) are as follows:

- Warts are not waxy.
- They are tan or brown.
- They have no central white core.

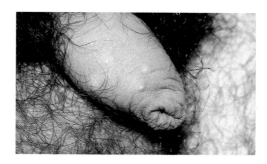

FIGURE 6.17 Molluscum contagiosum. Characteristic dome-shaped, shiny, waxy papules are present on the penis.

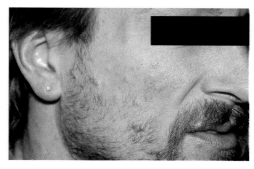

FIGURE 6.18 Molluscum contagiosum. Note the double and "giant lesions" on the face of a patient with acquired immunodeficiency syndrome.

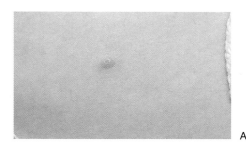

A

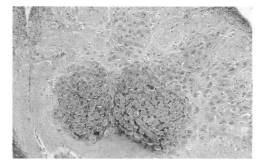

FIGURE 6.20 Molluscum contagiosum. "Molluscum bodies" (hematoxylin and eosin stain).

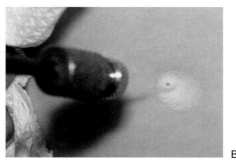

B

FIGURE 6.19 Molluscum contagiosum. *A:* Short application of liquid nitrogen (LN$_2$). *B:* LN$_2$ accentuates the central core.

Warts (Genital)
Condyloma acuminatum appears on the inner thighs, pubic area, vulvae, and penis.

- A biopsy may be necessary to differentiate these lesions from molluscum contagiosum.

Other Diagnoses
Disseminated cryptococcosis, toxoplasmosis, and histoplasmosis in HIV-infected patients should also be considered. A biopsy may be necessary to differentiate these infections from molluscum contagiosum.

MANAGEMENT

Home Treatment
Lesions may be ignored until they resolve spontaneously or molluscum contagiosum may be treated by the patient or caregiver with:

- A topical over-the-counter antiwart preparation, such as liquid salicylic acid in a rubber-based vehicle (DuoFilm), which is applied daily to the core of each lesion with a toothpick.
- Imiquimod 5% cream (Aldara cream) applied three times per week at bedtime.

Office Treatment
- They may be frozen lightly for 3 to 5 seconds with LN_2 applied with a cotton swab or a Cryogun.
- A topical vesicant (blistering agent), such as cantharidin, may be applied carefully with a toothpick to each lesion every 3 to 4 weeks.
- Electrodesiccation and curettage may be necessary for patients with refractory lesions.
- Trichloroacetic acid peels have been performed with some success in HIV-infected patients with extensive lesions.

Other Treatments
- For refractory lesions in HIV-infected patients, highly active antiretroviral therapy has been very effective in reducing the incidence of molluscum contagiosum in recent years.
- Systemic treatment with agents such as griseofulvin and cimetidine was anecdotally reported to be effective in the treatment of molluscum contagiosum; however, no controlled studies have been performed to confirm it.

POINTS TO REMEMBER

- Lesions on an infant or a young preschool child should not be treated aggressively.
- Molluscum contagiosum—particularly if it is located on the face of an adult—should alert the clinician to the possibility of HIV infection.
- Molluscum contagiosum in healthy, immunocompetent persons generally is self-limited and heals after several months or longer.

HELPFUL HINT

- For anxious children, a topical anesthetic such as EMLA (eutectic mixture of local anesthetics) cream can be applied under occlusion 1 hour before treatment to decrease the discomfort associated with procedures such as curettage, local anesthetic injections, or cryosurgery.

SEE PATIENT HANDOUT, PAGE 463

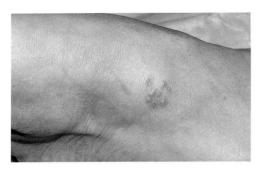

FIGURE 6.21 Herpes simplex virus. In this typical grouping, umbilicated vesicles overlie an erythematous base.

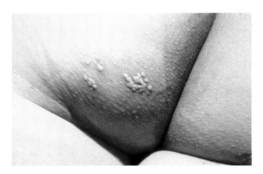

FIGURE 6.22 Herpes simplex virus. Here, most vesicles have evolved into pustules.

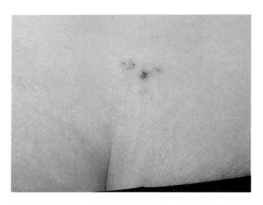

FIGURE 6.23 Herpes simplex virus (HSV). The presacral area is a common location for HSV-2 in women. This patient shows drying crusts (scabs) and erosions.

Overview

Herpes simplex virus (HSV) infections are caused by two virus types: HSV-1 and HSV-2. HSV-1 causes most nongenital infections. These highly contagious viruses are spread by direct contact with the skin or mucous membranes. After the primary infection resolves, the virus retreats to a dorsal root ganglion, where it becomes incorporated into the genetic material of the cell. The virus remains latent until it is reactivated by precipitating factors or triggers, such as sunlight exposure, menses, fever, common colds, and, possibly, stress.

Primary infections are acquired in infancy and early childhood; most are subclinical. Patients who have AIDS or who are taking immunosuppressant therapy for organ transplantation or cancer chemotherapy are at greatest risk for contracting severe recalcitrant HSV infections.

Nongenital HSV infection is extremely common. In fact, herpes-specific antibody (for type 1 and, less commonly, type 2) can be found in the serum of most lesion-free adults. Asymptomatic shedding probably accounts for the widespread transmission of this ubiquitous virus.

Since the 1980s, the public attention that genital herpes has attracted has led to misconceptions about HSV infection and to its overdiagnosis, especially in regard to lesions that occur within the oral cavity. For example, many people who suffer from recurrent nonherpetic painful intraoral mouth sores (aphthous stomatitis, or canker sores) are given a diagnosis of "herpes," and thus they may feel the stigma associated with sexually transmitted diseases. Because recurrent aphthous stomatitis—which has no known viral association—has a clinical appearance and course similar to those of recurrent herpes labialis, the two conditions are often confused by patient and clinician alike. HSV lesions, particularly recurrent ones, occur inside the mouth very infrequently, unless the virus is a primary infection or occurs in immunocompromised patients.

DESCRIPTION OF LESIONS

The following sequence of events describes the easily recognizable evolution of HSV "cold sores" or "fever blisters":

- A single vesicle or a group of vesicles overlies an erythematous base (Figure 6.21). Vesicles may sag in the center (umbilicate).
- The vesicles may become pustules (Figure 6.22), or they may dry and become crusts or erosions (Figure 6.23).
- The lesions generally heal without scarring (because they are intraepidermal).

PRIMARY HERPES SIMPLEX

DISTRIBUTION OF LESIONS

When symptoms are present during a primary HSV infection, the oral cavity (the lips, gums, buccal mucosa, fauces, tongue, and hard palate) is the area generally affected (Figure 6.24).

CLINICAL MANIFESTATIONS

Most cases of primary HSV are subclinical.

- Symptomatic primary HSV infections tend to be more severe than those of recurrent disease; they include gingivostomatitis, fever, lymphadenitis, and sore throat. Encephalitis and aseptic meningitis are rare complications.
- Distinguishing primary HSV infection from severe, recurrent disease can be difficult.

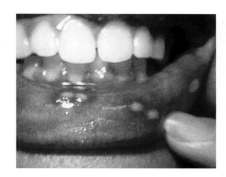

FIGURE 6.24 Primary herpes simplex virus infection. This patient has multiple erosions and gingivostomatitis.

RECURRENT HERPES SIMPLEX

DISTRIBUTION OF LESIONS

Lesions recur at the site innervated by the dorsal root ganglion inhabited by the virus.

- Recurrences are most often seen on or near the vermilion border of the lip *(herpes labialis)* (Figure 6.25).
- Lesions also tend to occur on the presacral area in women, but they may be found anywhere on the cutaneous surface.

CLINICAL MANIFESTATIONS

- Symptoms are generally milder and the number of lesions are fewer than those associated with primary HSV.
- Patients commonly experience a prodrome of itching, pain, or numbness.
- Infrequently, regional lymphadenopathy occurs.
- Over time, recurrences decrease in frequency and often stop altogether.
- Persistent ulcerative or verrucous vegetative lesions may be seen in immunocompromised patients.
- Most cases of recurrent erythema multiforme minor accompany, and appear to be caused by, recurrent (both clinical and subclinical) HSV episodes (see Chapter 18, "Diseases of Vasculature").

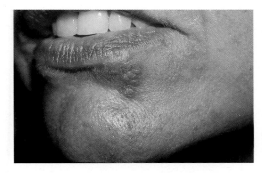

FIGURE 6.25 Recurrent herpes simplex virus infection (herpes labialis). Lesions are evident on the vermilion border of the lip and beyond.

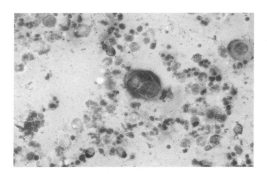

FIGURE 6.26 Positive Tzanck preparation. Note the typical multinucleated giant cells with large nuclei. This test does not distinguish between herpes simplex and herpes zoster. Note the presence of nuclei of normal sized keratinocytes, which are the size of neutrophils.

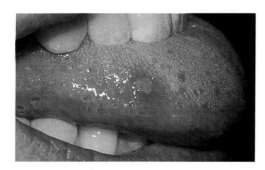

FIGURE 6.27 Aphthous stomatitis. This shallow erosion is surrounded by a ring of erythema.

DIAGNOSIS

The diagnosis of HSV is usually based on clinical appearance and history. At the time of an office visit, patients often present with only nonspecific crusted lesions or merely with a history consistent with recurrent HSV. When necessary, the following tests may be administered on fresh lesions:

- A Tzanck preparation, if positive, suggests HSV or varicella-zoster virus (VZV) infection. This test is used to rapidly determine the presence of HSV or VZV; it does not distinguish between these two viruses (Figure 6.26) (see the section on Tzanck procedure later in this chapter).
- HSV tissue culture using monoclonal antibodies requires only 24 hours. The test is 90% sensitive, but it is expensive.
- Polymerase chain reaction can be conducted; it also is expensive.
- Serologic tests for HSV are generally not very useful because so much of the general adult population has antibodies to herpes simplex; however, primary HSV infection can be documented by demonstration of seroconversion.

DIFFERENTIAL DIAGNOSIS

Aphthous Stomatitis
- Lesions of aphthous stomatitis are small, punched-out erosions that occur on the tongue and on the buccal, labial, and gingival mucosa (see Chapter 12, "Disorders of the Mouth, Lips, and Tongue") (Figure 6.27).
- Lesions typically consist of painful, shallow, gray or yellow 2- to 3-mm erosions.

Hand-Foot-and-Mouth Disease
- Oval erythematous erosions are most often seen on the soft palate and uvula (see Chapter 8, "Viral Exanthems").
- Lesions are asymptomatic
- Lesions may appear on the hands and feet.
- Lesions are shallower than those of primary HSV.

Squamous Cell Carcinoma
- A single, nonhealing crusted, erosive, or ulcerative lesion is noted.
- A biopsy should be performed.

Herpes Zoster
- Lesions of herpes zoster are unilateral, dermatomal, and often painful (see the discussion of herpes zoster later in this chapter).
- Lesions are also grouped and tend to vary in size.
- The condition may be clinically indistinguishable from HSV when lesions are located in a single focus.

CLINICAL VARIANTS OF CUTANEOUS HERPES SIMPLEX

Herpetic Whitlow

Painful herpetic whitlow results from the direct inoculation of the virus to the fingertip. Before the current stringent infection control measures were established, herpetic whitlow was an occupational hazard among dental and medical health care workers, whose fingertips came in contact with infected oral or respiratory excretions. Today, it is seen most frequently in infants, in whom spread is caused by thumb sucking (Figure 6.28).

Eczema Herpeticum (Figure 6.29)

Also known as *Kaposi's varicelliform* eruption, eczema herpeticum is an uncommon disseminated form of HSV infection. It occurs mainly in children who have severe atopic dermatitis.

MANAGEMENT

Topical Therapy

Skin symptoms may be eased by Burow's solution (aluminum acetate or aluminum sulfate) soaks two to three times daily. Alternatively, soaks with water or saline may help to dry the eruption and may prevent secondary infection.

- Topical acyclovir 5% (Zovirax) ointment, penciclovir 1% (Denivir) cream, and docosanol 10% (Abreva) cream are not very effective treatments, but they may help to reduce healing times.
- Patients in whom sun exposure incites recurrent HSV of the lips can apply an opaque sun-blocking agent before sun exposure.
- Patients can lessen the discomfort of oral HSV lesions by applying viscous lidocaine applications or over-the-counter "caine" products, taking oral analgesics, or sucking on ice cubes.

Systemic Therapy

Pharmacologic agents used for the treatment of HSV include acyclovir, valacyclovir, and famciclovir. Valacyclovir is rapidly converted to acyclovir, and its bioavailability is three to five times greater than that of acyclovir. For these reasons, acyclovir has been supplanted by valacyclovir in the treatment of HSV in adults. However, the use of valacyclovir is contraindicated in some patients (e.g., in some renal and bone marrow transplant recipients and in those infected with HIV) because of reports of thrombotic thrombocytopenic purpura and hemolytic uremia syndrome.

Treatment
Primary Herpes Simplex

- Acyclovir (200 mg five times daily or 400 mg three times daily for 10 days)
- Valacyclovir (1 g twice daily for 7 to 10 days)
- Famciclovir (250 mg three times daily for 7 to 10 days)

(continued)

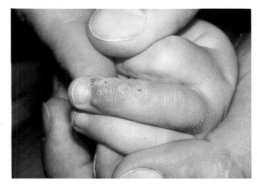

FIGURE 6.28 Primary herpes simplex virus infection in infancy. The spread of the infection from the mouth to the hand of this infant was likely caused by finger sucking.

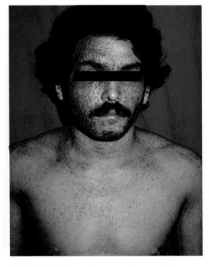

FIGURE 6.29 Eczema herpeticum (Kaposi's varicelliform eruption). This patient has an uncommon disseminated form of herpes simplex virus infection. He has underlying atopic dermatitis.

Recurrent Herpes Simplex

This treatment should be initiated at the first sign of prodrome, because it can often abort the lesions. Following are treatment options:

- Acyclovir (200 mg twice daily or 400 mg three times daily for 5 days)
- Valacyclovir (2 g twice a day for 1 day is a shorter, more economical course)
- Famciclovir (125 mg twice daily for 5 days)

For frequent recurrences (more than six recurrences per year), persistent HSV, severe disease, or recurrent erythema multiforme minor, long-term suppressive oral therapy may be used. After 1 year of treatment with these agents, the medication condition should be discontinued, to determine the recurrence rate, and the dosage can be adjusted as needed.

- Acyclovir (400 mg twice daily for 12 months)
- Valacyclovir (1 g daily for 6 to 12 months; afterward, the clinician should attempt to taper the dose to 500 mg or to discontinue the agent)
- Famciclovir (250 mg twice daily for 12 months)

Immunocompromised hosts, those with Kaposi's varicelliform eruption, or those with HSV encephalitis often require intravenous acyclovir therapy.

 POINTS TO REMEMBER

- Intraoral ulcers in immunocompetent patients are most likely canker sores (aphthous stomatitis).
- Recurrent HSV virus attacks can be aborted by treatment on a short-term basis with oral antivirals administered during the prodromal stage.
- Frequent recurrences can be aborted by treatment with suppressive oral antivirals.

 SEE PATIENT HANDOUT, PAGE 459

BASICS

Herpes zoster ("shingles") is caused by the same herpesvirus that causes varicella, or chickenpox. The virus first manifests as varicella (see Chapter 8, "Viral Exanthems"), a primary infection usually seen in childhood. Subsequently, when the same latent virus is reactivated, its second episode manifests as herpes zoster.

The infectious course of VZV is similar to that of HSV infection. After the primary infection resolves, the virus retreats to the dorsal root ganglion, where it remains in a dormant state. Reactivation—into dermatomal "shingles"—may be caused by severe illness or infection with HIV, but most often it occurs spontaneously, without an obvious precipitating cause. It is most likely a sign that immunity to VZV, which most people acquired in childhood, has decreased. The reemergence as a local vesicobullous eruption derives from the anterograde migration of virions, through the axon to the skin of a single dermatome or several adjacent ones. In immunocompetent patients, recurrent herpes zoster episodes are extremely uncommon; immunity to the virus is presumably boosted by the initial episode of herpes zoster.

The pain of herpes zoster is thought to result from nerve damage caused by the spread of the virus to the skin through the peripheral nerves. An inflammatory reaction leads to scarring of the peripheral nerves and dorsal root ganglia. **Postherpetic neuralgia** (PHN) presumably results from the consequent hyperexcitability of neurons, which tend to discharge spontaneously.

Reportedly, 75% of patients with herpes zoster are older than 75 years. However, herpes zoster also develops frequently in immunocompromised patients, such as transplant recipients and those with HIV infection or malignant disease, particularly lymphoproliferative malignancies (e.g., Hodgkin's disease). Elderly persons and immunocompromised patients also tend to have more severe disease, with complications such as PHN, disseminated zoster, and chronic zoster.

VZV infection occurs occasionally in pregnant women. A primary VZV infection (varicella) may result in severe fetal abnormalities; however, the development of herpes zoster during pregnancy does not appear to harm the developing fetus.

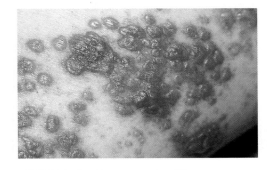

FIGURE 6.30 Herpes zoster. These grouped, umbilicated vesicles of various sizes are on an erythematous base.

DESCRIPTION OF LESIONS

The following sequence of events describes the evolution of herpes zoster:

- Lesions begin as "juicy" erythematous papules that rapidly mature into clustered vesicles or bullae on top of an erythematous base. They tend to vary more in size than do the lesions of HSV (Figure 6.30).
- Successive crops continue to appear for 6 to 8 days. The blisters sometimes umbilicate (sag in the middle); occasionally, they become pustular and hemorrhagic.
- In time, lesions dry into crusts or erosions that may heal and disappear completely or resolve with postinflammatory hyperpigmentation or hypopigmentation and, possibly, scarring.
- Lesions of herpes zoster in HIV-infected patients tend to be more verrucous and ulcerative, and they often heal with scars.
- Infrequently, dermatomal neuralgia may be accompanied or followed by nonbullous or urticarialike lesions (Figure 6.31). Rarely, skin lesions are absent ("zoster sine herpete").

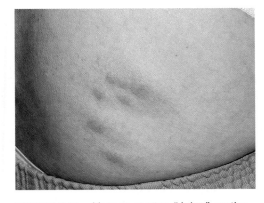

FIGURE 6.31 Herpes zoster. "Juicy," erythematous, urticarialike papules are seen here in a "zosteriform" distribution.

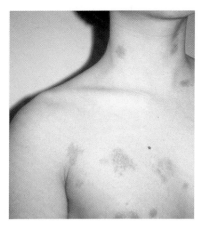

FIGURE 6.32 Herpes zoster. In this patient, lesions extend beyond the midline.

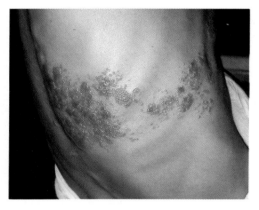

FIGURE 6.33 Herpes zoster. Drying hemorrhagic crusts appear in a "zosteriform" distribution. In this immunocompromised patient, the lesions will probably heal with scars.

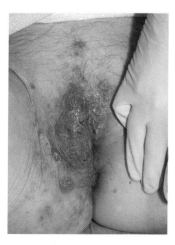

FIGURE 6.34 Herpes zoster. This patient has painful lesions of the vulva and perineum in a dermatomal distribution.

DISTRIBUTION OF LESIONS

Lesions of herpes zoster occur in a characteristic unilateral dermatomal ("zosteriform") distribution.

- Occasionally, lesions involve contiguous dermatomes or extend beyond the midline (Figure 6.32).
- Although it can affect any dermatome, herpes zoster is most commonly found on the thoracic (Figure 6.33), trigeminal, lumbosacral (Figure 6.34), and cervical areas.
- Immunocompromised patients have a greater risk for multidermatomal zoster, recurrent zoster, and dissemination beyond the skin (e.g., into the eyes or the lungs).

CLINICAL MANIFESTATIONS

- Several days before the cutaneous eruption, patients may experience the following focal (dermatomal) symptoms: numbness, pruritus, paresthesia, and skin tenderness or sensitivity *(tactile allodynia)*.
- In children, herpes zoster is often asymptomatic.
- In contrast to the disease in children, both the likelihood and severity of pain (acute and chronic) associated with herpes zoster are significantly increased in patients older than 50 years.

Pain and paresthesia in the affected dermatome may accompany the eruption or may precede it by 1 to 2 weeks. The neuropathic pain of some patients has been described as "boring," "burning," "crushing," or "stabbing." Some patients presenting with such pain have been thought to have a myocardial infarction or pleurisy, until the characteristic eruption of herpes zoster establishes the diagnosis.

Complications

- **PHN** is defined as pain persisting for more than 1 month after the eruption of the initial herpes zoster lesions. The pain may also develop after a pain-free interval. The frequency of PHN increases with age. It occurs more commonly in people with compromised immune systems, such as HIV-infected patients.
- In many elderly patients, PHN can cause chronic depression, anxiety, and social isolation.

- When herpes zoster occurs in the ophthalmic division of the fifth, or trigeminal, nerve, it is called *herpes zoster ophthalmicus* (Figure 6.35). Eye involvement, such as conjunctivitis, acute retinal necrosis, uveitis, and retinal arteritis, can lead to blindness. Ophthalmic zoster warrants an immediate ophthalmologic consultation.
- VZV involvement of the geniculate ganglion is called the Ramsay Hunt syndrome. This condition results in a motor and sensory neuropathy of the seventh cranial nerve.

Disseminated Herpes Zoster (see Figure 24.7)

In immunocompromised patients, the eruption usually begins with typical dermatomal herpes zoster. The lesions may then become widespread, with 25 or more lesions found outside the primary dermatome. The condition can become chronic and indistinguishable from varicella.

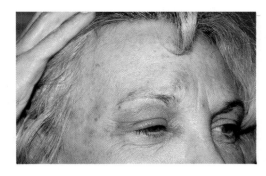

FIGURE 6.35 Ophthalmic herpes zoster. This condition affects the first branch of the fifth cranial nerve.

DIAGNOSIS

- Herpes zoster can most often be diagnosed on the basis of clinical appearance and the presence of pain in a dermatomal distribution.
- If necessary, a Tzanck smear should be obtained from the base of a fresh lesion (see the discussion of Tzanck preparation later in this chapter). A positive result suggests either HSV or VZV infection.
- A skin biopsy is generally unnecessary, but it can help to confirm the diagnosis.

 DIFFERENTIAL DIAGNOSIS

Herpes Simplex Virus Infection (Figure 6.36)

When HSV presents in a site usually occupied by herpes zoster, or when it occurs in a semidermatomal distribution, it may be clinically indistinguishable from herpes zoster. The vesicles of herpes simplex, however, tend to be more uniform in size and are much less painful than those seen in herpes zoster. Recurrence strongly suggests HSV infection.

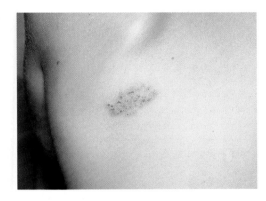

FIGURE 6.36 Herpes simplex virus infection. This patient has herpes simplex virus infection presenting in a site usually occupied by herpes zoster. Such manifestations may be clinically indistinguishable from herpes zoster.

Poison Ivy (Figure 6.37)

Also known as rhus dermatitis, poison ivy often occurs in a linear distribution of blisters that corresponds to, or suggests, a dermatome. Rhus dermatitis, however, is pruritic and painless. Most patients with rhus dermatitis offer a history of contact with poison ivy or poison oak.

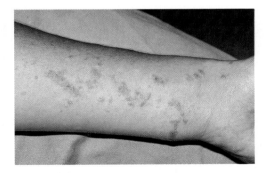

FIGURE 6.37 Poison ivy dermatitis. Also known as rhus dermatitis, poison ivy dermatitis often occurs in a linear distribution of blisters that may correspond to, or suggest, a dermatomal distribution.

MANAGEMENT

Topical Therapy

For the acute episode of herpes zoster, the following treatments are available without a prescription:

- Burow's solution. Wet dressings with Burow's solution (aluminum acetate or aluminum sulfate) are soothing and drying; so are moist soaks with water or saline.
- Topical anesthetic "caines" such as benzocaine may be helpful.

Systemic Therapy

Pain control is generally the paramount concern in herpes zoster.

- Oral analgesics, such as aspirin, acetaminophen, other nonsteroidal antiinflammatory drugs, and mild narcotics, are helpful in mild, self-limited cases.
- Both valacyclovir and famciclovir are most effective when they are given within 72 hours of the appearance of the zoster rash. They are equally effective in accelerating cutaneous healing, in shortening the duration of acute episodes, and in decreasing the chronic pain of PHN.
- Valacyclovir is much less expensive than famciclovir; however, its use is contraindicated in HIV-infected patients. Both valacyclovir and famciclovir are superior to acyclovir, which is reserved for use in children and for intravenous administration.

Note: Because most infections are first diagnosed more than 72 hours after the onset of skin eruptions—that is, after the infection is established—it is possible that the use of antivirals has no value. However, even after this 3-day window of opportunity, the elderly, the immunocompromised, and those with ophthalmic zoster should be treated with antivirals, because the drugs have very few adverse side effects.

Regimens

Following are the treatment options for immunocompetent adult patients with herpes zoster:

- Valacyclovir (1g [two 500-mg caplets] three times daily for 7 days)
- Famciclovir (500 mg three times daily for 7 days)
- Acyclovir (800 mg five times daily for 7 days)

Immunocompromised patients may require intravenous acyclovir. Intravenous foscarnet is used for acyclovir-resistant VZV infection.

Corticosteroids

The use of systemic corticosteroids in combination with oral acyclovir, valacyclovir, or famciclovir has been controversial. Anecdotal reports claim a faster resolution of acute pain and a decreased incidence of PHN. The rationale for adding corticosteroids is that they may decrease nerve inflammation.

However, elderly patients, in whom PHN more often occurs, are more likely to experience significant adverse side effects from systemic corticosteroids than are younger patients. Potential relative contraindications to the use of corticosteroids include hypertension, diabetes, glaucoma, and peptic ulcer disease.

Chronic Pain

Treatment of PHN is problematic. The following measures have met with varying degrees of success. Their great number reflects the finding that none of them appears to be totally satisfactory.

- Lidocaine patches. These bandages, impregnated with lidocaine, are the only treatment for PHN approved by the United States Food and Drug Association.
- Capsaicin (Zostrix). The active molecule in red hot chili peppers, capsaicin depletes substance P, a pain impulse transmitter. It is available over the counter and is applied three to five times daily. Unfortunately, many patients cannot tolerate the burning sensation that occurs after application.
- Low-dose tricyclic antidepressants. These agents (e.g., amitriptyline) may be helpful. Higher doses of tricyclic antidepressants—used alone or in combination with phenothiazines—may also be tried.
- Neurontin (gabapentin), an antiseizure drug, has been helpful in some patients.
- Neurosurgical procedures include nerve blocks with local anesthetics.
- Intralesional corticosteroids may be given as subcutaneous injections.
- Transcutaneous electrical nerve stimulation may be useful.
- Acupuncture may be tried.
- Biofeedback may be helpful.

Tzanck Preparation
Basics

A **Tzanck preparation** is used to aid in the diagnosis of herpes simplex, herpes zoster, and varicella.

(continued)

MANAGEMENT (*continued*)

Technique
This technique furnishes an inexpensive, efficient provisional diagnosis, but it does not enable one to distinguish HSV from VZV.

1. For best results, a fresh, intact vesicle or bulla usually present for less than 24 hours is preferred.
2. After swabbing the lesion with an alcohol preparation, the blister is unroofed by piercing it with a No. 11 blade or a needle, followed by blotting with a sponge.
3. The underlying moist base of the lesion is then scraped with a No. 15 scalpel blade, and a thin layer of material is spread onto a glass slide.
4. The specimen is then air-dried and is stained with a supravital stain such as Giemsa, Wright's, or methylene blue, which is left on for 1 minute.
5. The specimen is then gently flooded with tap water for 15 seconds to remove any remaining stain.
6. Examination initially under 40-power magnification and then 100-power oil immersion helps to identify the characteristic multinucleated giant cells (Figure 6.26).

Prevention
As noted earlier, a lasting cell-mediated immunity to VZV, which develops after the initial infection, may wane over time. Some researchers have hypothesized that the chickenpox vaccine, if administered to seropositive adults, will restimulate their immunity to VZV and thereby afford protection from, or attenuate the symptoms of, herpes zoster. This hypothesis currently is being investigated.

 POINTS TO REMEMBER

- Herpes zoster, particularly if it is recurrent or disseminated, may be an early indicator of an immunosuppressive disorder or a lymphoproliferative disease.
- An evolving herpes zoster eruption should be treated with antiviral drugs as early as possible.
- PHN is unusual in people younger than 50 years.
- Patients with herpes zoster can transmit the virus as chickenpox to persons who have not already been infected with this virus.

FORMULARY FOR HERPES SIMPLEX AND HERPES ZOSTER

ORAL AGENTS
Acyclovir (Zovirax): 200-mg capsule; 800-mg tablet
Valacyclovir (Valtrex): 500-mg caplet; 1-g caplet
Famciclovir (Famvir): 125-mg tablet; 500-mg tablet

TOPICAL AGENTS
Herpes simplex
Acyclovir (Zovirax) ointment
Penciclovir (Denavir) cream
Herpes zoster
Capsaicin (Zostrix) cream

CHAPTER 7

Superficial Fungal Infections

Clinical Presentations
Dermatophyte Infections
The term *tinea* refers to an infection by dermatophytes. Tinea is named according to the location on the body:

- **Tinea pedis and tinea manuum** (feet and hands)
- **Tinea cruris** (inguinal folds)
- **Tinea capitis** (scalp)
- **Tinea corporis and tinea faciale** (body and face)
- **Tinea unguium (onychomycosis)** (nails)

Tinea Versicolor
Tinea versicolor is an exception; in fact, it is not caused by a dermatophyte, but rather by a yeastlike organism. Tinea versicolor is referred to as *pityriasis versicolor* by many authors.

Candidiasis
Cutaneous candidiasis is also caused by yeast.

Overview

Superficial fungi are capable of germinating on the dead outer horny layer of skin. They produce enzymes (keratinases) that allow them to digest keratin, with resulting epidermal scale (e.g., **tinea pedis, tinea versicolor**), thickened, crumbly nails **(onychomycosis),** and hair loss **(tinea capitis).** In the dermis, an inflammatory reaction may result in erythema, vesicles, and, infrequently, a more widespread autoeczematous eruption known as an "id" reaction.

Infection may be acquired by the following means:

- Person-to-person contact
- Animal contact, especially with kittens and puppies
- Contact with inanimate objects (fomites)

Environmental and hereditary factors leading to fungal infections are as follows:

- Warm, moist, occluded environments such as the groin, axillae and feet
- Family history of tinea infections
- Lowered immune status of the host such as seen in patients with acquired immunodeficiency syndrome (AIDS), diabetes, collagen vascular diseases, or long-term systemic steroid therapy

DIAGNOSIS

- Diagnosis can often, but not always, be made on clinical grounds.
- A direct potassium hydroxide (KOH) examination or a fungal culture is necessary to make a definitive diagnosis.
- Periodic acid–Schiff stain on biopsy specimens can be helpful.
- Wood's lamp examination may be useful in some cases of tinea capitis and tinea versicolor.

TINEA PEDIS ("ATHLETE'S FOOT")

BASICS

Tinea pedis is an extremely common problem seen mainly in young men. Ubiquitous media advertisements for athlete's foot sprays and creams are testimony to the commonplace occurrence of this annoying dermatosis.

Most cases are caused by *T. rubrum*, which evokes a minimal inflammatory response, and less often by *T. mentagrophytes*, which may produce vesicles and bullae; less frequently, *Epidermophyton floccosum* may be responsible. There are three clinical types of tinea pedis.

TYPE 1: INTERDIGITAL TINEA PEDIS

BASICS

This is the most common type of tinea pedis. It is seen predominantly in men between the ages of 18 and 40 years.

DESCRIPTION OF LESIONS

- Scale, maceration, and fissures are characteristic (Figure 7.1).

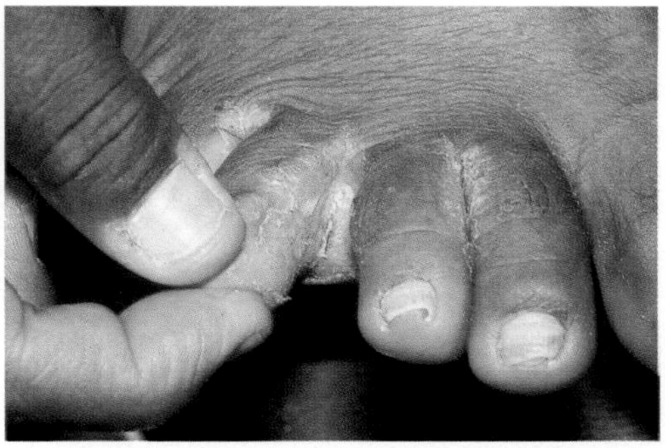

DISTRIBUTION OF LESIONS

- Toe web involvement is seen, especially between the third and fourth and the fourth and fifth toes.

CLINICAL MANIFESTATIONS

- It is often asymptomatic; however, it may itch intensely.
- Marked inflammation and fissures suggest bacterial superinfection.
- There may be coexistent yeast or saprophytic fungi present.

DIAGNOSIS

A positive KOH examination or fungal culture is diagnostic.

FIGURE 7.1 Interdigital tinea pedis (toe web infection). Note fissuring and maceration.

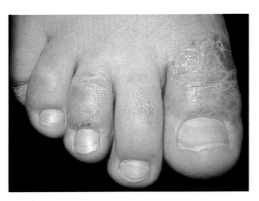

FIGURE 7.2 Atopic dermatitis versus contact dermatitis. Note the lichenification on the dorsal toes.

Atopic Dermatitis (Figure 7.2)

- Atopic dermatitis may be clinically indistinguishable from tinea pedis.
- There is a positive atopic history.
- It is seen especially in children on the dorsal or plantar surface of the feet (tinea pedis is unusual in preteens).

Contact Dermatitis

- This occurs most often on the dorsum of the feet.

MANAGEMENT

- For acute oozing and maceration, Burow's solution compresses are used two to three times daily.
- Broad-spectrum topical antifungal agents such as ketoconazole (Nizoral), ciclopirox (Loprox), or clotrimazole (Lotrimin) are applied once or twice daily. (See the formulary at the end of this chapter.)

Prevention consists of maintaining dryness in the area by:

- Using a hairdryer after bathing.
- Applying powders, such as miconazole (Zeasorb-AF) or talcum powder.

TYPE 2: CHRONIC PLANTAR TINEA PEDIS

BASICS

Tinea pedis ("moccasin" type) is relatively common.

DESCRIPTION OF LESIONS

- Lesions consist of diffuse scaling of the soles (Figure 7.3).

DISTRIBUTION OF LESIONS

- The entire plantar surface of the foot is usually involved.
- Borders are distinct.
- There is often nail involvement.

CLINICAL MANIFESTATIONS

- Symptoms are minimal, unless painful fissures occur.

DIAGNOSIS

- The KOH examination or fungal culture is positive.

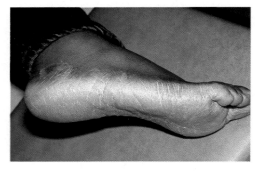

FIGURE 7.3 Tinea pedis. Chronic scaly infection of the plantar surface of the foot in a "moccasin" distribution.

DIFFERENTIAL DIAGNOSIS

Psoriasis
* Psoriasis has sharply demarcated plaques (Figure 7.4).

Atopic Dermatitis
* Atopic dermatitis usually is pruritic, whereas chronic plantar tinea pedis is generally asymptomatic.
* There is a positive atopic history.

CLINICAL VARIANT

"Two Feet One Hand" Tinea
* Tinea can present on one or both palms *(tinea manuum)*. Not infrequently, it appears in a "two feet one hand" distribution. This is pathognomic for tinea (Figure 7.5). This type of tinea infection represents a more widespread distribution of chronic tinea pedis. It is managed in a similar fashion.

MANAGEMENT

This is the most difficult type of tinea pedis to cure because topical agents do not effectively penetrate the thickened epidermis.

Treatment generally requires oral antifungal agents such as the following:

* Itraconazole (200 mg once daily for 14 days or longer)
* Terbinafine (250 mg once daily for 14 days or longer)
* Fluconazole (150 to 200 mg once daily for 4 to 6 weeks)

Nail involvement may require longer treatment because nails may serve as reservoirs for reinfection.

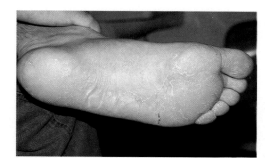

FIGURE 7.4 Psoriasis. A well-demarcated plaque that spares the instep is seen here.

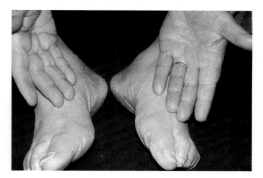

FIGURE 7.5 "Two feet, one hand" variant of tinea pedis. The scale is present on one hand only. Note the nail involvement. These findings are pathognomonic.

TYPE 3: ACUTE VESICULAR TINEA PEDIS

BASICS

This is the least common clinical variant.

DESCRIPTION OF LESIONS

* Vesicles and bullae generally occur on the sole, great toe, and instep of the foot.

CLINICAL MANIFESTATIONS

Acute vesicular tinea pedis is pruritic (Figure 7.6).

DIAGNOSIS

* For diagnosis, the specimen should be obtained from the inner part of the roof of the blister for KOH examination or culture.

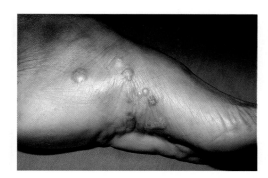

FIGURE 7.6 Acute vesicular tinea pedis. A potassium hydroxide/culture specimen is obtained from under the roof of a vesicle.

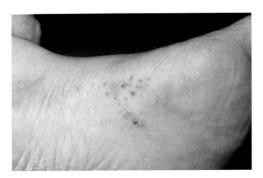

FIGURE 7.7 Dyshidrotic eczema. Note the small vesicles and the similarity to acute tinea pedis.

 DIFFERENTIAL DIAGNOSIS

Dyshidrotic eczema is easily confused with acute tinea pedis (Figure 7.7).

- Patients often have positive atopic history.
- It is KOH negative.

CLINICAL VARIANT

Uncommonly, an *id reaction* (dermatophytid) may occur. This is considered to be a hypersensitivity to fungal elements. Clinically, lesions consist of itchy, sterile (KOH and culture negative), vesicles on the hands similar to dyshidrotic eczema; it resolves when the primary acute process on the feet resolves.

 MANAGEMENT

- For symptomatic relief of severe inflammation and itching, a potent topical steroid, such as triamcinolone acetonide cream, may be used for 4 to 5 days. The resultant antiinflammatory effect also helps to increase the yield of obtaining organisms on KOH examination or culture.
- Treatment is similar to that of type 1, although systemic, as well as topical antifungals are often necessary.
- Prevention involves decreasing wetness, friction, and maceration. Absorbent powders, such as miconazole (Zeasorb-AF) powder, should be applied after the eruption clears to prevent recurrence.

 POINT TO REMEMBER

- Not all rashes of the feet are fungal. In fact, if a child younger than 12 years has what appears to be tinea pedis, it is probably another skin condition, such as eczema.

HELPFUL HINTS

- When the diagnosis is in doubt, a potent topical steroid may be applied to relieve the acute itch and burning.
- To increase positive yields, KOH examination or fungal cultures should be obtained only after the patient has not used topical therapy for at least 24 to 48 hours.
- Positive results of KOH examination and fungal cultures are not necessarily proof of pathogenesis because some organisms, especially yeasts and molds, may be saprophytes, or "contaminants."
- When there is a rash on the palms, the feet should *always* be examined.
- A common error is automatically to assume that a rash of the feet, or "athlete's foot," is fungal in origin. Often, these conditions are mistakenly treated with topical antifungal preparations alone or in combination with topical steroids with a "shotgun" approach. Careful observation and a positive KOH examination reveal the true nature of the problem. This caveat also applies to tinea cruris (see later).

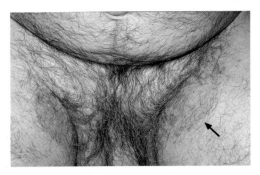

FIGURE 7.8 Tinea cruris. Note the scalloped shape with an "active border."

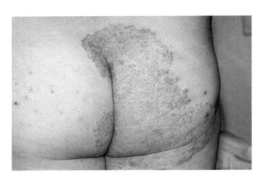

FIGURE 7.9 Tinea cruris. A large annular plaque involves the buttocks.

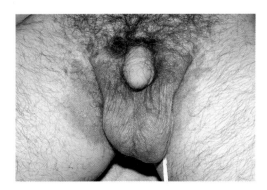

FIGURE 7.10 Inverse psoriasis. Note the well-demarcated plaques with no "active border."

BASICS

Tinea cruris ("jock itch") is a common infection of the upper inner thighs, most often occurring in postpubertal male patients. It is generally caused by the dermatophytes *T. rubrum* and *E. floccosum*. In contrast to candidiasis and lichen simplex chronicus, it generally spares the scrotum.

DESCRIPTION OF LESIONS

- Lesions are bilateral, fan-shaped, or annular plaques (plaques with central clearing), with a slightly elevated "active border" (Figure 7.8).

DISTRIBUTION OF LESIONS

- This involves the upper thighs, the crural folds, and possibly the pubic area and buttocks (Figure 7.9).
- It generally spares the scrotum and penis.

CLINICAL MANIFESTATIONS

- Generally, the lesions are pruritic or irritating.
- Frequently, the patient has tinea pedis as well.
- The condition may be chronic or recurrent, depending on environmental factors and exercise, for example.
- The likelihood of the spread of tinea cruris between sexual partners appears to be very small.

DIAGNOSIS

- A positive KOH examination or fungal culture is found most easily by sampling from the border of the lesions.

◆◆ DIFFERENTIAL DIAGNOSIS

Lichen Simplex Chronicus (Eczematous Dermatitis) (see Figure 2.16)
- It often involves the scrotum.
- KOH examination and fungal cultures are negative for fungus.
- Often, there is an atopic history.
- Lesions are confluent (no central clearing).
- Lichenification occurs as the condition becomes chronic.

Inverse Psoriasis (Figure 7.10)
- It often involves the scrotum.
- Evidence of psoriasis may be noted elsewhere.
- KOH examination and fungal cultures are negative for fungus.
- Lesions are confluent (no central clearing).

OTHER DIAGNOSES

Seborrheic Dermatitis, Candidiasis, Intertrigo, and Irritant Dermatitis

- All of these conditions may be clinically indistinguishable from one another.

MANAGEMENT

- Topical antifungal creams applied once or twice daily are often effective in controlling, and sometimes curing, uncomplicated, localized infections. Over-the-counter preparations of miconazole (Micatin), terbinafine (Lamisil), and clotrimazole (Lotrimin) are available.
- For severe inflammation and itching, a mild over-the-counter hydrocortisone 1% preparation or moderate-strength hydrocortisone valerate 0.2% (Westcort) may be used for 4 to 5 days for symptomatic relief.
- Systemic antifungal therapy may be necessary in cases that do not respond to topical therapy or for extensive chronic recurrent tinea cruris, particularly in immunocompromised patients:
  - Itraconazole (200 mg once daily for 7 days; pediatric dosage: 5 mg/kg per day for 7 days)
  - Terbinafine (250 mg once daily for 7 to 14 days)
  - Griseofulvin (330 mg twice daily for 30 days)

Prevention aims toward decreasing wetness, friction, and maceration by:

- Using an absorbent powder such as miconazole (Zeasorb-AF).
- Drying the area with a hairdryer after bathing.
- Wearing loose clothing; briefs are less frictional than boxer shorts.

HELPFUL HINT

- Tinea pedis, if present concurrently with tinea cruris, should also be treated to minimize reinfection.

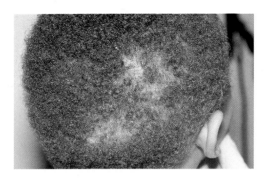

FIGURE 7.11 Tinea capitis. Scaly, alopecic patches mimic seborrheic dermatitis.

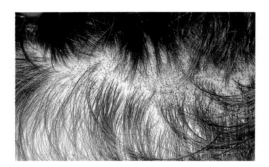

FIGURE 7.12 Tinea capitis. "Black dot" ringworm.

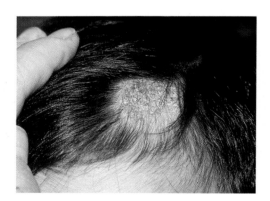

FIGURE 7.13 Tinea capitis. "Gray patch type." Note alopecia with broken off hairs close to scalp surface. *Microsporum canis* was found on culture, and the area fluoresced green with a Wood's lamp.

BASICS

Tinea capitis, or "ringworm," most commonly occurs in prepubertal children. In the United States, African-American children are disproportionately affected by this superficial fungal infection of the hair shaft. The incidence of tinea capitis has been increasing and presents a growing public heath concern, especially in overcrowded, impoverished, inner-city communities.

T. tonsurans is, by far, the most common etiologic agent; more than 90% of cases are caused by it. Other species, such as *Microsporum audouinii*, which is spread from human to human, and *M. canis*, which is spread from animals (cats and dogs), are more often seen in white children. Patients frequently have a family member, pet, or playmate with tinea.

Tinea capitis is quite contagious and is generally spread by person-to-person contact. Studies have demonstrated a 30% carrier state of adults exposed to a child with *T. tonsurans*. The organism has also been isolated from such inanimate objects as hairbrushes and pillows.

DESCRIPTION OF LESIONS

Clinical Types

There are essentially five clinical expressions of tinea capitis, with some overlapping physical presentations:

- Inflamed, scaly, often alopecic patches, mimicking seborrheic dermatitis, are especially common in infancy until the age of 6 to 8 months (Figure 7.11).
- A diffuse scaling is seen with multiple round areas, characterized by alopecia that occurs secondary to broken hair shafts, leaving residual black stumps ("black dot" ringworm) (Figure 7.12). It is seen uncommonly and is often mistaken for alopecia areata.
- The "gray patch" type (Figure 7.13) consists of round, scaly plaques of alopecia in which hairs are broken off close to the surface of the scalp.
- Tender pustular nodules or plaques called kerions may occur.
  - A kerion is a boggy, pustular, indurated, tumorlike mass, which represents an inflammatory hypersensitivity reaction to the fungus. A kerion can result in localized scarring.

– Secondary bacterial invaders such as *Staphylococcus aureus* and some gram-negative organisms may sometimes be recovered from a kerion. Often, there is accompanying nontender regional adenopathy (Figure 7.14).
- Occasionally, a pustular variety, with or without alopecia, can mimic a bacterial infection.

DIAGNOSIS

- A KOH preparation or fungal culture confirms the diagnosis.
  - When in doubt, or when a KOH preparation is negative, a fungal culture placed on Sabouraud's agar should be done. This can be performed by obtaining broken hairs and scale by stroking the affected area with a sterile toothbrush, a familiar object to a child and one that is less frightening than a surgical blade or forceps (see Chapter 26, "Basic Dermatologic Procedures"). The collected material is then tapped onto the surface of Sabouraud's agar.
  - An alternative method of harvesting broken hairs is by rubbing a moistened gauze pad on the involved area of scalp and then using forceps to place the hairs on the culture medium or slide. Pustules generally are sterile or grow bacterial contaminants.
- A biopsy is rarely necessary.
- In the past, Wood's light examination was a valuable screening tool to diagnose tinea capitis easily (because *Microsporum* species are usually fluorescent), but it has lost its usefulness because most cases are caused by the nonfluorescing *T. tonsurans*.

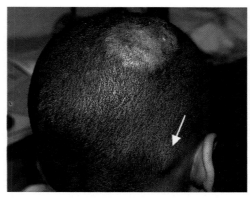

FIGURE 7.14 Tinea capitis with kerion. There is also a palpable, asymptomatic, nontender right occipital lymph node *(arrow).*

 DIFFERENTIAL DIAGNOSIS

Alopecia Areata (Figure 7.15)
- This has a well-demarcated, symmetric patch of alopecia.
- It is free of scales and is smooth.

Seborrheic Dermatitis
- Infants show "cradle cap" with thick scale.
- Alopecia is absent in adults who have scalp involvement.

Other Diagnoses
- Psoriasis
- Trichotillomania (a self-induced cause of hair loss) (see Chapter 10, "Hair and Scalp Disorders Resulting in Hair Loss")
- Tinea amiantacea, which is a KOH-negative local patch or plaque of adherent scale ("tinea" is a misnomer in this condition)
- Bacterial scalp infection
- Secondary syphilis
- Acute and chronic cutaneous discoid lupus erythematosus

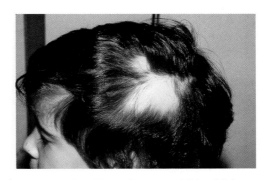

FIGURE 7.15 Alopecia areata. This child has smooth, well-demarcated, noninflammatory, asymptomatic patches of alopecia.

MANAGEMENT

- **Topical therapy** is of little or no value in treating tinea capitis, although an adjunctive antifungal shampoo such as ketoconazole 1% to 2% (Nizoral) or selenium sulfide 1% to 2.5% (Selsun) may be used by the infected person and contacts to prevent reinfection and spread.
- In children, **systemic therapy** with a liquid suspension of griseofulvin has been the mainstay of therapy.
  - The dosage of microsized griseofulvin is 20 to 25 mg/kg per day and is sometimes as high as 25 mg/kg per day in divided doses. Ultramicrosized griseofulvin is given as a dosage of 15 to 20 mg/kg per day. It should be given with milk or food, which increases its absorption. It should be continued until the patient is clinically cured, generally 6 to 8 weeks. Some patients may require longer therapy.
  - Occasionally, an "idlike" reaction occurs shortly after the initiation of griseofulvin therapy. This consists of multiple small sterile papules on the face or body, and it probably represents a hypersensitivity response.
  - Treatment failure, which is uncommon with griseofulvin, may indicate inadequate doses or duration of therapy, drug resistance, reinfection from another family member, poor compliance, or immune incompetence.

Newer Systemic Therapies

Itraconazole, terbinafine, and fluconazole are newer and more efficacious agents. They have been used in some cases of griseofulvin treatment failure.

Pediatric dosages are as follows:

- Itraconazole (Sporanox) (5 mg/kg per day). This drug is available as 100-mg capsules or as an oral solution (10 mg/mL).
- Terbinafine (Lamisil). Reduce dosage according to weight: Children weighing less than 20 kg should receive one fourth of a tablet (62.5 mg) per day; children 20 to 40 kg are given 125 mg per day; children weighing more than 40 kg receive 250 mg per day (available as 250-mg tablets only). Children reluctant to swallow tablets can be given terbinafine by crushing a tablet and mixing it in food.
- Fluconazole (Diflucan) (6 mg/kg per day for 2 weeks; repeat at 4 weeks if indicated). This drug is available as 100-, 150-, 200-mg tablets and as an oral solution (10 and 40 mg/mL).

POINTS TO REMEMBER

- The current standard of diagnosis is a positive KOH examination or culture.
- Topical therapy does not work.
- Systemic therapy must be in an adequate dosage and duration.

HELPFUL HINTS

- The pustular variety of tinea capitis can mimic a bacterial infection, and antibiotics are sometimes given before the correct diagnosis is made.
- When a child has scaling alopecia and enlarged lymph nodes in the posterior auricular or occipital area, obtain a fungal culture and consider starting empiric antifungal treatment.
- In many instances, therapy may have to be initiated in a patient with negative KOH examination and fungal cultures and based solely on clinical appearance.
- Occasionally, concomitant systemic steroid therapy is warranted in addition to griseofulvin, when the patient is experiencing a severe, tender, or painful kerion. A very short course (usually 3 or 4 days) of oral prednisone, 1 mg/kg per day, is sufficient.

TINEA CORPORIS ("RINGWORM")

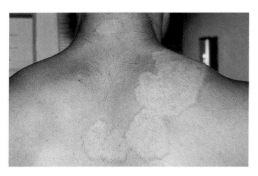

FIGURE 7.16 Tinea corporis. Multiple lesions are present, with a border of scale.

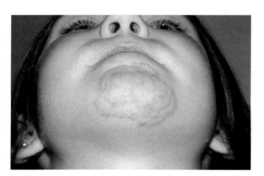

FIGURE 7.17 Tinea faciale. An erythematous scaly annular eruption is noted.

BASICS

Tinea corporis is commonly referred to as "ringworm," a term used by laypersons, and, frequently, many in the health care community, to describe practically any annular or ringlike eruption on the body. In fact, there are many nonfungal conditions that assume an annular "ringworm-like" configuration: granuloma annulare, erythema multiforme, erythema migrans (seen in acute Lyme disease), and figurate erythemas such as urticaria.

Tinea corporis (described as **tinea faciale** if it is located on the face) is most often acquired by contact with an infected animal, usually kittens and occasionally dogs. It may also spread from other infected humans, or it may be autoinoculated from other areas of the body that are infected by tinea such as tinea pedis or tinea capitis. Another common method of transmission of tinea corporis is noted in wrestlers (**tinea gladiatorum**). *M. canis, T. rubrum,* and *T. mentagrophytes* are the usual pathogens.

DESCRIPTION OF LESIONS

- Lesions are generally annular, with peripheral enlargement and central clearing. Odd gyrate or concentric rings may appear (Figures 7.16 and 7.17).
- The scaly, "active border" can sometimes be pustular or vesicular.
- Lesions are single or multiple.

DISTRIBUTION OF LESIONS

- If multiple lesions are present, their distribution is typically asymmetric.
- Lesions are found most often on the extremities, face, and trunk.

CLINICAL MANIFESTATIONS

- Lesions may be pruritic or asymptomatic.
- **Majocchi's granuloma** is a follicular deep form of tinea corporis. It may result when inappropriate therapy, such as topical steroids, or shaving drives the fungi into hair follicles.

DIAGNOSIS

- Diagnosis is confirmed by a positive KOH examination or fungal culture (it is especially easy to find hyphae in those patients who have been previously treated with topical steroids).
- A history of a newly adopted kitten, or of another infected contact, is helpful.

DIFFERENTIAL DIAGNOSIS

Urticaria (Figure 7.18)
- Erythema with no scale, i.e., epidermal involvement.

Acute Lyme Disease (Erythema Migrans) (Figure 7.19)
- Erythema with no scale
- Characteristic targetlike appearance

Granuloma Annulare (see Figure 4.9)
- Skin-colored or red firm papules
- Absence of scale
- Symmetric distribution of lesions
- Lesions slightly firm to palpation

Other Diagnoses
- Atopic dermatitis
- Psoriasis
- Subacute lupus erythematosus
- Mycosis fungoides (cutaneous T-cell lymphoma)

MANAGEMENT
- Topical antifungal agents are useful.
- Systemic antifungal agents (see the earlier discussion of tinea cruris) are sometimes necessary when multiple lesions are present or in areas that are repeatedly shaved, such as men's beards **(tinea barbae)** or, especially, women's legs, in which granulomatous lesions **(Majocchi's granuloma)** may appear.
- If pets appear to be the source of infection, they may also need antifungal treatment after evaluation by a veterinarian.

POINT TO REMEMBER
- Inquire about sports activities, such as wrestling.

HELPFUL HINT
- Tinea corporis is very often misdiagnosed and treated with topical steroids ("tinea incognito") (Figure 7.20).

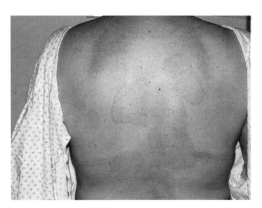

FIGURE 7.18 Urticaria. Dermal vasodilatation occurs, with no epidermal change (scale).

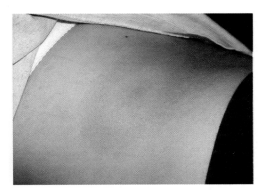

FIGURE 7.19 Acute Lyme disease (erythema migrans). Note the targetlike concentric rings with no scale.

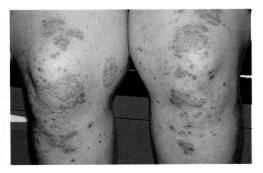

FIGURE 7.20 Tinea corporis ("tinea incognito"). This patient was treated with topical steroids for months until the correct diagnosis was made. The topical steroids modified the typical clinical appearance of tinea corporis; in fact, her lesions look more like psoriasis.

ONYCHOMYCOSIS (TINEA UNGUIUM)

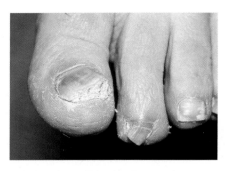

FIGURE 7.21 Distal subungual onychomycosis. The nail is dystrophic and discolored, and there is a buildup of keratin underneath it (subungual hyperkeratosis).

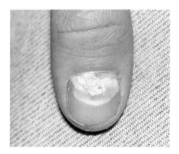

FIGURE 7.22 Superficial white onychomycosis. A potassium hydroxide specimen was easily obtained from the surface of this lesion.

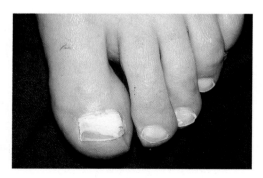

FIGURE 7.23 Proximal white subungual onychomycosis. Human immunodeficiency virus infection should be suspected in this patient.

BASICS

The term *onychomycosis* refers to an infection of the fingernails or toenails caused by various fungi, yeasts, and molds. In contrast, the term *tinea unguium* refers specifically to nail infections caused by dermatophytes. Onychomycosis is uncommon in children, but its prevalence increases with advancing age, with prevalence rates as high as 30% in those 70 years and older.

The major causes of onychomycosis are as follows:

- The dermatophytes *E. floccosum, T. rubrum,* and *T. mentagrophytes*
- Yeasts, mainly *C. albicans*
- Molds, such as *Aspergillus, Fusarium,* and *Scopulariopsis* species

DESCRIPTION OF LESIONS

Distal subungual onychomycosis (Figure 7.21) accounts for more than 90% of all cases of onychomycosis. It is usually characterized by the following:

- Nail thickening and subungual hyperkeratosis (scale buildup under the nail)
- Nail discoloration (yellow, yellow-green, white, or brown)
- Nail dystrophy
- Onycholysis (nail plate elevation from the nail bed)

CLINICAL MANIFESTATIONS

- Aside from footwear causing occasional physical discomfort and the psychosocial liability of unsightly nails, it is usually asymptomatic.
- Left untreated, onychomycotic nails, can, however, infrequently act as a portal of entry for more serious bacterial infections of the lower leg, particularly in patients with diabetes.
- Distal subungual onychomycosis is sometimes associated with chronic palmoplantar tinea (i.e., "two feet, one hand" variant of tinea).

CLINICAL VARIANTS

- In superficial white onychomycosis (Figure 7.22), the fungus is superficial, and material for scraping may be obtained from the dorsal surface of the nail.
- Proximal white subungual onychomycosis (Figure 7.23) may be seen in persons with human immunodeficiency virus (HIV) infection.

DIAGNOSIS

- A positive KOH examination or growth of dermatophyte, yeast, or mold on culture is diagnostic.

(See also Chapter 13, "Diseases and Abnormalities of Nails.")

Psoriasis of the Nails (Figure 7.24)
- This may be indistinguishable from, or coexist with, onychomycosis.
- Usually, evidence of psoriasis is found elsewhere on the body.
- The KOH examination is generally, but not always, negative.
- Characteristic nail pitting and nail discoloration ("oil spots," yellowish brown pigmentation) may be present.

Chronic Paronychia (Figure 7.25)
- This is seen in patients with an altered immune status (e.g., diabetic patients) and in people whose hands are constantly in water.
- Erythema and edema of the proximal nail fold are noted.
- The cuticle is absent.
- There is nail dystrophy.
- Culture may be positive for *Candida* and/or bacteria.

Pseudomonas Infection of the Nail (Green Nail Syndrome) (Figure 7.26)
- Onycholysis occurs, with secondary bacterial (pseudomonas) colonization.
- This is usually found in women with long finger nails.

Other Diagnoses
Onycholysis unrelated to a fungus or psoriasis can be idiopathic or associated with the following:

- Nail trauma, thyroid disease, use of nail polish or nail hardeners, and oral tetracyclines, especially demeclocycline (Declomycin) coupled with sun exposure

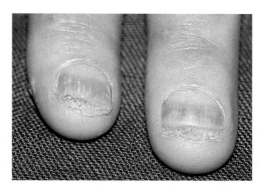

FIGURE 7.24 Psoriasis of nails. Subungual hyperkeratosis and "oil spots" are noted.

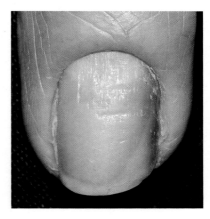

FIGURE 7.25 Chronic paronychia. Note the swelling of the proximal nail fold, the loss of the cuticle, and the dystrophy of the nail plate.

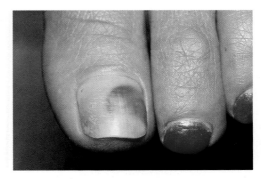

FIGURE 7.26 Green nail, onycholysis. The green color is the result of a secondary infection with *Pseudomonas*.

MANAGEMENT

Media attention has brought scores of patients to their health-care providers to have their unsightly nails treated with the newer oral antifungal agents, itraconazole (Sporanox) and terbinafine (Lamisil). These drugs have replaced griseofulvin, which is less effective and is associated with a high recurrence rate, and ketoconazole, which in a few instances has caused idiosyncratic hepatitis. Other treatments that are sometimes tried include surgical ablation and topical agents.

- Surgical ablation of nails is rarely indicated and is generally ineffective.
- Topical agents are generally ineffective because of poor nail penetration. In early distal subungual and superficial white onychomycosis, these drugs may be used as adjuvant therapy or to prevent recurrences after clearing with oral agents.
- Penlac Nail Lacquer Topical Solution, 8%, is a topical nail lacquer containing the antifungal agent ciclopirox; it is used in conjunction with oral antifungal agents or alone for the prevention of recurrent infection. The overall efficacy of this agent remains to be determined.
- Amorolfine nail lacquer (available in Europe) is reported to be effective when it is applied for at least 12 months.
- Carmol 40 Gel, a topical preparation that contains 40% urea, a keratolytic agent, is applied once daily to thickened nails. It may be used in conjunction with other topical antifungal agents.

Oral Therapy

Important factors to consider before starting oral therapy:

- Diagnostic confirmation by KOH examination or fungal culture
- Patient motivation and compliance
- Family history of onychomycosis
- Patient's age and health
- Drug cost
- Possible drug interactions and side effects (see "Antifungal Drug Formulary" at end of this chapter)

Oral Agents
Terbinafine (Lamisil) Tablets
- It is fungicidal, especially against dermatophytes.
- Long-term cure is probably no greater than 40% to 50%.
- Side effects are infrequent.
- This drug has a reservoir effect. Because it persists in the nail for up to 4 to 5 months, there is no need

to wait until the nail appears clinically normal; there is continued clearing even after cessation of therapy. Baseline liver function tests should be done, and the tests should be repeated in 6 to 8 weeks if therapy is long term.

Dosage
- 250 mg per day for 6 weeks for fingernails
- 250 mg per day for 12 weeks for toenails
- Pediatric dosage: children weighing 20 to 40 kg, 125 mg per day; children weighing more than 40 kg, 250 mg per day for 6 to 12 weeks

Baseline liver function tests are done, and the tests are repeated in 6 to 8 weeks.

Itraconazole (Sporanox) Capsules
- This is a broad-spectrum fungistatic agent.
- The primary drawback to the use of this drug is the risk for significant drug interactions.
- Long-term cure is probably no greater than 40% to 50%.
- Side effects are infrequent.
- This drug also has a reservoir effect.

Dosage
- 200 mg per day for 6 weeks for fingernails, 12 weeks for toenails
- Alternatively, pulse dosing with 200 mg twice daily, taken with full meals for 7 days of each month; for 3 months for fingernails, 4 months for toenails

Baseline liver function tests are done, and the tests are repeated in 6 to 8 weeks.

Fluconazole (Diflucan) Tablets
- This is a broad-spectrum fungistatic agent.
- It is more extensively used in patients with HIV infection.
- It has many fewer drug interactions than itraconazole.
- Side effects are minimal.

Dosage
- 150 to 400 mg daily for 1 to 4 weeks or 150 mg once per week for 9 to 10 months

Liver toxicity must be monitored if the drug is used long term.

POINTS TO REMEMBER

- Onychomycosis should be confirmed before initiating oral therapy.
- Nails that appear abnormal do not always have a fungal infection.
- Onychomycosis is generally asymptomatic, and treatment with the newer systemic antifungal agents is expensive and not always curative.
- Preexisting liver disease is a relative contraindication to the use of antifungal agents for onychomycosis.
- A patient with a family history of onychomycosis is less likely to have a successful treatment outcome than persons without such a history.

 HELPFUL HINTS

The following important questions must be answered before oral therapy is prescribed:

- What are the patient's age and health status?
- Can the patient afford the cost of the drug?
- Is the patient taking any other medications that could interact adversely with the antifungal agent?

CUTANEOUS CANDIDIASIS

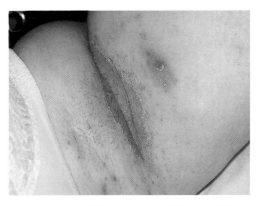

FIGURE 7.27 Cutaneous candidiasis of the axillae. This patient has diabetes. Note the satellite pustules.

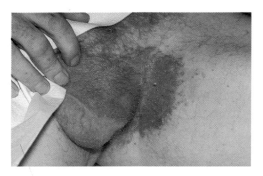

FIGURE 7.28 Cutaneous candidiasis of the groin. A "beefy red" plaque and satellite pustules are seen here.

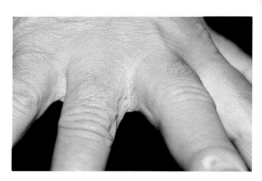

FIGURE 7.29 Cutaneous candidiasis ("erosio interdigitalis blastomycetes"). Candidal infection of the web spaces of the fingers is present.

BASICS

Cutaneous candidiasis is a superficial fungal infection of the skin and mucous membranes caused by *Candida albicans.* It is seen much less commonly than tinea infections. *C. albicans* thrives on moist occluded sites, particularly as a secondary invader. It occurs in the following:

- People who continually expose their hands to water (e.g., dishwashers, health care workers, florists)
- Obese persons
- Infants (in the diaper area, mouth)

It is also found on hosts with an altered immune status such as:

- Patients with diabetes
- Patients taking long-term systemic steroid therapy
- Patients with AIDS
- Patients with polyendocrinopathies

DESCRIPTION OF LESIONS

- The appearance of lesions varies according to the location.

Candidal Intertrigo
- Initially, pustules appear, followed by well-demarcated erythematous plaques with small papular and pustular lesions at the periphery ("satellite pustules") (Figure 7.27).
- Erythematous areas later become eroded and "beefy red" (Figure 7.28).
- Lesions are not annular (they have no central clearing), as seen in tinea infections.

DISTRIBUTION OF LESIONS

- Lesions are seen in intertriginous areas, such as under pendulous breasts, the axillae, the groin, the intergluteal fold, the perineal region including the scrotum, and at the corners of the mouth *(perlèche).*

Other Locations and Descriptions of Clinical Variants
- **"Erosio interdigitalis blastomycetes."** Superficial interdigital scaly, erythematous erosions or fissures occur in the web spaces of the fingers (Figure 7.29).

- **Candidal diaper dermatitis** occurs in the area occluded under diapers.
- **Candidal folliculitis** is characterized by follicular pustules.
- **Candidal balanitis** is seen in men with diabetes. Erythema, edema, and moist curdlike accumulations occur on the glans penis, with possible fissuring and ulceration of the foreskin.
- **Candidal vulvitis/vulvovaginitis** consists of erosions, pustules, and erythematous plaques (Figure 7.30).
- **Candidal paronychia** is characterized by edema, erythema, and purulence of the proximal nail fold with secondary nail dystrophy (see Chapter 13, "Diseases and Abnormalities of Nails").
- **Oral candidiasis ("thrush")** is characterized by white, creamy exudate or plaques, which, when removed, appear eroded and beefy red. Oral candidiasis appears in infants ("thrush") and in the clinical settings of immunosuppression and diabetes (see Chapter 24, "The Cutaneous Manifestations of HIV").

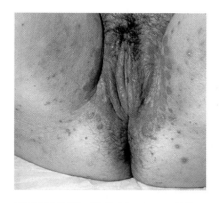

FIGURE 7.30 Cutaneous candidiasis. Note the "beefy" erythematous plaques and satellite pustules.

CLINICAL MANIFESTATIONS

- Cutaneous candidiasis is characterized by itching and burning.

DIAGNOSIS

- The organism is KOH positive for **pseudohyphae, budding yeast,** or **mycelia** (see Chapter 26, "Basic Dermatologic Procedures").
- Fungal culture on **Sabouraud's media** reveals creamy dull-white colonies.

 DIFFERENTIAL DIAGNOSIS

- Inverse psoriasis (Figure 7.31)
- Tinea infections
- Irritant intertrigo
- Atopic dermatitis
- Seborrheic dermatitis

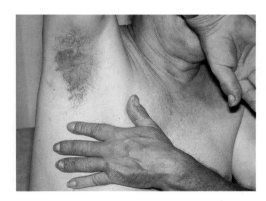

FIGURE 7.31 Inverse psoriasis. Close inspection of this patient reveals typical psoriasis on his hands. Note the great similarity to Figure 7.27.

MANAGEMENT

Cutaneous Candidiasis

- Burow's solution in cool wet soaks two to three times daily are helpful. This solution can be applied to decrease moisture and maceration.
- The intertriginous area should be kept dry with powders, such as miconazole (Zeasorb-AF) powder, and by drying with a hairdryer after bathing.
- Topical broad-spectrum antifungal creams, such as prescription ketoconazole (Nizoral) cream or the over-the-counter preparations of clotrimazole (Lotrimin) and miconazole (Micatin), can be applied.
- Systemic antifungal agents, such as itraconazole or fluconazole, are used for widespread involvement or recalcitrant infections.

POINT TO REMEMBER

- Cutaneous candidiasis is frequently confused with inverse psoriasis and irritant intertrigo; thus, documentation of candidal organisms should be made.

BASICS

Tinea versicolor, also known as *pityriasis versicolor*, is a very common superficial yeast infection caused by the hyphal form of *Pityrosporum ovale*. The organism is also known as *P. orbiculare* and *Malassezia furfur*. Seen mostly in young adults, it is unusual in very young and elderly persons. Tinea versicolor is primarily of cosmetic concern and is generally asymptomatic. The term "versicolor" refers to the varied coloration that tinea versicolor can display. The color of the lesions may vary from a whitish to pink to tan or brown (Figures 7.32 to 7.34). It is a chronic relapsing condition because the causative fungus is part of the skin's normal flora. It is ubiquitous in tropical and subtropical countries.

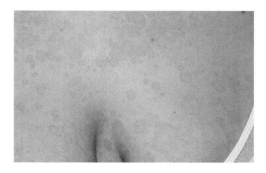

FIGURE 7.32 Tinea versicolor. This patient has light tan (faun-colored) tinea versicolor.

DESCRIPTION OF LESIONS

The primary lesions are well-defined round or oval macules with an overlay of fine scales; the lesions often coalesce to form larger patches. The condition is more common in consistently hot climates and recurs during the summer in more temperate zones. It is also seen more commonly in immunocompromised patients.

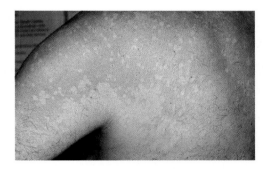

FIGURE 7.33 Tinea versicolor. Here the lesions are brown and confluent.

DISTRIBUTION OF LESIONS

Lesions are most often distributed on the trunk, upper arms, and neck; however, they may also be seen on the face.

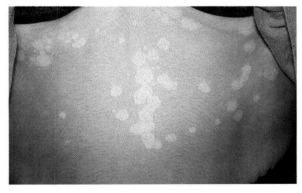

FIGURE 7.34 Tinea versicolor. This patient has hypopigmented lesions. Note the similarity to vitiligo.

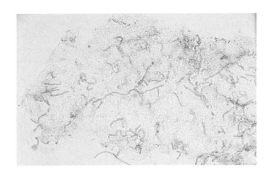

FIGURE 7.35 Tinea versicolor. In this photomicrograph of a potassium hydroxide examination, note the short, wavy hyphae ("spaghetti") and several clusters of spores ("meatballs").

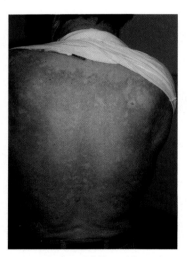

FIGURE 7.36 Vitiligo. Note the complete depigmentation and the lack of scale.

DIAGNOSIS

If scale is present, KOH examination is positive, and the typical "spaghetti and meatball" hyphae are abundant and easily found (Figure 7.35; and see Figure 26.7). Wood's light examination is used to demonstrate the extent of the infection and may help to confirm the diagnosis, because lesions often fluoresce an orange mustard color when the Wood's light is held close to lesions in a dark room.

 ## DIFFERENTIAL DIAGNOSIS

Tinea versicolor is usually easily recognized, but the whitish (hypopigmented) variety is frequently mistaken for **vitiligo** (Figure 7.36).

 ## MANAGEMENT

Topical Agents
- For mild, limited tinea versicolor, topical therapy is applied in the shower. Daily applications of selenium sulfide (Selsun Blue) shampoo, pyrithione zinc (Head & Shoulders) shampoo, and ketoconazole (Nizoral) cream or shampoo are inexpensive over-the-counter methods that often clear the eruption.
- In addition, application of topical antifungals such as miconazole (Micatin), clotrimazole (Lotrimin), or terbinafine (Lamisil) sprays (Micatin and Lamisil sprays allow for easy application on the back). The topical agents are used once or twice daily.
- This treatment regimen may be repeated for 3 or 4 weeks. It is also a good idea to repeat this regimen before the next warm season or before a tropical vacation.

Systemic Therapy
- For stubborn or widespread disease, systemic therapy with itraconazole (Sporanox) or fluconazole (Diflucan) for 7 to 10 days may be prescribed. Although administered short-term, systemic therapy should not be given routinely for this essentially cosmetic problem.

POINTS TO REMEMBER

- Patients should be advised that the uneven coloration of the skin may take several months to disappear after the fungus has been successfully eliminated.
- Recurrences are very common, especially in warm weather.

HELPFUL HINTS

- Prophylactic application of ketoconazole cream or shampoo once or twice weekly may prevent recurrences.
- Topical therapy can be repeated 1 week before the next exposure to warm weather.

SEE PATIENT HANDOUT, PAGE 469

FORMULARY: TINEA VERSICOLOR

AGENT	DOSAGE
TOPICAL AGENTS: OVER-THE-COUNTER	
Selenium sulfide 1% (Selsun Blue) shampoo	Apply daily to wide area for 10 minutes, followed by a shower
Selenium sulfide 1%, zinc pyrithione (Head & Shoulders) shampoo	Apply daily to wide area for 10 minutes, followed by a shower
Miconazole 2% (Micatin) spray	Spray on once daily for 2 weeks
Clotrimazole (Lotrimin) 1% cream	Apply once daily for 2 weeks
TOPICAL AGENTS: PRESCRIPTION REQUIRED	
Terbinafine (Lamisil) 1% solution	1 to 4 weeks, twice daily
Ketoconazole 2% (Nizoral) shampoo	Apply daily to wide area for 10 minutes, followed by a shower
Selenium sulfide 2.5% (Selsun 2.5%) shampoo	Apply daily to wide area for 10 minutes, followed by a shower
SYSTEMIC AGENTS	
Itraconazole (Sporanox)	100 mg for 10 days
Fluconazole (Diflucan)	150 mg for 7–10 days

ANTIFUNGAL DRUG FORMULARY

AGENT	APPLICATION	FORMS	COMMENTS
TOPICAL AGENTS: OVER-THE-COUNTER			
Terbinafine 1% (Lamisil)	1 to 4 weeks, twice daily	Cream, solution, spray	Tinea (not indicated for *Candida*)
Clotrimazole 1% (Lotrimin)	Twice daily	Cream lotion, solution	Tinea, *Candida,* tinea versicolor
Miconazole 2% (Micatin)	Twice daily	Cream, lotion, spray	Tinea, *Candida,* tinea versicolor
Tolnaftate 1% (Tinactin)	Twice daily	Cream	Tinea
Selenium sulfide 1% (Selsun Blue)	Apply daily to wide area for 10 minutes, followed by a shower	Shampoo	Tinea versicolor
Miconazole 2% (Zeaborb A-F powder)	As needed	Powder	Tinea, *Candida,* tinea versicolor; antifungal, antifriction/drying agent
TOPICAL AGENTS: PRESCRIPTION			
Ketoconazole 2% (Nizoral)	Once daily	Cream	Tinea, *Candida,* tinea versicolor
Econazole 1% (Spectazole)	4 weeks, once daily	Cream	Tinea, *Candida,* tinea versicolor, gram-positive bacteria
Ciclopirox 0.77% (Loprox)	4 weeks, as needed	Cream, lotion	Lotion preferred for nail penetration
Naftifine 1% (Naftin)	Once daily	Cream, gel	Tinea; has antiinflammatory activity
Sulconazole (Exelderm)	4 weeks, twice daily	Cream, solution	Tinea, *Candida,* tinea versicolor
Miconazole (Monistat-Derm)	4 weeks, twice daily	Cream	Tinea, *Candida,* tinea versicolor
Oxiconazole 1% (Oxistat)	4 weeks, once to twice daily	Cream, lotion	Tinea, *Candida,* tinea versicolor

SYSTEMIC ANTIFUNGAL AGENTS

AGENT	BRAND NAME(S)	FORMS	COMMENTS
Griseofulvin	Fulvicin, Grisactin, Gris-PEG	Microsized: 250-, 500-mg tablets; ultramicrosized: 125-, 250-, 333-mg tablets Pediatric: Microsized: 125 mg/tsp pediatric suspension	Effective only against dermatophytes Contraindicated in pregnancy Fungistatic Take with fatty meals Alcohol should be avoided Occasional headache Gastrointestinal upset Photosensitivity Elevation of liver function tests Significant drug interactions (phenobarbital, warfarin, other drugs metabolized in liver)
Terbinafine	Lamisil tablets	250-mg tablets	Side effects minimal: includes rare hepatotoxicity, reversible taste loss Many fewer drug interactions than with itraconazole; blood levels decreased by cimetidine and terfenadine; and increased by rifampin; lowers cyclosporine levels **Severe hepatotoxicity including liver failure** has been reported in patients with no preexisting liver disease. A baseline

AGENT	BRAND NAME(S)	FORMS	COMMENTS
			hepatic profile (alanine and aspartate aminotransferase) levels is recommended for all patients before initiating therapy with this agent. These tests should be monitored in patients receiving continuous treatment for more than 1 month or patients who develop signs or symptoms suggestive of liver disease.
Itraconazole	Sporanox	100-mg capsules Oral solution (10 mg/mL)	Side effects minimal; rare hepatotoxicity Significant drug interactions and contraindications: drugs not to be taken with itraconazole include astemizole, cisapride, terfenadine, triazolam, midazolam, lovastatin, and simvastatin **Studies report a risk for developing congestive heart failure** (CHF) from negative inotropic effects of this drug. Because of this risk, itraconazole should not be used in the treatment of onychomycosis in patients with ventricular dysfunction such as CHF or a history of CHF.
Fluconazole	Diflucan	50-, 100-, 150-, 200-mg tablets; oral solution 10 mg/mL, 40 mg/mL	Side effects minimal: rare hepatotoxicity Liver toxicity must be monitored if used long term Not to be taken with cisapride

CHAPTER 8

Viral Exanthems

Kenneth Howe

Overview

Viral exanthems are the cutaneous manifestation of an acute viral infection. In most exanthems, viral particles are present within the visible lesions, having reached the skin through the bloodstream. It is unclear whether the observed exanthem results from active viral infection of the skin, the immune response to the virus, or a combination of these two.

Most common in children, viral exanthems may present as distinct, clinically recognizable illnesses such as measles or chickenpox. More frequently, however, a nonspecific eruption is seen that makes an exact diagnosis elusive. More than 50 viral agents are known to cause exanthems, and many of these rashes are indistinguishable from one another. Because most viral illnesses are benign and self-limited, a specific diagnosis is often not made.

In some situations, however, determining the precise etiology may be of vital importance. Examples include the appearance of a viral exanthem during pregnancy or in an immunocompromised patient. It is also important to distinguish viral exanthems from rashes caused by treatable bacterial or rickettsial infections and from hypersensitivity reactions to medications.

BASICS

- Varicella, or chickenpox, is an infection caused by the varicella-zoster virus (VZV). Transmission occurs by aerosolized droplet spread, with initial infection occurring in the mucosa of the upper respiratory tract. Traveling through the blood and lymphatics (primary viremia), a small amount of virus reaches cells of the reticuloendothelial system, where the virus replicates during the remainder of the incubation period. Nonspecific host defenses contain the incubating infection at this point, but in most cases these defenses are eventually overwhelmed, and a large secondary viremia results. It is through this secondary viremia that VZV reaches the skin. The viremia occurs cyclically over a period of approximately 3 days and results in successive crops of lesions.
- Most cases occur during childhood, and half of the patients are younger than 5 years.
- Epidemics have a peak incidence during late winter and spring.

DESCRIPTION OF LESIONS

- The characteristic lesions begin as red macules and progress rapidly from papules to vesicles to pustules to crusts. The entire cycle may occur within 8 to 12 hours. The typical vesicles are superficial and thin walled, and they are surrounded by an irregular area of erythema, giving them the appearance of "a dewdrop on a rose petal" (Figure 8.1).
- The lesions are usually pruritic.
- Involvement of the oral mucous membranes **(enanthem)** occurs as well, most commonly on the palate. Because vesicles in these sites quickly rupture, it is common to observe shallow erosions.
- Because the lesions appear in successive crops, a characteristic feature of varicella is the simultaneous presence of **lesions in varying stages of development.** In any given area, macules, vesicles, pustules, or crusts may be seen (Figure 8.2).
- Crusts usually fall off within 1 to 3 weeks, depending on the depth of involvement.
- Large blisters can also be seen in varicella, often resulting from superinfection with *Staphylococcus aureus*. Hemorrhagic lesions may occur in patients with thrombocytopenia.
- Scarring is not unusual in uncomplicated varicella. Facial "punched-out" scars are common.

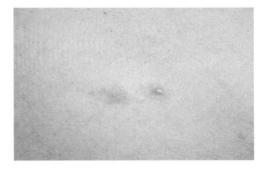

FIGURE 8.1 Varicella. "Dewdrops on rose petals."

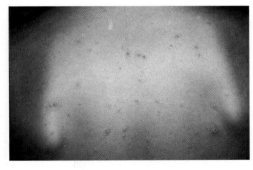

FIGURE 8.2 Varicella. Vesicles and crusts.

DISTRIBUTION OF LESIONS

- The eruption typically begins on the face, scalp, and trunk and then spreads to involve the extremities.
- Successive crops appear over 3 to 5 days and result in a diffuse, widespread eruption of discrete lesions.

CLINICAL MANIFESTATIONS

Incubation Period
- The duration typically is 2 weeks (range, 10 to 21 days).
- During this period, children are usually asymptomatic, with the onset of the rash being the first sign of illness.
- In older children and adults, symptoms are typically more severe. The rash is frequently preceded by 2 to 3 days of fever and flulike symptoms, which often persist during the acute illness.

Complications
- Complications in healthy children are rare; complications are more common in infected adults.
- Varicella pneumonia is a relatively uncommon complication that usually occurs in adults. It begins 1 to 6 days after onset of the rash, with pulmonary symptoms such as cough, dyspnea, and pleuritic chest pain. The severity of the symptoms is out of proportion to the findings on physical examination. Chest radiographs typically reveal diffuse nodular densities.

DIAGNOSIS

- The diagnosis of varicella is usually straightforward, based on the characteristic presentation and clinical findings.
- A **Tzanck smear** can be helpful in confirming the diagnosis (see Chapter 6, "Superficial Viral Infections"). When the test is positive, it reveals characteristic multinucleated giant cells. Identical findings are seen in herpes zoster or herpes simplex virus infections.

Laboratory Testing
- Smears obtained from active lesions can be tested by the direct immunofluorescence technique, which uses fluorescent-labeled antibodies to detect the presence of VZV. This technique has a sensitivity and specificity nearly equal to those of culture, with the advantage of providing rapid results.
- Active lesions can also be cultured for VZV.

◆◆ DIFFERENTIAL DIAGNOSIS

Other Viral Exanthems
- Vesicular exanthems of coxsackievirus and echovirus infections may be mistaken for varicella.
- These exanthems may show a characteristic distribution, as in hand-foot-and-mouth disease.

Disseminated Herpes Zoster (see Figure 24.7)
- Patients have a previous history of primary varicella.
- There is often a typical vesicular eruption accentuated in one unilateral dermatome in a typical "zosteriform" pattern. This is seen in addition to a widespread rash indistinguishable from varicella.
- The patient is generally immunocompromised, secondary to medications, malignant disease, or human immunodeficiency virus infection.

Eczema Herpeticum (Kaposi's Varicelliform Eruption) (see Figure 6.29)
- Preexisting skin disease such as atopic dermatitis becomes secondarily infected with herpes simplex virus.
- Direct immunofluorescence or culture results indicative of herpes simplex virus infection.

Atypical Measles
- This occurs in adults who received killed measles virus vaccine from 1963 to 1967.
- The eruption begins on the palms and soles and then spreads proximally.
- Pneumonia is a common feature.
- The diagnosis can be confirmed by a rise in measles antibody titers.

Impetigo
- The patient generally feels well.
- Typical moist, honey-colored crusts are present, often in a periorificial distribution.

MANAGEMENT

Acute Varicella

- Uncomplicated varicella in otherwise healthy children is generally treated with supportive care such as antipruritics and antipyretics. Aspirin should be avoided because of the risk for Reye's syndrome.
- **Oral acyclovir** is warranted in patients at increased risk for the development of complications, and, in general, it should be started within 24 hours of the onset of the rash. These patients include:
  - Otherwise healthy, nonpregnant patients 13 years of age or older.
  - Children older than 12 months with chronic skin or pulmonary conditions or who are receiving long-term salicylate therapy.
  - Children receiving short, intermittent or aerosolized courses of corticosteroids.
- **Intravenous acyclovir** is indicated in immunocompromised patients or in patients with virally mediated complications of varicella.

Varicella Vaccine

The VZV vaccine (Varivax) is recommended for universal immunization in all children.

- It is optimally given between 12 and 18 months of age; it may be administered in a single dose at any time before 13 years of age.
- In older adolescents or adults, two doses of vaccine should be administered 4 to 8 weeks apart.

Varicella and Pregnancy

- Peripartal maternal varicella poses a particular risk to the newborn. Neonates born 2 days before or 5 days after the onset of maternal varicella should be given varicella immunoglobulin (VZIG). Those newborns who develop varicella should be treated with intravenous acyclovir.
- Oral acyclovir is not recommended in pregnant women with uncomplicated varicella because the risk or benefit to the fetus is unknown.
- Pregnant patients who develop varicella in the first trimester have a 2.3% to 4.9% risk for delivering a child with the *fetal varicella syndrome*.
  - This syndrome is a congenital malformation complex with features such as intrauterine growth retardation, prematurity, cicatricial lesions in a dermatomal distribution, limb paresis and hypoplasia, chorioretinitis, and cataracts.
  - It is not known whether the administration of acyclovir will prevent these complications.

POINT TO REMEMBER

- Patients remain contagious until all cutaneous lesions are crusted.

BASICS

- Hand-foot-and-mouth disease is an acute viral infection that manifests as a vesicular eruption with a characteristic distribution. The infection is caused by enteroviruses, most commonly coxsackievirus A16. The virus is spread from person to person by the fecal-oral route.
- Outbreaks are typically in the summer or early fall, and epidemics may occur. Transmission is more likely in crowded environments.
- Young children (ages 1 to 5 years) are most commonly infected.
- The incubation period ranges from 4 to 6 days.

DESCRIPTION OF LESIONS

- Oral lesions (enanthem) are the first manifestation of hand-foot-and-mouth disease. Although initially vesicular, it is more common to see multiple shallow erosions, because the vesicles are very fragile.
- Individual lesions may range in size from 1 to 5 mm in diameter, and they may exhibit a rim of erythema. These oral lesions may be painful, and they frequently interfere with eating (Figure 8.3).
- The exanthem consists of round or angulated, grayish white vesicles that are typically 3 to 7 mm in diameter.
- These vesicles, which are located on the palms and soles, have a characteristic oval or linear shape and tend not to rupture (Figure 8.4).

DISTRIBUTION OF LESIONS

- The enanthem appears most commonly on the tongue and buccal mucosa and occasionally on the lips, palate, and gums.
- The exanthem is characteristically present on the hands and feet. Lesions occur on the dorsal or lateral aspects of the fingers and toes and on the palms and soles. All three sites may not be involved at the time of presentation.
- The diaper area in infants may show a greater concentration of lesions.
- Occasionally, an eruption of erythematous papules on the proximal extremities may occur, in addition to the acral lesions.

CLINICAL MANIFESTATIONS

- The illness most frequently begins as a sore throat or mouth. In young children, refusal to eat is often a presenting sign.
- Occasionally, a 1- to 2-day prodrome of fever and abdominal pain may be seen.
- The acral eruption follows the development of oral lesions. It is usually not pruritic, although it may be painful.
- In contrast to most viral illnesses, lymphadenopathy is absent to minimal.
- Although in general complications are rare, the one seen most frequently is aseptic meningitis.

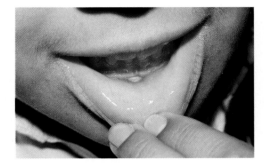

FIGURE 8.3 Hand-foot-and-mouth disease. Oral lesion: note the oval shape and rim of erythema.

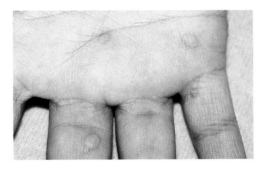

FIGURE 8.4 Hand-foot-and-mouth disease. Oval intact vesicles are noted on the palm.

DIAGNOSIS

- Diagnosis is made on the basis of the characteristic clinical presentation.
- Although not routinely indicated, laboratory testing can confirm the diagnosis. Virus can be cultured from throat washings or stool, with the latter giving a higher yield. Acute and convalescent sera will show an elevation in antibody titer to the causative virus.

 DIFFERENTIAL DIAGNOSIS

Primary Oral Herpes Simplex
- Usually, the lips and gingiva are affected, and the back of the throat is spared.
- There are recurrent outbreaks.
- The Tzanck smear and culture are positive for herpes simplex virus.

Aphthous Ulcers
- Lesions are painful.
- As with herpes simplex, the lips and gingiva are usually affected, and the back of the throat is spared.

 MANAGEMENT

- Treatment is with supportive care. Antipyretics and a clear liquid diet while the throat is sore are typically all that is necessary.

 POINT TO REMEMBER

- The course of the illness is self-limited, lasting less than a week in most cases.

BASICS

- Erythema infectiosum is a common viral illness caused by infection with parvovirus B19. Transmission is from person to person, probably through respiratory secretions.
- It occurs most commonly in the late winter and spring. Epidemics are frequently seen, particularly among school-age children.
- The incubation period lasts 4 to 14 days, but it may be as long as 3 weeks.
- By the time the characteristic exanthem appears, the patient is unlikely to be infectious.

DESCRIPTION OF LESIONS

- Erythema infectiosum is most commonly identified in children by its characteristic facial erythema. Bright red and tending to involve the malar surfaces, this eruption is described as having a "slapped cheek" appearance (Figure 8.5).
- An exanthem also appears on the extremities and trunk. This develops 1 to 4 days after the facial erythema, and it begins as a macular or macular and papular erythema that later clears centrally to produce a characteristic reticular ("lacy") pattern (Figures 8.6 and 8.7).
- Although the exanthem usually resolves in 1 to 2 weeks, the reticular erythema may show a recrudescent course in some patients. In these cases, the erythema tends to flare in response to physical stimuli, such as exercise, excitement, sunlight, or warm baths.

DISTRIBUTION OF LESIONS

- The facial erythema favors the malar surfaces. The "slapped cheek" appearance is further accentuated by a tendency to spare the nasal bridge and the periorbital and perioral areas.
- The reticular erythema most commonly affects the extensor surfaces of the extremities and the buttocks. The palms and soles are usually spared.

CLINICAL MANIFESTATIONS

- Although facial erythema is the most common initial presentation, some patients experience a mild prodrome of low-grade fever, malaise, upper respiratory or gastrointestinal symptoms, and myalgias.
- It can be associated with joint symptoms in adults, particularly in women. **A symmetric polyarthropathy** develops, involving the hands, feet, elbows, and knees.
- The illness is benign and self-limited, with the exanthem resolving within 1 to 2 weeks.
- Although joint symptoms generally resolve within 2 to 3 weeks, it is not uncommon for them to persist for several months.

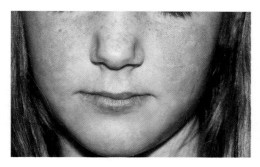

FIGURE 8.5 Erythema infectiosum. "Slapped cheeks:" the erythema favors the malar surfaces. The slapped cheek appearance is further accentuated by a tendency to spare the nasal bridge and the periorbital and perioral areas.

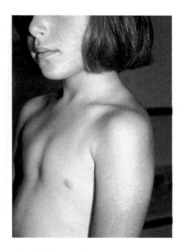

FIGURE 8.6 Erythema infectiosum. This child has "slapped cheeks" in addition to the characteristic reticular ("lacy") pattern on her arms.

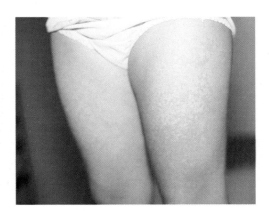

FIGURE 8.7 Erythema infectiosum. Lesions on legs.

- Erythema infectiosum during pregnancy may result in fetal death because of the development of **hydrops fetalis.** The risk for fetal death with maternal infection is estimated at 4.2% to 9%, with greater risk when the infection occurs during the first 20 weeks of pregnancy.
- Infection with parvovirus B19 can lead to **aplastic crisis** in patients with chronic anemias such as sickle cell disease, hereditary spherocytosis, and thalassemia intermedia.
- Immunocompromised patients who develop chronic parvovirus B19 infection are at risk for **chronic red cell aplasia** or more **generalized bone marrow failure.**

DIAGNOSIS

- The diagnosis is based on the characteristic clinical presentation.
- Although usually unnecessary, serologic testing is the most accurate method of confirming infection. The presence of immunoglobulin M (IgM) antibodies to parvovirus B19 is indicative of recent infection. These antibodies appear approximately 3 days after the onset of the exanthem and begin to decline 1 to 2 months later.

 DIFFERENTIAL DIAGNOSIS

Systemic Lupus Erythematosus
- This may be difficult to differentiate from erythema infectiosum with associated joint symptoms.
- The patient often has history of photosensitivity.
- Positive antinuclear antibodies are present.
- Other signs of systemic involvement such as serositis, renal disease, and central nervous system involvement are noted.

MANAGEMENT
- Supportive care is all that is required for uncomplicated cases.
- No effective antiviral therapy exists for parvovirus B19.

POINTS TO REMEMBER
- Facial erythema is often absent in infected adults.
- Because they are at risk for aplastic crisis, all patients with erythema infectiosum who have chronic anemia should have a complete blood cell count evaluated.

BASICS

- Roseola infantum, or *exanthem subitum,* is an acute viral illness marked by a high fever that characteristically resolves with the onset of the rash (Figure 8.8).
- It is caused by infection with herpesvirus type 6 (HHV-6).
- Although the exact route of transmission is not known, it is probably spread through oral or respiratory secretions.
- After HHV-6 exposure, there is an incubation period of 7 to 15 days before the onset of symptoms.
- As with other herpesvirus infections, it is likely that HHV-6 establishes a latent infection after the acute illness. The isolation of HHV-6 from the saliva of healthy adults supports this view.

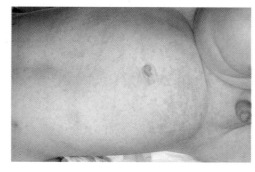

FIGURE 8.8 Roseola. (Courtesy of Bernard A. Cohen, http://dermatlas.org.)

DESCRIPTION OF LESIONS

- The exanthem appears 1 day before to 1 day after defervescence.
- It consists of discrete macules or papules, 1 to 5 mm in diameter, often with a surrounding rim of pallor. The color of these lesions has been described as "rose pink." Frequently, the individual lesions coalesce to form areas of confluent erythema.
- The exanthem typically clears within 1 to 2 days, although it may persist for up to 10 days.

DISTRIBUTION OF LESIONS

- A widespread distribution is seen, with lesions appearing on the trunk, buttocks, neck, and, occasionally, the face and limbs.

CLINICAL MANIFESTATIONS

- A febrile illness typically precedes the exanthem by 3 to 5 days. Characteristically, this prodrome is marked by a high fever in an otherwise well child.
- On occasion, the fever is accompanied by coryza, cough, headache, or abdominal pain.
- Occipital, cervical, and postauricular lymphadenopathy is commonly present.
- Complications are uncommon and include seizures, encephalitis, and thrombocytopenia.

DIAGNOSIS

- The characteristic clinical presentation is usually sufficient for diagnosis.
- Although rarely necessary, the diagnosis can be confirmed by laboratory studies demonstrating either the presence of IgM to HHV-6 or a fourfold rise in IgG titers to the virus.

 ## DIFFERENTIAL DIAGNOSIS

Other Febrile Viral Exanthems
- Other conditions such as enterovirus, rubella, and measles must be excluded.

Scarlet Fever
- This has severe constitutional symptoms and characteristic oral changes. It resolves with acral desquamation.

Drug Reaction
- This is typically not preceded by high fever.
- The rash is usually of longer duration.

 ### MANAGEMENT

- During the prodromal phase of illness, antipyretics are often useful, particularly because they may reduce the risk for febrile seizures.

 ### POINT TO REMEMBER

- Infection with HHV-6 is one of the most common causes of febrile illness in young children.

BASICS

- Rubella is a mild viral illness that, because of its devastating effects on the developing human fetus, is recognized as a major public health issue.
- Maternal infection may lead to fetal death or permanent damage. The consequences are more severe when the infection occurs during the first 8 weeks of gestation. Fetal damage is rare after 5 months of gestation.
- Sensory neural hearing loss, cataracts, and cardiac anomalies are the most common defects of congenital rubella.
- The rubella virus is an RNA virus of the Togaviridae family. Humans are the only known natural hosts. The initial infection occurs in the nasopharyngeal mucosa.
- The incidence of rubella has declined markedly since mass immunization for rubella began in 1969.

DESCRIPTION OF LESIONS

- The eruption consists of pink to red macules with faint pinpoint papules.
- Initially discrete, the lesions may coalesce to form an erythematous rash reminiscent of scarlet fever.
- The eruption may be pruritic, particularly in adults.

DISTRIBUTION OF LESIONS

- The eruption begins on the face and spreads within 24 hours to the trunk and extremities (Figure 8.9).
- The exanthem of rubella is characteristically short-lived, with resolution beginning on the first or second day of the rash. Resolution proceeds in a cephalocaudad direction, and it may be accompanied by fine, branny desquamation.

CLINICAL COURSE

- A mild prodromal illness is the earliest clinical feature of infection.
- A mild fever develops, accompanied by lymphadenopathy. The lymphadenopathy, which most commonly affects the postauricular, suboccipital, and posterior cervical lymph nodes, may be impressive.
- In older patients, the prodrome may be longer and more severe.
- Constitutional symptoms usually resolve within 24 hours of the onset of the rash. In some cases, however, the lymphadenopathy persists for weeks.
- Complications are rare.

DIAGNOSIS

- The clinical features of rubella are not distinctive enough to allow one to make the diagnosis with certainty based on the clinical presentation alone.
- Acute and convalescent antibody titers can confirm the diagnosis. Although unnecessary in most cases, these tests are important in pregnant women exposed to rubella.

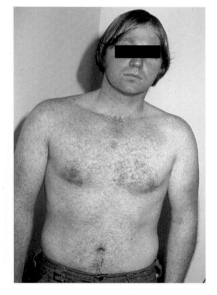

FIGURE 8.9 Rubella. This patient has a viral exanthem. This rash is not distinctive enough to allow one to make the diagnosis with certainty based on the clinical presentation alone.

Measles
- Prodromal symptoms are of greater severity.
- Koplik's spots are present.
- The rash lasts longer.

Roseola
- A high prodromal fever occurs in the absence of other symptoms.
- The morphologic appearance and duration of the exanthem are similar to those of rubella.

Mononucleosis
- Prominent lymphadenopathy, hepatosplenomegaly, and exudative pharyngitis are noted.
- Atypical lymphocytes and heterophile antibodies are found in the blood.

Erythema Infectiosum
- Patients have a distinctive "slapped cheek" erythema.
- A lacy, reticular eruption occurs on the extremities.
- The exanthem lasts longer than in rubella.

Enterovirus Infection
- This is distinguished by a prominent enanthem.

Scarlet Fever
- Severe constitutional symptoms and pharyngitis are noted.
- Patients have a "strawberry tongue."
- A "sandpapery" exanthem occurs.
- Marked desquamation is associated with resolution.

Drug Reaction
- It may be associated with marked pruritus.
- The exanthem lasts longer than in rubella.

 MANAGEMENT

- No specific therapy is available. When necessary, supportive care should be provided. Such care includes antipyretics or antiinflammatory medications for arthralgias.
- Infected patients should be isolated from susceptible persons.

 POINT TO REMEMBER

- Rubella immunization should be well documented in young women; if antirubella antibiotic titers are negative, rubella immunization should be given.

BASICS

- Measles is a viral illness characterized by a distinctive **exanthem** and **enanthem.** The primary site of infection is the respiratory epithelium of the oropharynx.
- The measles virus is a single-stranded RNA virus of the Paramyxoviridae family. Humans are the natural host for the virus, although other primates may be infected as well.
- Transmission occurs by the respiratory aerosol route. The incubation period lasts from 9 to 11 days.
- The incidence of measles in the United States has decreased dramatically since the introduction of the measles vaccine.
- Measles has been all but eradicated in the Western Hemisphere. Almost all the cases most recently reported in the United States can be traced to immigrants form other nations where measles is more common.
- The disease still rages outside the West. It kills more than 800,000 children worldwide each year, more than half of them in central Africa.

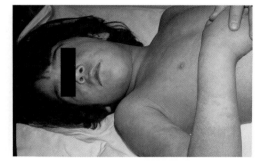

FIGURE 8.10 Rubeola (measles). The typical exanthem (morbilliform rash) of measles.

DESCRIPTION OF LESIONS

- The exanthem appears 3 to 5 days after the onset of the prodromal illness. Lesions begin as discrete erythematous macules and papules, which soon coalesce into areas of confluent erythema (Figure 8.10). Pruritus is usually absent.
- The rash lasts 4 to 7 days before resolving, often with fine desquamation.
- A characteristic enanthem known as **Koplik's spots** (Figure 8.11) appears 2 days before the onset of the exanthem. The lesions are 1-mm bluish white macules that develop on a background of erythematous oral mucosa. These lesions are pathognomonic for measles and, because they develop before the rash, provide an opportunity for early diagnosis.

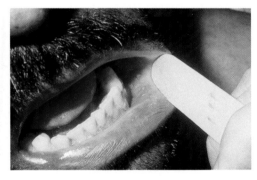

FIGURE 8.11 Rubeola (measles). Koplik's spots: this patient has the pathognomonic enanthem opposite his premolar teeth.

DISTRIBUTION OF LESIONS

- The rash most characteristically begins on the forehead or behind the ears. It then spreads to involve the remainder of the face, the trunk, and the arms and legs over 2 to 3 days. It follows a cephalocaudad order in its development, and it later resolves in the same direction.
- Koplik's spots are most prominent on the buccal mucosa opposite the molars, although they may appear on the labial and gingival mucosa as well.

CLINICAL FEATURES

- The illness begins with a 2- to 4-day prodrome of fever, hacking, barklike cough, coryza, conjunctivitis, and photophobia. These patients appear acutely ill, and they often have cervical and preauricular lymphadenopathy on examination.
- In most cases, measles is a benign and self-limited infection. Recovery is usually complete within 14 days of the onset of the prodrome.

Complications

- Pneumonia is the most common complication. In children, this most frequently takes the form of primary measles pneumonitis, whereas in adults, secondary bacterial pneumonias are more common. Measles pneumonia is particularly severe in immunosuppressed patients.
- Encephalitis occurs in 1 to 2 patients per 1,000 cases of measles.
- Patients vaccinated with the killed virus vaccine, which was in use from 1963 to 1967, are at risk for developing *atypical measles*. After a 2- to 3-day prodrome of fever, dry cough, headache, and abdominal pain, a macular and papular exanthem appears. In contrast to classic measles, this eruption begins on the palms and soles and then spreads proximally. Pneumonia is often present in these patients as well.

DIAGNOSIS

- The diagnosis of measles is usually made on clinical grounds.
- Although usually unnecessary, serologic testing is available. A fourfold or greater rise in antibody titers between acute and convalescent sera confirms the diagnosis.

 ## DIFFERENTIAL DIAGNOSIS

- Atypical measles
- Rubella
- Erythema infectiosum
- Scarlet fever
- Roseola
- Drug hypersensitivity reaction

 ### MANAGEMENT

- No specific therapy for measles virus infection exists. Supportive care should be provided, and patients should be isolated from susceptible persons.
- Passive immunization should be given to pregnant women, infants younger than 1 year, and immunocompromised patients who lack antibodies to the measles virus. Immunoglobulin preparations containing a high antimeasles titer should be administered within 6 days of exposure.
- Routine immunization is recommended for all children 15 months of age or older.

 ### POINTS TO REMEMBER

- A patient with measles becomes contagious 3 days before onset of the rash and remains so until desquamation of the rash.
- All cases should be reported to local public health officials.

CHAPTER 9

Bacterial Exanthems

Kenneth Howe and Herbert P. Goodheart

SCARLET FEVER

BASICS

- Scarlet fever is a streptococcal infection of the pharynx associated with widespread mucocutaneous changes that are caused by an erythrogenic exotoxin-producing strain of group A beta-hemolytic streptococci. In the past, scarlet fever was a major public health threat; its morbidity, mortality, and incidence have declined markedly, both because of the development of antibiotics and because of a reduction in the virulence of the streptococci causing the condition.
- The cutaneous manifestations of scarlet fever represent a delayed hypersensitivity response to streptococcal products. Thus, prior exposure to streptococci is a necessary precondition for scarlet fever.

Etiology
- Usually, group A beta-hemolytic *Streptococcus pyogenes* is the pathogenic organism. Uncommonly, exotoxin-producing *Staphylococcus aureus* may be responsible.

DESCRIPTION OF LESIONS

- A finely popular, erythematous rash appears on the trunk and extremities. This rash may be referred to as "sandpapery" or "scarlatiniform."
- The skin around the mouth may show a characteristic pallor *(circumoral pallor)*. Linear streaks of petechiae called *Pastia's lines* may develop in flexural areas such as the antecubital fossae, the axilla, and the inguinal region.
- Mucosal findings include erythema and edema of the pharyngotonsillar area, punctate erythematous macules and petechiae on the palate, and "strawberry tongue." The last is a characteristic finding, caused by prominence of the papillae on the surface of the tongue.
- During the convalescent phase of the illness, the skin of the palms and soles frequently desquamates. This desquamation may be sheet-like, and the original infection may have passed unnoticed. In such instances, the patient may seek medical attention solely for the desquamation (Figure 9.1).

DISTRIBUTION OF LESIONS

- The scarlatiniform eruption is widespread and symmetric, primarily affecting the trunk and extremities.

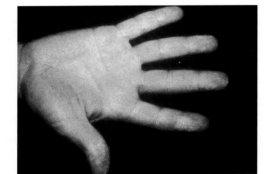

FIGURE 9.1 Scarlet fever. Skin peeling from fingertips. This desquamation occurred during the convalescent phase of the illness.

CLINICAL MANIFESTATIONS

- Scarlet fever typically begins with the abrupt onset of fever, sore throat, headache, and chills.
- Complications of this illness are uncommon, but they may include pneumonia, pericarditis, meningitis, hepatitis, glomerulonephritis, and rheumatic fever. Erythema nodosum and acute guttate psoriasis may also follow or accompany an infection with group A beta-hemolytic streptococci (see Chapter 25, "Cutaneous Manifestations of Systemic Disease," and Chapter 3, "Psoriasis").
- Scarlet fever can recur, with recurrence rates as high as 18% having been reported.

DIAGNOSIS

- The diagnosis of scarlet fever is often made on clinical grounds.
- The isolation of group A streptococci from the pharynx, or the presence of serologic tests such as an elevation of antistreptolysin-O titers, can help to confirm the diagnosis.

 DIFFERENTIAL DIAGNOSIS

- Streptococcal or staphylococcal toxic shock syndromes are distinguished by hypotension and multiorgan system involvement.
- Kawasaki's syndrome (KS) is characterized by prominent lymphadenopathy.
- Febrile drug reactions cause a blotchy, erythematous rash. Pastia's lines and strawberry tongue are not present.
- Viral exanthem is a possible diagnosis.
- Flaccid bullae are the predominant feature of *staphylococcal scalded-skin syndrome*, which occurs in newborns and in infants younger than 2 years.

 MANAGEMENT

- First-line treatment is with penicillin. Alternatives include erythromycin, cephalosporins, ofloxacin, rifampin, and newer macrolide antibiotics.
- Emollients can be used to soothe the scarlatiniform eruption.

TOXIN-MEDIATED STREPTOCOCCAL AND STAPHYLOCOCCAL DISEASE

Overview

- Some streptococcal and staphylococcal species are capable of producing circulating toxins. Patients infected with these toxin-producing bacteria exhibit clinical manifestations distant from the site of local infection. Several distinct syndromes related to these toxins have been recognized, including toxic shock syndrome (TSS) and, rarely, streptococcal toxic shock syndrome (STSS). The principal features of STSS are the same as those of classic TSS: a local infection leads to various clinical manifestations in distant organ systems, resulting from the action of a toxin produced by the infecting bacteria. In most cases of STSS, group A streptococci are isolated from the local infection.
- The responsible toxins act as superantigens, bypassing the normal sequence of immune system activation, to stimulate an immune response in a general, nonspecific manner. This nonspecific immunologic activation leads to damage in various organ systems. Certain physical signs—such as strawberry tongue, acral erythema with subsequent desquamation, and an erythematous eruption with perineal accentuation—are shared in common by several of the toxin-mediated syndromes.

TOXIC SHOCK SYNDROME

BASICS

- TSS is a systemic illness caused by infection with toxin-producing strains of *S. aureus*. Originally described in association with tampon use, TSS now occurs more commonly with a local wound infection, particularly in the postoperative setting.

DESCRIPTION OF LESIONS

- A diffuse macular erythema is often present, which may be scarlatiniform (i.e., "sandpapery" to the touch) and may show accentuation in the flexures.
- Erythema and edema of the palms and soles are often seen.
- Desquamation of the palms and soles, as seen in many bacterial toxin-mediated disorders, occurs 1 to 2 weeks after the onset of the illness.
- Hyperemia of the conjunctiva and mucous membranes and "strawberry tongue" are often present.

DISTRIBUTION OF LESIONS

- The erythematous eruption is diffuse, with accentuation in flexures such as the antecubital folds.
- The mucous membranes, palms, and soles are also sites of characteristic changes.

CLINICAL MANIFESTATIONS

- Patients with TSS have a high fever.
- Multiorgan involvement is a hallmark of this condition. Systemic manifestations may include hypotension, elevated blood urea nitrogen and creatinine levels, abnormal liver function test results, leukocytosis and thrombocytopenia, and increased serum creatine kinase levels.
- In nonmenstrual TSS, the classic signs of erythema, tenderness, and purulence may be absent in the local infection, thereby making its identification difficult.

DIAGNOSIS

- Diagnosis is made when the characteristic clinical findings of fever, rash, and hypotension are present in patients who have an infection with *S. aureus* or in menstruating women who use tampons.
- Diagnosis also is made when laboratory tests such as Gram's stain and cultures of vaginal exudate or wounds are positive for *S. aureus* or, rarely, group A streptococci.

 DIFFERENTIAL DIAGNOSIS

- Hypotension does not occur in **scarlet fever.**
- **A febrile drug reaction** is not associated with hypotension.
- **Kawasaki's syndrome** (see later) usually occurs in children and causes prominent lymphadenopathy.
- **Staphylococcal scalded-skin syndrome** occurs in newborns and in infants younger than 2 years.

 MANAGEMENT

- Treatment of TSS includes the administration of penicillinase-resistant antibiotics and drainage of any abscesses.
- Supportive care may include hydration and vasopressors for hypotension.
- Management of STSS is similar to that of classic TSS.
- Intravenous γ-globulin has been reported to be effective in treating STSS, but it is not yet in widespread use.

 HELPFUL HINTS

- Look for a cutaneous site of infection or for a forgotten or retained vaginal tampon.
- STSS may be clinically identical to TSS, but it is usually distinguished by a more marked soft tissue infection at the site of origin, with localized pain in an extremity the most frequent initial complaint.
- Blood cultures are positive in more than 50% of patients with STSS.
- Antibiotic coverage for both staphylococci and penicillin-resistant streptococci should be given.

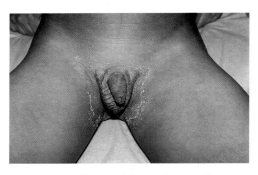

FIGURE 9.2 Kawasaki's syndrome. Desquamation in the genital area. This sheetlike desquamation occurred 2 weeks after the original infection.

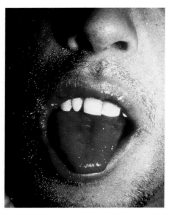

FIGURE 9.3 Kawasaki's syndrome. "Strawberry tongue."

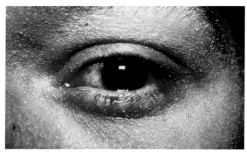

FIGURE 9.4 Kawasaki's syndrome. Ocular involvement.

BASICS

- Kawasaki's syndrome (KS), also known as **mucocutaneous lymph node syndrome,** is an acute, febrile, multisystem illness that primarily affects young children. Its most serious complications are the result of systemic vasculopathy.
- The peak incidence of KS is between 1 and 2 years of age. It is more common in boys.
- In the United States, children of Asian ancestry are affected six times more often than are white children.
- KS occurs sporadically and in epidemics. A seasonal predilection has been observed, with cases occurring more often in the winter and spring.
- Although the exact cause of KS is unknown, it is most likely the result of a superantigen produced by an infectious agent such as *S. aureus*, resulting in massive cytokine release.

DESCRIPTION OF LESIONS

- The truncal rash of KS is polymorphous and may be scarlatiniform, morbilliform, or targetoid.
- Changes of the hands and feet are distinctive. An intense erythema appears on the palms and soles on days 3 to 5 of the illness, followed by an indurated edema. A sharp demarcation may be seen at the wrists and the sides of the hands and feet. As noted in scarlet fever, during the convalescent phase of the illness, the skin of the fingertips and toes peels off in sheets (see Figure 9.1). During the convalescent phase of the illness, the skin of the fingertips and toes peels off in sheets.
- The presence of scarlatiniform erythema in the perianal or inguinal area (Figure 9.2) may be a useful diagnostic sign. The rash in this area progresses to desquamation before the palms and soles begin to peel.
- Characteristic findings are present in the mouth, on the lips, and on the tongue. The earliest manifestations are seen on the lips, with bright red erythema accompanied by fissuring and swelling. Prominent papillae create the appearance of a "strawberry tongue" (Figure 9.3). Examination of the oropharynx reveals a diffuse erythema without vesicles, erosions, or ulcers.
- Eye involvement (Figure 9.4) consists of bilateral, nonpurulent conjunctival injection. Patients may exhibit signs of photophobia.

DISTRIBUTION OF LESIONS

- The polymorphic eruption favors the trunk and proximal extremities, but it may be generalized.

CLINICAL MANIFESTATIONS

- **Fever** usually marks the onset of KS. Elevated temperature shows a remittent pattern, with spikes to 103° and even up to 105°. The average duration of the fever is 11 days.
- Seen in 75% of patients, **cervical lymphadenopathy** is the least common diagnostic feature of KS. It usually manifests as a single, enlarged, nonsuppurative lymph node on the side of the neck.

- **Cardiac involvement** is the most worrisome complication of KS. During the acute phase of the illness, tachycardia may develop, with gallop rhythm, subtle electrocardiographic changes, pericardia effusion, tricuspid insufficiency, or mitral regurgitation. Coronary artery aneurisms may result in thrombosis with subsequent infarction.

DIAGNOSIS

The diagnosis of KS is based on recognition of its clinical features and is supported by compatible laboratory findings; however, laboratory findings are nonspecific. None of the following diagnostic guidelines are in themselves diagnostic, but their presence may be helpful:

- Fever persisting 5 days or more
- Polymorphous rash
- Bilateral conjunctival injection
- Oral mucous membrane changes
- Cervical lymphadenopathy
- Changes of peripheral extremities: erythema of palms and soles, indurative edema of the hands and feet, desquamation of the fingertips

 ### DIFFERENTIAL DIAGNOSIS

- Staphylococcal or streptococcal toxic shock syndrome (see earlier)
- Scarlet fever (see earlier)
- Measles
- Febrile viral exanthems
- Hypersensitivity reactions (including Stevens–Johnson syndrome)

 ### MANAGEMENT

- Most children with KS are hospitalized for a complete workup and supportive care. Because high temperatures and irritability make feeding difficult, intravenous fluids are often needed for hydration.
- Children with evidence of cardiac disease may require intensive support.
- Once the diagnosis of KS has been established, therapy with intravenous γ-globulin and aspirin should be started.

 ### POINTS TO REMEMBER

- All patients with KS should have an echocardiogram during the acute illness and 3 to 6 weeks after the onset of fever.
- Prompt treatment with aspirin and intravenous γ-globulin significantly decreases the risk for cardiac complications.

 ### HELPFUL HINT

- KS should be considered in children with an unexplained fever lasting more than 5 days who have a polymorphous rash that may look like scarlet fever or measles and conjunctivitis without pus.

CHAPTER 10

Hair and Scalp Disorders Resulting in Hair Loss

Overview

Common baldness, or androgenic alopecia **(male- or female-pattern baldness),** is not a disease but a normal consequence of aging. In most, if not all, cultures, hair plays a powerful role in a person's psychosexual identity and self-image. It is not surprising that in our youth- and image-driven society, hair replacement and retention methods have taken on almost the status of a subspecialty in health care.

BASICS

Androgenic alopecia is a common noninflammatory, nonscarring condition that is seen more frequently in men than in women. It tends to be less apparent in women because hair loss in women is generally incomplete and begins at a later age.

The condition is genetically influenced (autosomal dominant with variable penetrance), and it is more common in whites than in Asians or blacks. Androgenic alopecia is caused by an androgenic action on hair follicles that shortens the anagen (growth) phase of the hair cycle and thus produces thinner, shorter hairs in a process known as miniaturization.

CLINICAL MANIFESTATIONS

- **In men,** this type of alopecia usually begins in late adolescence, with hair loss often starting at the parietal hairline (Figure 10.1).
- **In women,** the loss of hair is more subtle, and it tends to begin later, most often after menopause, but occasionally in the third or fourth decade of life (Figure 10.2).

DESCRIPTION AND DISTRIBUTION OF LESIONS

Androgenic alopecia produces two typical patterns of hair loss.

- **In men,** the process usually begins in an M-shaped pattern on the front and vertex of the head (this is often referred to as male-pattern baldness).
- **In women,** a "Christmas-tree," midparietal pattern (female-pattern baldness) is usually noted initially.

Hair loss may progress in both sexes but is often more extensive in men. Thus, in the end stages of androgenic alopecia, many men have only a fringe of remaining hair, whereas women tend to maintain the frontal hairline and do not become frankly bald.

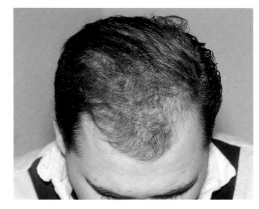

FIGURE 10.1 Male-pattern baldness is characterized by an M-shaped pattern of hair loss on the front and vertex of the head.

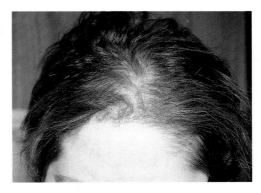

FIGURE 10.2 Female-pattern baldness occurs in a "Christmas-tree," midparietal pattern of decreasing hair loss toward the vertex (the "widened part"). The integrity of the frontal hairline is maintained.

DIAGNOSIS

The diagnosis of androgenic alopecia is generally based on the clinical pattern of baldness coupled with an absence of clues pointing to a specific disease that may cause hair loss.

 DIFFERENTIAL DIAGNOSIS

Other processes, however, should be considered. The differential diagnosis of androgenic alopecia in women includes the following:

Telogen Effluvium
- Patients have sudden, **diffuse shedding** of hair.
- There may be a history of an acute event, such as an illness or childbirth **(postpartum effluvium).**

Anagen Effluvium (Shedding of Growing Hairs)
- This may be associated with various agents, including anticancer drugs, anticoagulants, beta-blockers, angiotensin-converting enzyme inhibitors, oral contraceptives, oral retinoids, and radiation therapy (of the scalp).

Self-Induced Alopecia
- This may occur secondary to the use of hair straighteners or hot combs or as a result of trichotillomania *(compulsive hair pulling)*.

Other Diagnoses
Thyroid Disease
- Hair loss in association with thyroid disease is generally diffuse and may be seen on all parts of the body.
- In hypothyroidism, hair may become dull, coarse, and brittle.
- In hyperthyroidism, hairs are often fine and soft.

Androgen Excess
- Loss of hair on the head in association with hirsutism on other areas (face, chest, groin) in a male pattern, menstrual irregularities, infertility, or the sudden onset of acne may suggest a hormonal origin, such as an androgen-secreting tumor. (For a full discussion of this condition, see Chapter 11, "Hirsutism".)

Diffuse Alopecia Areata and Iron Deficiency Anemia and Insufficient Calories, Protein, or Vitamins
- These are rare causes of hair loss and should be considered in the appropriate clinical context.

MANAGEMENT

The following are components of the management of androgenic alopecia.

Women
- Ongoing emotional support is important.
- **Minoxidil** (2% solution, applied twice daily) may reduce shedding and may possibly contribute to some regrowth. (The 5% solution of minoxidil may be more effective, but it has not yet been approved for use in women.)
- Women with excess androgen may benefit from **systemic antiandrogen therapy** with agents such as spironolactone or oral contraceptives that decrease ovarian and adrenal androgen production, especially agents with a nonandrogenic progestin.
- **Hair transplantation,** using a micrografting technique in which a small incision is used to insert one or more donor hairs, is particularly effective in women, because they (unlike men) rarely become completely bald.

Men
- Minoxidil 5% solution **(Rogaine),** applied twice daily, may reduce shedding and may possibly contribute to some regrowth.
- Finasteride **(Propecia),** 1 mg per day, an agent which is also used for benign prostatic hypertrophy, is intended for use in men only.
- **Hair transplantation** may be helpful.

POINTS TO REMEMBER

Women and Hair Loss
- Evaluation of a female patient with androgenic alopecia may include a complete blood count and testing of thyroid-stimulating hormone and serum iron levels.
- Women with symptoms or signs of virilization should undergo a careful history and evaluation for an androgen-excess syndrome. These patients require hormonal studies and may need referral to an endocrinologist.

HELPFUL HINT

- A patient's anxiety regarding hair loss should be taken seriously by his or her health care provider. Hair loss should not simply be "brushed off" as an insignificant cosmetic complaint.

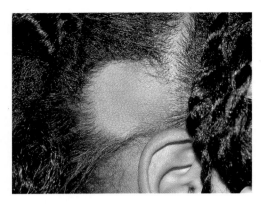

FIGURE 10.3 Alopecia areata. The hair loss is a round patch. Note the absence of scales or inflammation.

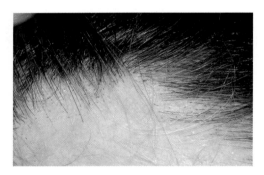

FIGURE 10.4 Alopecia areata. Note black, flecklike "exclamation mark" hairs at the periphery.

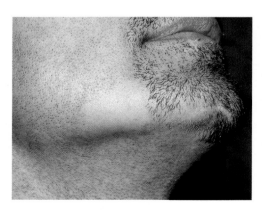

FIGURE 10.5 Alopecia areata. This man's alopecia areata is limited to his beard.

BASICS

A common, noninflammatory, idiopathic disorder, alopecia areata (AA) is characterized by well-circumscribed round or oval areas of nonscarring hair loss. Alopecia totalis is a loss of all or almost all scalp hair and eyebrows. Alopecia universalis refers to a total loss of body hair.

AA most commonly affects young adults and children. Occasionally, a family history of AA exists; often, onset is attributed to recent stress or a major life crisis.

The origin of AA is generally considered autoimmune, because biopsy findings demonstrate T-cell infiltrates surrounding the hair follicles and because AA is sometimes associated with other putative autoimmune disorders, such as the following:

- **Vitiligo**
- **Thyroid disease (Hashimoto's disease)**
- **Pernicious anemia**

DESCRIPTION OF LESIONS

- AA most commonly presents as oval, round, or geometric patches of alopecia (Figure 10.3).
- On occasion, a hand lens may reveal tiny "exclamation mark" hairs at the periphery of lesions (Figure 10.4).
- Increased friction (not the expected smoothness) is felt on palpation of lesional skin because of the loss of vellus hairs.

DISTRIBUTION OF LESIONS

- Lesions are most often found on the scalp, eyebrows, eyelashes, and areas of the face that bear hair, such as the beard (Figure 10.5) or mustache on men.
- The entire scalp **(alopecia totalis)** may be involved, or even the entire body **(alopecia universalis),** including pubic, axillary, and nasal hair (Figure 10.6).
- Nails may demonstrate a characteristic pitting ("railroad tracks").

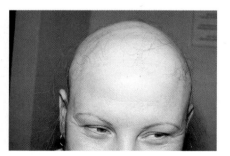

FIGURE 10.6 Alopecia areata (alopecia universalis). This patient has lost most of her eyebrows, which she colors in with an eyebrow pencil. She also lacks eyelashes, pubic hair, axillary hair, and hair on her extremities.

CLINICAL MANIFESTATIONS

- There is usually asymptomatic shedding of hair, which is often discovered by the patient's hairdresser or a family member.
- Frequently, hair spontaneously regrows; however, a recurrence of hair loss may be seen in 30% of patients who had experienced regrowth. Regrowing hair is initially thin and sometimes white (vitiliginous) (Figure 10.7).
- A poorer prognosis is associated with extensive alopecia, an atopic history, and chronicity.
- Alopecia universalis is generally refractory to therapy and usually lasts a lifetime; spontaneous regrowth is rare.

DIAGNOSIS

The diagnosis of AA is generally based on its clinical appearance; however, a scalp biopsy may be performed if the diagnosis is in doubt.

 DIFFERENTIAL DIAGNOSIS

Tinea Capitis (see Chapter 7, "Superficial Fungal Infections")

- This is seen most frequently in African-American children.
- The scalp is often scaly, itchy, and inflamed.
- The diagnosis is confirmed when the potassium hydroxide examination or fungal culture is positive.

Androgenic Alopecia

- The hair loss is gradual and has a characteristic male or female pattern.

Telogen Effluvium (see later)

- The hair loss is diffuse.
- There is often a history of antecedent illness or childbirth, for example.

Traction Alopecia and Hot-Comb Alopecia

Both conditions are discussed later in this chapter.

Other Diagnoses

Trichotillomania

Trichotillomania is also known as compulsive hair pulling (Figure 10.8).

- This is seen most often in young girls.
- Hairs tend to be broken at different lengths.
- There is an asymmetric loss of scalp hair.

Secondary Syphilis (see Figure 19.19)

This should always be considered in cases of unexplained hair loss.

- The hair loss is referred to as "moth-eaten" in appearance.
- Serologic tests for syphilis are generally reactive.

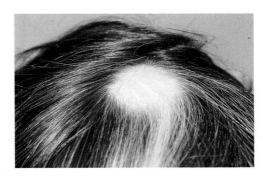

FIGURE 10.7 Alopecia areata (regrowing hair). In this patient with alopecia areata, clusters of hair regrew after intralesional triamcinolone acetonide injections. Some of the regrown hairs are white (vitiliginous).

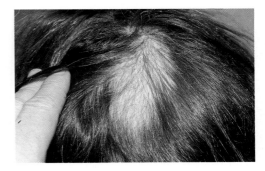

FIGURE 10.8 Trichotillomania. This condition is seen most often in young girls. Hairs tend to be broken at different lengths. The areas of alopecia are not completely devoid of hair.

MANAGEMENT

- Because mild cases of AA often show spontaneous regrowth, therapy is often unnecessary.
- The daily application of superpotent **topical steroids,** such as clobetasol cream 0.05%, may speed hair regrowth. For increased drug penetration, potent topical steroids, such as fluocinonide cream 0.05%, may be applied, occluded with a plastic shower cap, and left on overnight.
- If necessary, **intralesional steroid injections** into the alopecic patches with triamcinolone acetonide may be administered every 6 to 8 weeks.

Further Treatment Modalities

The numerous treatment modalities for severe AA that have been tried over the years are a reflection of the finding that few are very effective. The success rates associated with the following measures have ranged from no response to varying degrees of partial success:

- **Irritant therapy** involves using a topical anthralin (a coal tar derivative) preparation.
- **Topical minoxidil** in a 2% or 5% concentration, scalp massage, heat, aloe vera, vitamins, hypnotherapy, PUVA (oral psoralens combined with exposure to ultraviolet light in the A range), topical cyclosporine, and immunotherapy by induction of contact dermatitis with chemical compounds have all been tried.
- The most important part of widespread AA management is providing **emotional support** to the patient.

POINTS TO REMEMBER

- Alopecia totalis and universalis, the most severe forms of AA, generally spark great emotional problems in patients and their families.
- Consider workup for other diseases (e.g., thyroid disease) that may be suggested by the history or examination.

HELPFUL HINT

- The National Alopecia Areata Foundation is an excellent resource for information and can direct patients to AA support groups and information about wigs, for example. It can be reached at the following address:

  National Alopecia Areata Foundation
  710 C Street, Suite 11
  San Rafael, CA 94901-3853
  (415) 456-4644; fax: (415) 456-4274
  http://www.alopeciaareata.com

SEE PATIENT HANDOUT, PAGE 471

BASICS

Hair follicles show intermittent activity. Each hair grows to a maximum length and is retained for a period without further growth **(telogen).** It then goes through a **catagen** phase, is shed, and is replaced by a growing **anagen** hair (see Illustration 11.1).

Telogen effluvium is a temporary sudden, diffuse, shedding of "resting hairs." Its causes include major illness, trauma, surgery, "crash" dieting, and emotional stress. When telogen effluvium occurs in women, it may be associated with giving birth *(postpartum effluvium)*, aborted pregnancy, or the discontinuation of oral contraceptives.

The precipitating event usually precedes hair loss by 6 to 16 weeks, which is the time required for a catagen hair to become a telogen hair. The marked loss of hair can manifest as a blockage of a bathtub drain, or it may be more subtle and chronic.

DESCRIPTION OF LESIONS

- This diffuse (nonpatterned) alopecia is usually not obvious to the clinician.

DISTRIBUTION OF LESIONS

- Alopecia is diffuse.

CLINICAL MANIFESTATIONS

- Patients have noninflammatory, asymptomatic, and rapid shedding of hair.
- Hair is seen on pillows, in combs and brushes, and in the bathtub (Figure 10.9).
- Hair regrowth occurs within 1 year, but hair may not grow back completely.

DIAGNOSIS

- This diagnosis is made by history, because the diffuse loss of telogen effluvium is barely perceptible to the clinician.
- There is a loss of 400 or more hairs per day (normal shedding is 40 to 100 hairs a day).

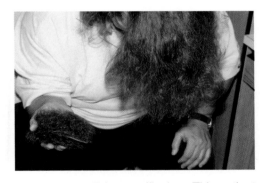

FIGURE 10.9 Telogen effluvium. This patient presented with a small plastic bag full of hair that had been shed over the course of one month.

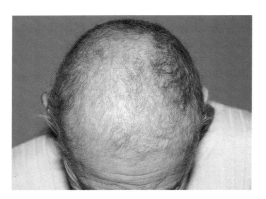

FIGURE 10.10 Anagen effluvium. This patient's alopecia resulted from chemotherapy for lung cancer. Her hair loss was diffuse, and her hair is now regrowing.

Androgenic Alopecia
• This has a patterned distribution.

Anagen Effluvium Secondary to Drugs
• It is more diffuse and more rapid than telogen effluvium (Figure 10.10).
• Cancer chemotherapy and immunotherapy drugs are causes.

MANAGEMENT
• The underlying cause is treated, if possible.
• The patient should be reassured that hair tends to grow back normally.

POINT TO REMEMBER
• A careful history should be taken, to look for antecedent illness, recent childbirth, ingestion of drugs, or trauma 3 to 4 months before the onset of rapid alopecia.

HELPFUL HINTS
• Anticoagulants, thyroid medications, beta-blockers, angiotensin-converting enzyme inhibitors, heavy metals, oral contraceptives, lithium, and retinoids may also be associated with hair loss.
• When the cause of telogen effluvium is not apparent, a complete blood count and thyroid-stimulating hormone, VDRL, and antinuclear antibody tests should be obtained.

BASICS

Some African-American women use grooming techniques to straighten the natural kinkiness of their hair. Traumatic alopecia is a common cause of hair loss in these women. It may result from the use of hair reshaping products (e.g., relaxers, straighteners, hot combs, foam rollers, and permanent wave products) or hair braiding methods (e.g., cornrows) that are popular in the black community.

It is a common misconception that these techniques are used solely to make hair more becoming and stylish; in fact, they are used as much to make hair more manageable. **Traction alopecia, chemical alopecia,** and **hot-comb alopecia** (also known as **follicular degeneration syndrome**) may be caused by the use any of these methods alone or in combination and may ultimately result in permanent alopecia.

The persistent physical stress of traction injury caused by tight rollers and tight braiding or ponytails causes hair loss. In addition, using hair dryers (with resultant overheating of hair shafts), vigorous combing or brushing, and bleaching can also contribute to hair breakage.

Chemicals such as thioglycolates, which are found in commercial styling products, create curls by destroying the disulfide bonds of keratin. These chemicals may also have irritant effects on the scalp that can result in hair shaft damage, as well as inflammation of the scalp and loss of hair roots. Hot-comb alopecia results from the excessive use of pomades with a hot comb or iron. (Hot combs or pomades alone do not cause permanent alopecia.) On contact with the hot comb or hot iron (i.e., marcelling iron), the pomade liquefies and drips down the hair shaft into the follicle, and it results in a chronic inflammatory folliculitis that, in time, can lead to scarring alopecia and permanent hair loss.

DESCRIPTION OF LESIONS

- **Traction alopecia** is manifested by a symmetric pattern of hair loss, with broken hairs. A characteristic border of residual hairs is often at the distal margin of the hair loss (Figures 10.11 and 10.12). Traction alopecia may result in permanent scarring alopecia.
- **Chemical or hot-comb alopecia** may cause scaling, pustules, and itching. Either disorder may result in temporary or permanent alopecia.

DISTRIBUTION OF LESIONS

- **Traction pattern:** Alopecia is evident at the temples and along the frontal hairline. Hair loss later extends to the vertex and occipital areas.
- **Chemical or hot-comb pattern:** Hair loss is more irregular (less symmetric) and reflects the areas where the chemicals and hot comb were applied (Figure 10.13).
- **A combination of these patterns** may be seen if both traction and hot combs or chemicals are used.

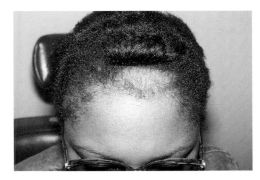

FIGURE 10.11 Traction alopecia. This woman's alopecia is the result of the use of tight curlers: Note the symmetric loss of hair in a frontotemporal distribution. Also note the "relaxed" curl that was chemically straightened.

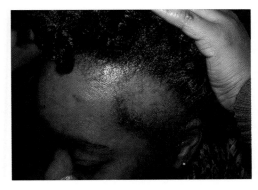

FIGURE 10.12 Traction alopecia. Note the fringe of residual hairs at the distal margin of alopecia. These hairs were too short to be "grabbed" by the hair curlers.

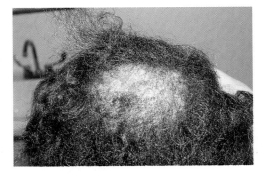

FIGURE 10.13 Chemical or hot-comb pattern of alopecia. The continuous use of a hot comb and chemical relaxers resulted in permanent hair loss at the vertex of this woman's scalp.

CLINICAL MANIFESTATIONS

Early hair loss is usually asymptomatic and gradual. Later, particularly if chemical relaxers and hot combs are used, scaling, pustules, and itching may occur and may result in scarring alopecia. The diagnosis is based on the clinical appearance, a history of hair reshaping techniques, and a scalp biopsy, if necessary.

 DIFFERENTIAL DIAGNOSIS

Systemic Lupus Erythematosus
- There is a diffuse, sudden loss of hair.
- The patient's antinuclear antibody test generally is positive, and other signs and symptoms of lupus are evident.

Discoid Lupus Erythematosus (see Chapter 25, "Cutaneous Manifestations of Systemic Disease")
- The patient has focal areas of scarring alopecia.

Sarcoidosis
- Hair loss may closely resemble that of traumatic alopecia.
- However, other signs and symptoms of sarcoidosis are usually apparent. A scalp biopsy of lesional skin may be necessary to distinguish sarcoidosis from traumatic alopecia.

Other Diagnoses
Alopecia Areata
- Hair loss occurs in round or oval patches that are smooth and non-inflamed (see the description earlier).

Secondary Syphilis
- Hair loss has a "moth-eaten" appearance.
- Serologic tests for syphilis are generally reactive.

Tinea Capitis
- This is more commonly seen in African-American children.

MANAGEMENT

Discontinuance of styling practices may result in an abatement of hair loss and partial hair regrowth, depending on the length of insult to the roots; even complete regrowth is possible if the hair loss is managed early in its course. If the patient decides to continue with her styling practices, she should:

- Use chemicals only on the hair and not directly on the scalp.
- Use looser wrapping, to produce less tension on the hair roots.
- Fix hair into braids that are larger and looser.
- Unbraid the hair every 2 weeks.

POINTS TO REMEMBER

- Traumatic alopecia is common in African-American and Afro-Caribbean women.
- It is frequently misdiagnosed as alopecia areata by health care providers who are unfamiliar with their patients' styling practices.
- Other conditions, such as cutaneous lupus and sarcoidosis, may closely resemble or occur concomitantly with traumatic alopecia.
- Clinicians should always ask patients with hair loss what they routinely do to style and manage their hair.

PSEUDOFOLLICULITIS BARBAE AND ACNE KELOIDALIS

Overview

Hair follicle problems are very common in men and women of African-American and Hispanic origin who have tightly curled hair. Postadolescent black men, in particular, experience "shaving bumps" (**pseudofolliculitis barbae**) and a characteristic acnelike, scarring condition located on the occiput referred to as **acne keloidalis**. Less commonly, severe, scarring alopecia can occur on the scalp (**folliculitis decalvans**).

These follicular disorders are believed to be the result of a delayed hypersensitivity reaction targeting the hair follicle that often results in scarring alopecia (**cicatricial alopecia**). The diagnosis of these conditions is generally made on the basis of their clinical appearance.

PSEUDOFOLLICULITIS BARBAE

BASICS

Tightly coiled hairs emerge from curved hair follicles (Illustration 10.1). When shaved, the hair becomes a sharp tip that curves downward as it grows and reenters the epidermis, or the sharpened hair may grow parallel to the skin and penetrate it. Furthermore, newly erupting hairs from below may pierce and aggravate areas that are already inflamed. Thus, growing hairs act as traumatic vehicles that produce an inflammatory foreign body–like reaction.

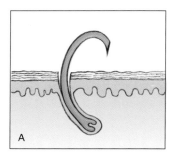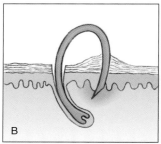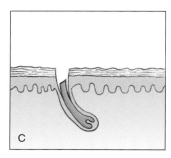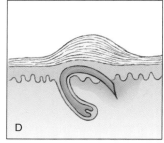

Illustration 10.1   Pseudofolliculitis barbae: "razor bumps." *Left:* Extrafollicular penetration. A curly hair grows from a sharply curved follicle. When shaved, the hair is left with a sharp point. As this hair grows, the sharp tip curves back and pierces the skin. *Right:* Transfollicular penetration. Alternatively, when hairs are cut too closely, the hairs penetrate the side of the follicle. Both types of follicular reentry cause a foreign body–like reaction (papule). (Modified from Crutchfield CE 3rd. The causes and treatment of pseudofolliculitis barbae. *CUTIS* 1998; 61:351–356, with permission.)

DESCRIPTION OF LESIONS

- On close inspection, tight, curly hairs that have been sharpened by shaving penetrate the skin are noted.
- Inflammatory papules and pustules ensue (Figure 10.14).
- Ultimately, persistent flesh-colored papules that represent hypertrophic scars and postinflammatory pigmented lesions become prominent clinical features.

DISTRIBUTION OF LESIONS

- Lesions are seen on the beard, particularly on the neck and the submental areas.

 DIFFERENTIAL DIAGNOSIS

- Acne vulgaris
- Bacterial folliculitis

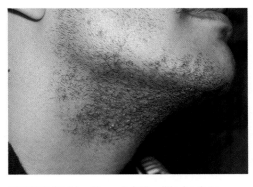

FIGURE 10.14 Pseudofolliculitis barbae. Tight, curly hairs that have been sharpened by shaving penetrate the skin. Inflammatory papules and pustules that resemble acne are evident.

 MANAGEMENT

Prevention

- Discontinuance of shaving is only partially helpful; however, this is generally not a choice desired by most patients.
- Avoid close shaving by using a guarded razor ("PFB Bump Fighter"). This razor is covered with a plastic coating that prevents the razor from contacting the skin directly. The use of an electric razor is another method that reduces the closeness of the shave.
- Hairs may be lifted with a fine needle or a toothpick before they penetrate the skin (Figure 10.15).
- Patients should be advised not to pluck hairs because new hairs will again grow from below and will penetrate a site that is already inflamed.

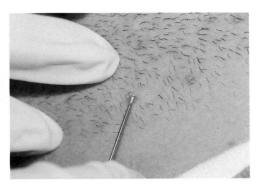

FIGURE 10.15 Pseudofolliculitis barbae. A curled hair is lifted with a fine needle after it had penetrated the skin.

Treatment

- Nonfluorinated topical steroids are used for inflammation and itching.
- Used once daily, topical antibiotics such as erythromycin 2% (Akne-mycin) ointment or Benzaclin (a combination of clindamycin and benzoyl peroxide) gel often reduce inflammation.
- Systemic antibiotics such as minocycline are helpful when marked inflammation and pustulation are present.
- Chemical depilatories such as Magic Shave and Royal Crown powders are effective in removing and softening hairs; the main disadvantages are that they are irritating and they have an unpleasant odor.
- Hair destruction using an extended pulse-width laser has been shown to be effective.
- Eflornithine hydrochloride 13.9% (Vaniqa) is an enzyme inhibitor that slows hair growth (see Chapter 11, "Hirsutism").
- Electrolysis is difficult to use on inflammatory foci, but it can be partially effective as an adjunctive treatment method.

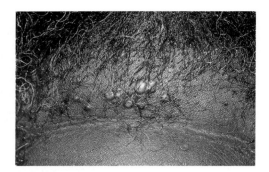

FIGURE 10.16 Acne keloidalis. Hypertrophic scarring and flesh-colored papules are seen in this patient.

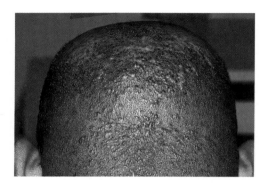

FIGURE 10.17 Acne keloidalis and scalp folliculitis. Here the problem extends to the adjacent scalp.

ACNE KELOIDALIS (FOLLICULITIS KELOIDALIS)

BASICS

The name acne keloidalis is actually a misnomer. It has nothing to do with acne—it is actually a type of folliculitis. The pathogenesis of acne keloidalis is similar to that of pseudofolliculitis barbae, in which coiled hairs produce a **reentry phenomenon** that results in characteristic features.

DESCRIPTION OF LESIONS

- Initially, inflammatory papules and pustules are noted.
- Ultimately, hypertrophic scarring occurs, characterized by flesh-colored papules (Figure 10.16) and possibly keloid formation.

DISTRIBUTION OF LESIONS

- This condition is characteristically seen in the occipital area, but it can extend to the adjacent or the entire scalp and thus may be indistinguishable from **folliculitis decalvans** (Figure 10.17).

MANAGEMENT

- Potent topical or intralesional steroids (5 to 10 mg/mL) help to decrease itching and inflammation.
- Topical antibiotics are used when papules and pustules are present.
- A systemic antibiotic such as minocycline seems to be helpful because of its antiinflammatory effect.
- Surgical treatment is reserved for extreme cases and may result in worse scarring.

POINTS TO REMEMBER

- When present in these patients, bacterial folliculitis is usually the result of secondary, not primary, pathogens.
- Prevention of these disorders depends on avoidance of close "clipper" shaves and haircuts.

CHAPTER 11

Hirsutism

Overview

Hirsutism is defined as the excessive growth of thick, dark hair in locations where hair growth in women is normally minimal or absent. Such male-pattern growth of terminal body hair usually occurs in androgen-stimulated locations, such as the face, chest, and areolae.

Although the terms *hirsutism* and *hypertrichosis* are often used interchangeably, hypertrichosis actually refers to excess hair (terminal or vellus) in areas that are not predominantly androgen dependent. Whether a given patient is hirsute is often difficult to judge because hair growth varies among individual women and across ethnic groups. What is considered hirsutism in one culture may be considered normal in another. For example, women from the Mediterranean and Indian subcontinents have more facial and body hair than do women from Asia, sub-Saharan Africa, and Northern Europe. Dark-haired, darkly pigmented whites of either sex tend to be more hirsute than blond or fair-skinned persons.

BASICS

Hirsutism, by itself, is a benign condition primarily of cosmetic concern. However, when hirsutism in women is accompanied by masculinizing signs or symptoms, particularly when these arise well after puberty, it may be a manifestation of a more serious underlying disorder, such as an ovarian or adrenal neoplasm. Fortunately, such disorders are rare.

Pathogenesis

Hirsutism can be caused by abnormally high androgen levels or by hair follicles that are more sensitive to normal androgen levels. Therefore, increased hair growth is often seen in patients with endocrine disorders characterized by hyperandrogenism. These disorders may be caused by abnormalities of either the ovaries or the adrenal glands.

Cycles of Hair Growth

Hair grows in long cycles over many months: an **anagen** (active) phase (Illustration 11.1) is followed by **catogen** (degenerative phase), then **a telogen** (resting) phase, with different hairs alternating phases. The anagen and telogen phases are hormonally regulated. During the telogen phase, the hair shaft eventually separates from the follicle and falls out.

The amount of free testosterone—the biologically active androgen that, after conversion to dihydrotestosterone, causes hair growth—is regulated by sex hormone-binding globulin (SHBG). Lower levels of SHBG increase the availability of free testosterone. SHBG decreases in response to the following:

- Exogenous androgens
- Certain disorders that affect androgen levels, such as polycystic ovary syndrome (PCOS)
- Cushing's syndrome
- Obesity
- Hyperinsulinemia
- Hyperprolactinemia
- Excess growth hormone

Conversely, SHBG increases with higher estrogen levels, such as those that occur during oral contraceptive therapy. The resulting increased SHBG levels lower the activity of circulating testosterone.

For circulating testosterone to exert its stimulatory effects on the hair follicle, it must first be converted into its more potent follicle-active metabolite, dihydrotestosterone. This conversion is performed by the enzyme 5-α-reductase, which is found in the hair follicle.

Testosterone stimulates growth, thereby increasing size and intensifying the pigmentation of hair. Estrogens act in an opposite manner, by slowing growth and producing finer, lighter hairs. Progesterone has minimal effect on hair growth.

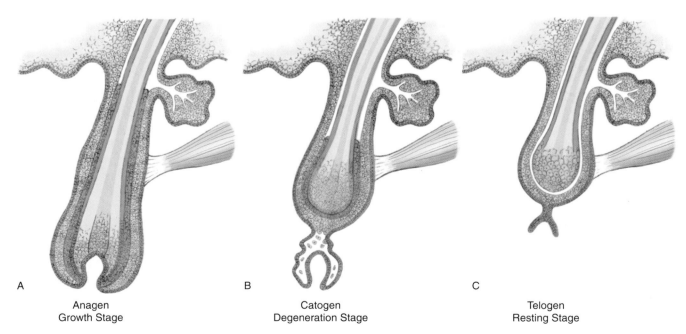

A Anagen Growth Stage

B Catogen Degeneration Stage

C Telogen Resting Stage

Illustration 11.1 (Modified from Sams WM Jr., Lynch PJ, eds. Structure and function of the skin. In: *Principles and Practice of Dermatology.* New York: Churchill Livingstone, 1990:8, with permission.)

DISORDERS ASSOCIATED WITH HIRSUTISM

Polycystic Ovary Syndrome (PCOS)

The most common cause of androgen excess and hirsutism is PCOS. Virilization is minimal and hirsutism is often prominent in patients with this disorder. PCOS is characterized by **menstrual irregularities, dysmenorrhea, occasional glucose intolerance** and **hyperinsulinemia,** and, often, **obesity.** The hyperinsulinemia is believed to hyperstimulate the ovaries into producing excess androgens.

Women with PCOS may show other cutaneous manifestations of androgen excess in addition to hirsutism, such as **recalcitrant acne** (Figure 11.1), **acanthosis nigricans,** and **alopecia** on the crown area of the scalp (a pattern that contrasts with the bitemporal and vertex androgenic alopecia seen in men).

Hirsutism may also be seen in the following ovarian conditions, most of which are associated with virilization:

- Luteoma of pregnancy
- Arrhenoblastomas
- Leydig cell tumors
- Hilar cell tumors
- Thecal cell tumors

Familial Hirsutism

This type of hirsutism is not associated with androgen excess. Familial hirsutism is both typical and natural in certain populations, such as some women of Mediterranean or Middle Eastern ancestry (Figure 11.2).

Drug-Induced Hirsutism

Drugs that can induce hirsutism by their inherent androgenic effects include dehydroepiandrosterone sulfate (DHEAS), testosterone, danazol, and anabolic steroids. The current low-dose oral contraceptives are less likely to cause hirsutism than were previous formulations.

Adrenal Causes

- Children with **congenital adrenal hyperplasia,** the classic form of adrenal hyperplasia, may exhibit hirsutism. Such children may be born with ambiguous genitalia and symptoms of salt wasting and failure to thrive, and they may develop masculine features.
- **Late-onset congenital adrenal hyperplasia** affects about 1% to 5% of hyperandrogenic women. Although these patients have clinical features that resemble PCOS, they manifest no salt-wasting symptoms and may not develop signs of virilization and menstrual irregularities until puberty or adulthood (Figure 11.3).
- **Cushing's syndrome** is a noncongenital form of adrenal hyperplasia. It is characterized by an excess of adrenal cortisol production.
- **Androgen-producing adrenal tumors** are extremely rare.

Other Associated Disorders

Other less common but potentially serious disorders associated with hirsutism include anorexia nervosa, acromegaly, hypothyroidism, porphyria, and cancer.

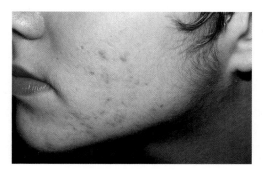

FIGURE 11.1 Hirsutism related to polycystic ovary syndrome. This is the most common cause of androgen excess and hirsutism. Note the lesions of acne.

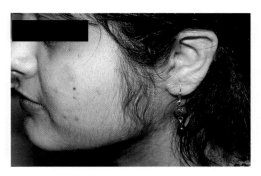

FIGURE 11.2 Familial hirsutism. As seen in this Pakistani woman, familial hirsutism is both typical and natural in certain populations.

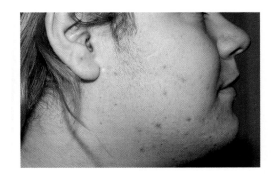

FIGURE 11.3 Hirsutism in an 18-year-old woman with late-onset congenital adrenal hyperplasia. Clinical features are similar to those of polycystic ovary syndrome: acne, hirsutism, menstrual irregularities, and obesity.

Idiopathic Hirsutism

The few hirsute women who do not have a familial form of hirsutism or any detectable hormonal abnormality are usually given a diagnosis of idiopathic, or end-organ, hirsutism. Such patients have normal menses, normal-sized ovaries, no evidence of adrenal or ovarian tumors or dysfunction, and no significant elevations of plasma testosterone or androstenedione.

Antiandrogen therapy may improve hirsutism in some idiopathic cases. This suggests that this form of hirsutism may be androgen induced. It is believed that many of these women may have mild or early PCOS and androgen levels in the upper normal ranges.

CLINICAL MANIFESTATIONS

The onset of hirsutism can take one of the following forms:

- For example, in women with familial hirsutism, it often appears during puberty.
- Excess growth of facial hair is seen in elderly postmenopausal women and may be caused by unopposed androgen.
- It appears rather abruptly when an androgen-secreting tumor arises.

DESCRIPTION OF LESIONS

Excess terminal hair grows in a masculine pattern. Other accompanying signs and symptoms to be looked for may include the following:

- Acanthosis nigricans
- Obesity
- Pelvic mass
- Signs or symptoms of virility
- Signs or symptoms of Cushing's syndrome
- Acne
- Alopecia

DISTRIBUTION OF LESIONS

A woman with hirsutism has excess terminal hair in a masculine pattern in key anatomic sites, including the following:

- Face, particularly the moustache, beard, and temple areas
- Chest, areolae, linea alba, upper back, lower back, buttocks, inner thighs, and external genitalia

DIAGNOSIS

Workup for Hirsutism

After familial and drug-induced causes for hirsutism have been ruled out, hirsutism resulting from androgen excess is considered.

Testosterone Levels

- Initial screening for total or free testosterone often determines whether further testing is necessary.
- Total testosterone is mostly protein bound and poorly reflects the fluctuations of androgen metabolism, but its level does suggest the amount of SHBG present. Low levels of SHBG occur in the presence of excess androgen and insulin.
- There is no direct correlation between the level of total testosterone and the degree of hirsutism, because hirsutism is caused by the action of dihydrotestosterone, the more potent testosterone metabolite.
- Elevated free serum testosterone levels (greater than 80 ng/dL) are found in most women with anovulation and hirsutism. In most cases, when total testosterone is greater than 200 ng/dL (greater than 100 ng/dL in postmenopausal women), a tumor workup is indicated.
- This workup includes a pelvic examination and an ultrasound scan, which are usually adequate to diagnose PCOS. If these tests are negative, an adrenal computed tomography scan is obtained.

Dehydroepiandrosterone and Its Sulfate Form, Dehydroepiandrosterone Sulfate, and Androstenedione

- In many patients with hirsutism, DHEAS is elevated. (Serum DHEAS determinations are generally used as a marker of adrenal androgen output because serum DHEAS concentrations fluctuate less with the menstrual cycle and diurnal changes in serum cortisol levels than do concentrations of dehydroepiandrosterone.) Moderate elevations suggest an adrenal origin of the hirsutism. A tumor workup is indicated in most patients with DHEAS levels greater than 700 µg/dL (400 µg/dL in postmenopausal women). An increase of this magnitude is usually the result of adrenal hyperplasia, rather than the extremely rare adrenal carcinomas.
- A serum androstenedione level greater than 100 ng/dL suggests an ovarian or adrenal neoplasm.
- These tests, in combination with a testosterone measurement, may provide clues to the source of excessive androgen production. For example, high levels of testosterone and androstenedione that are accompanied by normal levels of DHEAS indicate that the ovaries, and not the adrenals, are producing the excess androgen.

Further Testing

Expensive hormonal laboratory tests for a woman with simple hirsutism are usually not cost-effective. However, if a woman shows a constellation of virilizing signs or symptoms, such as infrequent or absent menses, acne, deepening of the voice, male-pattern balding, increased muscle mass, increased libido, and clitoral hypertrophy, she should be referred to an endocrinologist.

 DIFFERENTIAL DIAGNOSIS

- **Drug-induced hirsutism** should be distinguished from drug-induced hypertrichosis, in which a uniform growth of fine hair appears over extensive areas of the trunk, hands, and face. This growth is not dependent on androgen.
- **Precipitating drugs** include phenytoin, minoxidil, diazoxide, cyclosporine, penicillamine, high-dose corticosteroids, phenothiazines, acetazolamide, and hexachlorobenzene. The exact mode of action is not known, but presumably these agents exert their effects independent of androgens.

MANAGEMENT

Overview

Treatment of hirsutism is unnecessary if no abnormal origin can be diagnosed and if the patient does not find the hirsutism cosmetically objectionable. Treatment should be offered, however, if an underlying disorder is identified or if the patient is troubled by the hair growth.

Management depends on the underlying cause. For example, non–androgen-dependent excess hair, such as hypertrichosis, is treated primarily with physical hair removal methods. In contrast, those patients who have androgen-dependent hirsutism may require a combination of physical hair removal and medical antiandrogen therapy.

As an alternative to hair removal, simple bleaching of hair is an inexpensive method that works well when hirsutism is not too excessive. Bleaches lighten the color of the hair so that it is less noticeable.

Hair Removal
Depilation

Depilatories remove hair from the surface of the skin. Depilatory methods include ordinary shaving and the use of chemicals, such as thioglycolic acid.

Shaving removes all hairs, but it is immediately followed by growth of hairs that were previously in anagen; as these hairs grow in, they produce rough stubble. There is no evidence that shaving increases the growth or coarseness of subsequent hair growth. Most women, however, prefer not to shave their facial hair.

Chemical depilation may be best suited for treatment of large hairy areas in patients who are unable to afford more expensive treatments, such as electrolysis and laser epilation. Chemical depilatories separate the hair from its follicle by reducing the sulfide bonds that are found in abundance in hairs. Irritant reactions and folliculitis may result.

Temporary Epilation

Epilation involves the removal of the intact hair with its root. **Plucking or tweezing** is widely performed. This method may result in irritation, damage to the hair follicle, folliculitis, hyperpigmentation, and scarring.

Waxing entails the melting of waxes that are applied to the skin. When the wax cools and sets, it is abruptly peeled off the skin, and embedded hair is removed with it. This method is painful and sometimes results in folliculitis. Repetitive waxing may produce miniaturization of hairs, and, over the long run, it may permanently reduce the number of hairs.

Certain natural sugars, long used in parts of the Middle East, are becoming popular in place of waxes. They appear to epilate as effectively as, but less traumatically than, waxing.

Threading, a method used in some Arab countries, is a technique in which cotton threads are used to pull out hairs by their roots. Home epilating devices that remove hair by a rotary or frictional method are available. Both methods may produce traumatic folliculitis.

Radiation therapy was a popular method of hair removal in the past. However, it has fallen out of favor and is no longer acceptable.

Permanent Epilation

Techniques of permanent epilation include **electrolysis, thermolysis,** and **laser epilation.**

Electrolysis and Thermolysis

Hair destruction by electrolysis, thermolysis, or a combination of both is performed with a fine, flexible electrical wire that produces an electrical current after it is introduced down the hair shaft. Thermolysis (diathermy) uses a high-frequency alternating current and is much faster than the traditional electrolysis method, which uses a direct galvanic current. Electrolysis and thermolysis are slow processes that can be used on all skin and hair colors, but multiple treatments are required. Electrolysis and thermolysis can be uncomfortable and may produce folliculitis, pseudofolliculitis, and postinflammatory pigmentary changes in the skin.

Laser Epilation

Lasers can treat larger areas and can do so faster than electrolysis and thermolysis. They have skin-cooling mechanisms that minimize epidermal destruction during the procedure. Skin and hair color often determine

(continued)

MANGEMENT *(continued)*

whether a laser should be used. Lasers are most effective on dark hairs on fair-skinned people. In such patients, lighter skin does not compete with darker hairs for the laser, which selectively targets the pigment, melanin. In dark-skinned people, a newer approach that delivers more energy to the hairs over a longer period may prove safe and effective.

As with electrolysis and thermolysis, multiple treatments are necessary for long-term hair destruction. Folliculitis, pseudofolliculitis, discomfort, and pigmentary changes may result from laser therapy. It remains to be proved whether lasers are more effective in permanent hair removal than the more traditional methods. They are certainly more costly.

Pharmacologic Treatment

In general, pharmacologic treatments of hirsutism are selected based on the underlying cause. Medications (antiandrogens) are often administered while cosmetic hair removal techniques are being used. All these drugs must be given continuously because when they are stopped, androgens will revert to their former levels. The following medications are all absolutely contraindicated for use during pregnancy because of the risk for feminization of a male fetus:

- Ovarian suppression (oral contraceptives)
- Androgen receptor blockade and inhibition (spironolactone, flutamide, and cyproterone acetate)
- Adrenal suppression (oral corticosteroids)
- 5-α-reductase inhibition (finasteride)

These agents can be used singly or in combination.

New Treatments

- **Eflornithine hydrochloride** cream 13.9% (Vaniqa) is a prescription topical cream that acts as a growth inhibitor, not a depilatory. The agent inhibits ornithine decarboxylase, an enzyme required for hair growth. It is indicated for the reduction of unwanted facial hair in women. Continued twice-daily use for at least 4 to 8 weeks is necessary before effectiveness is noted.
- **Metformin (Glucophage)** reduces insulin levels, and this change, in turn, reduces the ovarian testosterone levels by competitive inhibition of the ovarian insulin receptors. This drug is effective in treating hirsutism in women with PCOS.

  POINT TO REMEMBER

- Androgen-stimulated excessive hair growth may be a marker for androgen excess and may occasionally signal a potentially serious underlying metabolic disorder or potentially fatal neoplasm.

Disorders of the Mouth, Lips, and Tongue

Overview

Oral mucous membrane lesions are often clues to the presence of systemic illnesses, such as acquired immunodeficiency syndrome (AIDS), syphilis, and systemic lupus erythematosus. They may also be helpful in diagnosing dermatologic conditions, including lichen planus and pemphigus. Lesions such as "canker sores" are often seen as isolated phenomena, but may also be an accompaniment or a precursor to a symptom complex, such as seen in Behçet's syndrome or ulcerative colitis.

It is often difficult to make a clinical diagnosis in the oral cavity. Lesions may resemble normal variants, or they may look like each other. Common manifestations include:

- Blisters, erosions, and ulcers
- Whitish plaques
- Pigmentary changes
- Neoplasms
- Cystic lesions

Inflammatory oral lesions—particularly those that are bullous—rarely remain intact and unruptured. Instead, such lesions usually become erosions and ulcers by the time clinicians see them, adding to the difficulty of diagnosis.

APHTHOUS STOMATITIS

BASICS

Commonly known as *canker sores*, aphthous stomatitis lesions (aphthous ulcers) are a common, recurrent problem consisting of shallow erosions of the mucous membranes. They are seen in children and adults and appear to be more common in women than men. Aphthous stomatitis has no known cause, but an immune mechanism is considered the most likely contributory factor.

Most cases heal spontaneously, only to recur unexpectedly. Patients often ascribe recurrences to psychological stress or local trauma. Oral erosions that are indistinguishable from aphthous stomatitis are sometimes seen in primary HSV infections.

DESCRIPTION OF LESIONS

- The lesions of aphthous stomatitis are small (2 to 5 mm), shallow, well-demarcated, punched-out erosions.
- Lesions typically have a ring of erythema, with a gray or yellowish center (Figure 12.1).

DISTRIBUTION OF LESIONS

- Lesions may be seen on the buccal, labial, and gingival mucosa and the tongue.

CLINICAL MANIFESTATIONS

- The lesions are usually painful.
- They tend to heal in 4 to 14 days, a duration similar to that of HSV lesions.
- Patients with human immunodeficiency virus (HIV) or Behçet's disease may develop aphthous stomatitis lesions that are larger and more persistent, painful, and extensive than are those seen in other patients (Figure 12.2).

DIAGNOSIS

- The diagnosis is made clinically.
- Most intraoral ulcers in immunocompetent patients are canker sores, not HSV lesions.

 ### DIFFERENTIAL DIAGNOSIS

- The differential diagnosis of aphthous stomatitis is similar to that of intraoral HSV infections (see Chapter 6, "Superficial Viral Infections").

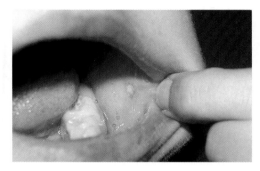

FIGURE 12.1 Aphthous stomatitis. A small punched-out erosion has erythema surrounding a yellow-white center.

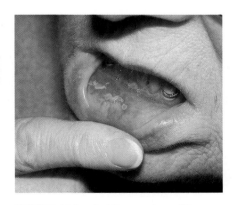

FIGURE 12.2 Aphthous stomatitis. Larger, more extensive aphthae are seen in this woman, who has Behçet's syndrome.

Recurrent (HSV) infections and aphthous stomatitis, which they resemble, are often mistaken for each other by patient and physician alike, whereas with the exception of primary herpes simplex, recurrent herpes simplex infection rarely occurs inside the mouth.

MANAGEMENT

Therapeutic options for aphthous stomatitis lesions include:

- Symptomatic therapy with topical anesthetic viscous lidocaine (Xylocaine).
- Vanceril (beclosmethasone dipropionate) aerosol sprayed directly on lesions.
- Superpotent topical steroids applied directly to lesions and held there by pressure with a finger.
- Tetracycline suspension (250 mg/tsp)—"swish and swallow."
- Diphenhydramine suspension—"gargle and spit."
- Tacrolimus ointment 0.1% applied at bedtime may accelerate healing.
- Silver nitrate applied directly to lesions sometimes promotes healing.
- Intralesional corticosteroid injections or a brief course of systemic corticosteroids are effective in reducing pain and healing lesions in patients with large, persistent, painful ulcers.
- Recently, thalidomide has been used with some success in healing large, painful, persistent aphthae in persons with HIV infection.

However, even a single dose of thalidomide has been known to cause fetal malformation; consequently, women of childbearing potential should use thalidomide only if they receive counseling and use effective contraception.

POINTS TO REMEMBER

- Most intraoral ulcers in immunocompetent patients are canker sores, not HSV lesions.
- Persistent erosions should alert one to the possibility of Behçet's disease, ulcerative colitis, erosive lichen planus, systemic lupus erythematosus, or a primary blistering disease such as pemphigus vulgaris or bullous pemphigoid.

HELPFUL HINTS

- Tacrolimus (Protopic) ointment 0.03% or 0.1% applied at bedtime may promote more rapid healing of lesions.
- Application of silver nitrate directly to lesions sometimes promotes healing.
- A single, nonhealing ulcer (lasting more than 2 months) should undergo biopsy to rule out squamous cell carcinoma.

Perlèche (derived from the French, "to lick") is also known as *angular cheilitis* (Figure 12.3).

It is an erythematous eruption that occurs at the corners of the mouth. Perlèche is sometimes seen in young patients who have atopic dermatitis. It also appears in the elderly and may be caused by aging and atrophy of the muscles of facial expression that surround the mouth which results in "pocketing" at the corners of the mouth. These pockets become macerated and serve as nidi for the retention of saliva resulting in the secondary overgrowth of microorganisms such as yeast forms and/or bacteria.

Other factors such as poor-fitting dentures, malocclusion, edentia, and bone resorption may lead to drooling or vertical shortening of the face, thus accentuating the melolabial crease. Lip licking in children, mouth breathing, and orthodontic devices are also risk factors. Vitamin deficiency is often blamed but rarely proved as a cause of perlèche.

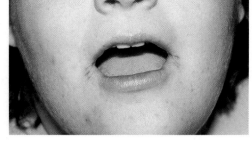

FIGURE 12.3 Perlèche *(angular cheilitis).* This patient has scaling, fissuring, and crusting at the corners of her mouth. She has atopic dermatitis elsewhere on her skin.

CLINICAL MANIFESTATIONS

- Redness, scaling, fissuring, and crusting at the corners of the mouth.
- Patients may have evidence of atopic dermatitis elsewhere on the body.

MANAGEMENT

- A mild topical steroid such as desonide (DesOwen), 0.05% or Elocon ointment often helps to resolve the inflammation.
- Petrolatum or other ointments are used to protect and moisturize the area.
- Topical anticandidal (ketoconazole, clotrimazole, nystatin) and antibacterial agents (mupirocin), alone or in combination with a topical hydrocortisone ointment, are often effective.
- Topical immunomodulators such as Protopic ointment or Elidel cream may also be tried.
- If necessary, a dental referral is suggested to correct potential causative factors mentioned earlier.
- Injection of collagen into the responsible skin folds has been beneficial in some selected patients.

OTHER EROSIONS AND ULCERS

Mucous Patches of Secondary Syphilis

The lesions of **secondary syphilis** on the tongue are known as mucous patches (Figure 12.4). For a full discussion of this condition, see Chapter 19, "Sexually Transmitted Diseases."

- This is characterized by asymptomatic round or oval eroded lesions or papules that are devoid of epithelium.
- The lesions teem with spirochetes.
- A reactive VDRL is noted.

FIGURE 12.4 Mucous patches of secondary syphilis. These mucous patches result from eroded epithelium of the tongue.

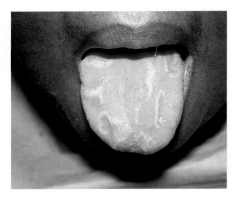

FIGURE 12.5 Geographic tongue. Shiny, red patches are devoid of papillae (resembles mucous patches in Figure 12.4).

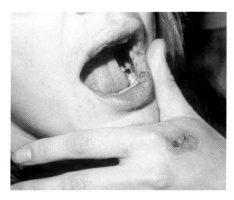

FIGURE 12.6 Erythema multiforme major (Stevens–Johnson Syndrome). Bullae and crusts are noted on the lips, and targetoid lesions are seen on the hand.

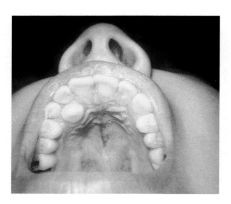

FIGURE 12.7 Systemic lupus erythematosus. Ulceration is present on the hard palate.

Geographic Tongue

Geographic tongue, or **benign migratory glossitis,** is a common idiopathic finding (Figure 12.5).

- The lesions of geographic tongue are areas that are shiny, red, and devoid of papillae and resemble mucous patches. These lesions seem to move about on the surface of the tongue and change configurations from one day to the next, thus accounting for the bizarre shifting patterns. Reports have suggested an association of geographic tongue with psoriasis; however, its 2% incidence in patients with psoriasis is no greater than would be expected in the otherwise healthy population.
- No treatment is necessary.

Erythema Multiforme (see Chapter 18, "Diseases of Vasculature")

Erythema Multiforme Minor

- Erythema multiforme minor is a self-limited eruption characterized by symmetrically distributed erythematous papules, which develop into the characteristic target-like lesions consisting of concentric color changes with a dusky central zone that may become bullous. It is not a disease but a syndrome with multiple causes including recurrent herpes virus infection.
- One may see a crusted lesion of recurrent HSV present on the vermillion border of the lip.

Erythema Multiforme Major

- This is the more serious variant of erythema multiforme. It has extensive mucous membrane involvement, systemic symptoms, and widespread lesions. Erythema multiforme major is often accompanied by fever, malaise, myalgias, and severe, painful mucous membrane involvement. Hemorrhagic crusts on lips and other mucous membranes are seen in addition to the extensive targetoid lesions elsewhere (Figure 12.6).

Systemic Lupus Erythematosus

- Erosions or ulcerations are present on the hard palate (Figure 12.7).
- This is discussed in Chapter 25, "Cutaneous Manifestations of Systemic Disease."

LICHEN PLANUS

For a full discussion of this condition, see Chapter 4, "Inflammatory Eruptions of Unknown Cause."

- A white, lacy network of lesions is present on the buccal mucosa, tongue, or gums (Figure 12.8).
- The lesions may be erosive, ulcerative, and painful.
- Typical lesions of lichen planus may or may not be present elsewhere on the body.

ORAL LEUKOPLAKIA

This white macular or plaquelike lesion is considered a precursor to squamous cell carcinoma of the mucous membranes. Smoking, chewing tobacco, and ethanol abuse are all contributing factors.

- White adherent plaques are present.
- Lesions occur on the tongue (Figure 12.9), buccal mucosa, hard palate, and gums.
- **Oral leukoplakia** may resemble oral lichen planus, and **oral hairy leukoplakia** or white plaques due to trauma.
- Less than 5% become squamous cell carcinoma.

ORAL HAIRY LEUKOPLAKIA

Oral hairy leukoplakia is associated with the Epstein–Barr virus (Figure 12.10). It is seen in the following:

- Patients with HIV infection (see Chapter 24, "Cutaneous Manifestations of HIV Disease" and transplant recipients
- Filiform papules on sides of tongue that resemble white hairs are seen
- Lesions are usually asymptomatic

CANDIDIASIS ("THRUSH") (SEE CHAPTER 24, "CUTANEOUS MANIFESTATIONS OF HIV DISEASE")

- Oral candidiasis is seen in immunocompromised patients and in neonates.
- Curd-like or erosive lesions are easily removed with gauze.
- Lesions may involve the tongue, the oropharynx, and the angles of mouth *(angular cheilitis)*.
- The potassium hydroxide examination or fungal culture is positive.

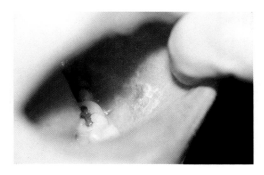

FIGURE 12.8 Lichen planus. A white, lacy network of lesions and erosions is present on the buccal mucosa. Note erosions.

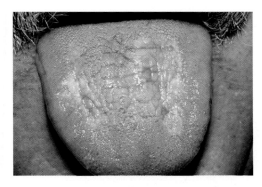

FIGURE 12.9 Leukoplakia. This patient actually has lichen planus which in this case is clinically indistinguishable from leukoplakia.

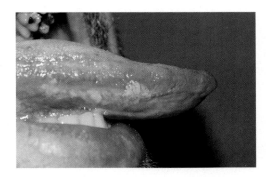

FIGURE 12.10 Oral hairy leukoplakia. This patient has acquired immunodeficiency syndrome. Note the papules on sides of the tongue that resemble white hairs.

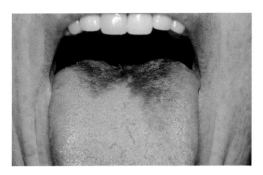

FIGURE 12.11 Black hairy tongue. A velvety, hairlike thickening of the tongue's surface is noted. The color can range from a yellowish brown or green to jet black.

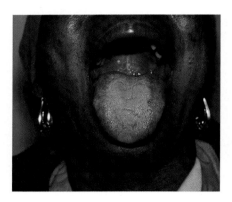

FIGURE 12.12 Antimalarial hyperpigmentation. Pigmentation of this patient's tongue is secondary to antimalarial therapy with hydroxychloroquine.

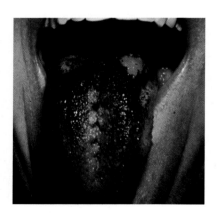

FIGURE 12.13 Pigment artifact. The black pigmentation on this patient's tongue was due to the deposition of bismuth, the active ingredient in Pepto Bismol. It was easily removed.

BLACK HAIRY TONGUE

Black hairy tongue is more than just a pigmentary change. Actually, it represents benign, asymptomatic hyperplasia (an accumulation of keratin) of the filiform papillae of the tongue. The pigmentation results from the normal pigment-producing bacterial flora that colonize the keratin. It has been debatably associated with smoking, excessive coffee or tea drinking, and the prolonged use of oral antibiotics, and it is considered by some clinicians as a possible marker for AIDS.

CLINICAL MANIFESTATIONS

- A velvety, hairlike thickening of the tongue's surface is noted (Figure 12.11).
- The color can range from a yellowish brown or green to jet black.

MANAGEMENT

- Brushing with a dilute hydrogen peroxide solution may bleach the pigmentation.
- A toothbrush can be used to scrape off the excess keratin.

PIGMENTATION FROM DRUGS

Oral mucous membrane pigmentation has been noted to result from the following agents:

- Antimalarials (Figure 12.12), chlorhexidine, doxorubicin, doxycycline, fluoxetine, ketoconazole, lomefloxacin, propranolol, risperidone, terbinafine, zidovudine, and all tetracyclines.
- Artifactual pigmentation has been noted to result from amalgam tattoos, dental fillings, and bismuth deposition from oral medications (Figure 12.13).

LONGITUDINAL RIDGING

This is a common, normal variant in elderly persons (Figure 13.1). Occasionally, longitudinal ridging is seen in younger persons. It is not indicative of any trauma or nutritional deficiency.

ONYCHOSCHIZIA

Split (onychoschizia) and brittle nails are common in adults (Figure 13.2). In some people, nails become fragile and easily break off at the free edge. Peeling fingernails are usually a sign of nail plate dehydration.

MANAGEMENT

Distal nail splitting is comparable to scaly, dry skin elsewhere. Thus, many treatment recommendations are similar to those for dry skin:

- Avoid excessive contact with water.
- Wear gloves in cold weather.
- Apply moisturizing creams or ointments (e.g., lactic acid creams in 5% to 12% concentrations) at bedtime or after bathing or washing.
- Keep the nails short; trim them when they are well hydrated and less likely to be frayed.
- Consider taking the B_2-complex vitamin, biotin (2.5 mg per day). Some observers claim to have had some success in increasing nail integrity and thickness with this regimen.

ONYCHOLYSIS

This finding represents a separation of the nail plate from the underlying pink nail bed (Figure 13.3). The separated portion is white and opaque, in contrast to the pink translucence of the attached portion. Physiologic onycholysis is seen at the distal free margin of healthy nails as they grow.

When separation is more proximal, the onycholysis becomes more obvious and is often cosmetically objectionable. In some patients, the nail takes on a green or yellow tinge (see the discussion of green nail syndrome later in this chapter).

Onycholysis is most frequently seen in women, particularly those with long fingernails. It may become painful and may interfere with routine function of the nails (e.g., picking up small objects, such as coins and paper clips).

Etiology

Whereas onycholysis may sometimes result from onychomycosis *(tinea unguium)*, fungal nail infection is only one cause of onycholysis. The causes of this disorder can be divided into two main areas.

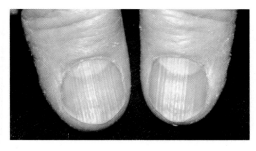

FIGURE 13.1 Longitudinal ridging. Parallel elevated ridges are characteristic of this normal variant.

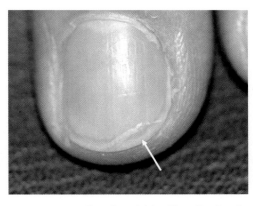

FIGURE 13.2 Onychoschizia. The distal nail splits into layers parallel to the nail's surface.

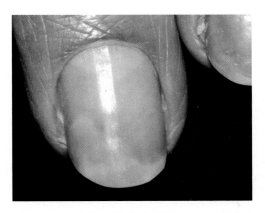

FIGURE 13.3 Onycholysis. The separated portion of the nail is white and opaque; the attached portion is pink and translucent.

External Causes

- Irritants, such as nail polish, nail wraps, nail hardeners, and artificial nails can cause the problem. Onycholysis may also be seen in persons who frequently come into contact with water, such as bartenders, hairdressers, manicurists, citrus fruit handlers, and domestic workers.
- Trauma, especially habitual finger sucking, athletic injuries to the toes, wearing of tight shoes, and the use of fingernails as a tool, can all cause the disorder.
- Fungal infections (e.g., chronic paronychia or onychomycosis) are another cause.
- Some drugs can act as phototoxic agents to induce onycholysis. These include diuretics, sulfa drugs, tetracycline, doxycycline, and, particularly, demethylchlortetracycline.

Internal Causes

- Psoriasis is the most common cause. Patients generally have evidence of psoriasis elsewhere on the body, or there may be other psoriatic nail findings, such as pitting.
- Inflammatory skin diseases of the nail matrix (root), such as eczematous dermatitis or lichen planus, can cause the disorder.
- Neoplasms and subungual warts are possible causes, especially if only one nail is involved.
- Other possible internal causes include thyroid disease, pregnancy, and anemia.

MANAGEMENT AND PREVENTION

- Keep nails dry and cut closely.
- Use nail polish sparingly.
- Avoid unnecessary manipulation of nails.
- Treat or avoid the underlying cause of the problem, if known.

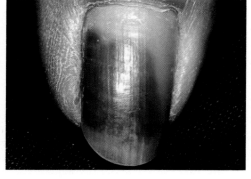

FIGURE 13.4 Green nail syndrome. The "dead space" under the nail often harbors *Pseudomonas* species.

GREEN NAIL SYNDROME

This is a consequence of onycholysis. Green nail syndrome is a painless discoloration under the nail and should not be confused with a subungual fungal infection (Figure 13.4).

Etiology

The "dead space" under the onycholytic nail serves as an excellent breeding ground for microbes. Often, *Pseudomonas* species are present; their presence usually accounts for the green or green–black nail color.

MANAGEMENT AND PREVENTION

- Soak the affected nail twice daily in a mixture either of one part chlorine bleach and four parts water or of equal parts acetic acid (vinegar) and water. This generally eliminates the discoloration.
- If possible, avoid or minimize the underlying cause (i.e., the factor that led to onycholysis, as described earlier).

BASICS

Injuries to the nail root (the matrix that directly underlies the proximal nail fold) may be caused by microbes (e.g., fungi), inflammatory conditions (e.g., eczema), or a digital myxoid cyst (see Figure 21.27). These disorders sometimes result in characteristic deformities; for example, nail pitting, "oil spots," and onycholysis may be seen in patients with psoriasis. At other times, the deformities are nonspecific, such as those resulting from eczema in the proximal nail fold.

TRAUMATIC LESIONS

Trauma is the most common cause of nail disorders.

Subungual Hematoma

This condition results from trauma to the nail matrix or nail bed, such as repeated minor injuries (e.g., tight shoes, sports injuries) or substantial impact (as from a hammer). An acute subungual hematoma that results from rapid accumulation of blood under the nail plate can be very painful, whereas small lesions may be painless and may go unnoticed for some time (Figure 13.5).

 DIFFERENTIAL DIAGNOSIS

- Junctional nevus (see Figures 13.19 and 22.37)
- Acral lentiginous melanoma should be considered (see Figure 22.38).

 MANAGEMENT

An acute, painful, swollen subungual hematoma may be incised and drained by placing the red-hot end of a heated paper clip on the area elevated by the hematoma. The small hole created with this procedure allows the blood to drain and thus quickly relieves the pain. (Note: This technique is best left to a health professional. Patients with hematomas should not be encouraged to try it for themselves.) Twirling a 27-gauge needle to create a similar hole is an alternative method for draining the blood.

POINT TO REMEMBER

- If there is a strong suspicion of melanoma, the nail bed should undergo biopsy.

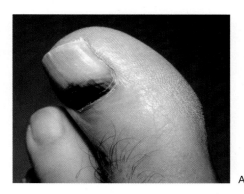
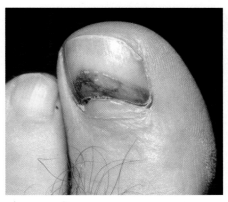
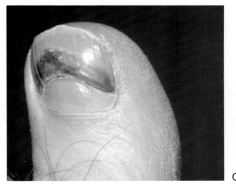

FIGURE 13.5 *A:* Acute subungual hematoma. The result of rapid blood accumulation, this can often be painful. *B:* Chronic subungual hematoma. This is the same nail after 3 months. *C:* Even 6 months after injury, the coagulated bloodstain can persist.

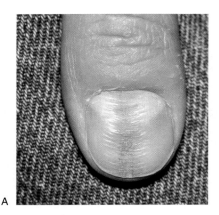

A

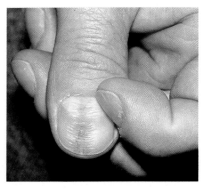

B

FIGURE 13.6 Median nail dystrophy.
A: Note the vertical ridging this habitual tic causes in the nails. After repeated trauma to the proximal nail
fold, median nail dystrophy can result.
B: Most often, the patient habitually
presses the nail of the adjacent finger
against the proximal nail fold.

HELPFUL HINT

- A quick method to substantiate the presence of a hematoma is to pare the nail plate gently with a No. 15 scalpel blade or to file it down until the coagulated blood can be visualized.

Median Nail Dystrophy

This condition results from a compulsive habit tic—repeated trauma to the proximal nail fold of the thumb, usually inflicted by the nail of the adjacent index finger (Figure 13.6). Some patients may do this with both hands, and this causes bilateral damage. The resultant nail deformity is analogous to an injury to the root of a tree that deforms the growing tree trunk.

Diagnosis

- The patient can sometimes be observed performing the repeated action without being aware of it. (This is particularly true in children.)

MANAGEMENT

- Treatment of any habit tic is difficult; the habit and resultant nail deformity are usually chronic by the time medical attention is sought.
- It can be suggested to patients that breaking this habit may be aided by an alternative activity, such as knitting or needlepoint.

POINTS TO REMEMBER

- Fingernail and toenail problems are commonly caused by minor injuries or repeated trauma.
- Proper trimming (along the contour) on a regular basis can protect the nails from injury.

HELPFUL HINT

- Wearing well-fitted shoes with low to moderately high heels may also prevent injury to toenails.

INFLAMMATORY DISORDERS

Inflammatory disorders that involve the nail matrix, such as psoriasis, can result in distinctive deformities of the nails. Whereas other conditions, such as eczema of the proximal nail fold, result in nonspecific deformities.

Psoriasis
- For a complete discussion, see Chapter 3, "Psoriasis."
- The typical nail changes are pitting (Figure 13.7), onycholysis, thickening (subungual hyperkeratosis), and "oil spots."

Eczematous Dermatitis with Secondary Nail Dystrophy
Nail deformity secondary to eczematous dermatitis is a problem that is often overlooked in patients with severe atopic dermatitis (Figure 13.8). It results when eczematous dermatitis involves the distal extensor surface of the fingers, and the associated inflammation also involves the matrix, or "root," of the nail. The inflamed matrix, which underlies the proximal nail fold, consequently gives rise to a dystrophic nail plate. The resultant nail deformity is analogous to a damaged root of a tree that deforms the growing tree trunk.

DESCRIPTION OF LESIONS

- Eczematous dermatitis is located on the dorsum of the distal part of the finger (the proximal nail fold).
- The nails generally have a ripplelike deformity that corresponds to the time of activity of the inflammation.

MANAGEMENT

- Improvement of the appearance of the nail plate follows control of inflammation of the proximal nail fold skin with the use of topical steroids or topical immunomodulators.

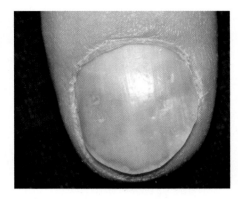

FIGURE 13.7 Psoriasis. Pitting, onycholysis, and "oil spots" are evident in this nail.

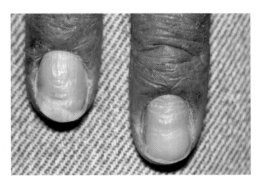

FIGURE 13.8 Eczematous dermatitis. The eczema of the proximal skin also affects the matrix (root) of the nail; this results in nail dystrophy.

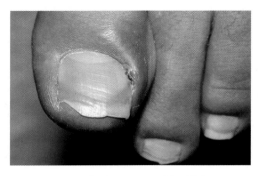

FIGURE 13.9 Acute paronychia. Note erythema and edema of the proximal nail fold.

ACUTE PARONYCHIA

The term *paronychia* refers to inflammation of the nail folds surrounding the nail plate (Figure 13.9). The condition can be either acute or chronic.

Acute paronychia usually results from an infection caused by *Staphylococcus aureus;* less commonly, it may be caused by streptococci or *Pseudomonas* species. Generally, only one nail is involved. The condition may occur spontaneously, or it may follow trauma or manipulation, such as nail biting, a manicure, or removal of a hangnail.

CLINICAL MANIFESTATIONS

- Acute paronychia is heralded by the rapid onset of bright red swelling of the proximal or lateral nail fold behind the cuticle. A throbbing, tender, and intensely painful lesion often results.

 ### DIAGNOSIS AND DIFFERENTIAL DIAGNOSIS

Acute bacterial paronychia can be confused with herpetic whitlow. Thus, a Tzanck preparation, bacterial culture, or both must be performed when the diagnosis is in doubt.

MANAGEMENT

- Mild cases may require only warm saline or aluminum acetate (Domeboro 1:40) soaks for 10 to 15 minutes two to four times daily.
- In more severe cases, simple incision and drainage (with a No. 11 surgical blade) usually afford rapid relief of pain.
- Occasionally, systemic therapy with antistaphylococcal antibiotics, such as dicloxacillin, or a cephalosporin, may be needed.

CHRONIC PARONYCHIA

This condition primarily results from a combination of chronic moisture, irritation, and trauma to the cuticle and proximal nail fold (Figure 13.10). It occurs much more often in women than in men, and it is particularly common in persons whose hands are frequently exposed to a wet environment, such as housewives, domestic workers, bartenders, janitors, bakers, dishwashers, dentists, dental hygienists, and children who habitually suck their thumbs. It is also seen more often in diabetic patients and in persons who manicure their cuticles.

The predisposing factor is usually trauma or maceration that produces a break in the barrier (cuticle) between the nail fold and nail plate. This allows moisture to accumulate and microbial colonization to follow.

Although *Candida* is frequently isolated from the proximal nail fold of patients with chronic paronychia, a primary pathogenesis for this organism has never been proven. In fact, evidence indicates that this condition is not a fungal infection at all, but is actually an eczematous process. For this reason, topical steroids are often more effective

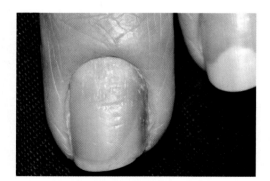

FIGURE 13.10 Chronic paronychia. In addition to erythema and edema, you can also observe nail dystrophy, the absence of a cuticle.

as therapy than topical or even systemic antifungal agents. Instances in which *Candida* may play a primary pathogenic role include patients who are diabetic and in those individuals with primary mucocutaneous candidiasis.

CLINICAL MANIFESTATIONS

- Chronic paronychia usually develops slowly and asymptomatically.
- Secondary nail plate changes often occur, including onycholysis (a lifting of the nail plate from the underlying nail bed), greenish or brown discoloration along the lateral borders, and transverse ridging.
- One or more fingers may be involved.

 DIAGNOSIS AND DIFFERENTIAL DIAGNOSIS

- The diagnosis can generally be established based on the typical clinical appearance of the fingers and the patient's history.
- Various pathogens and contaminants—including *Candida sp*, gram-positive or gram-negative organisms, or mixed flora—may be cultured from the pus obtained from under the proximal nail fold.

 MANAGEMENT

- Avoid prolonged exposure to moisture and trauma, especially frequent hand washing and manicures.
- Wear gloves (the cotton-under-vinyl variety is best) when performing tasks such as washing dishes.

In addition, one or more of the following treatments should be considered:

- A superpotent topical steroid such as clobetasol cream 0.05% applied once or twice daily to the proximal nail fold. In addition, Cordran tape may be applied nightly to this area.
- Alternatively, 1 to 2 drops daily of 3% thymol in 70% ethanol (compounded by a pharmacist) can be placed under the proximal nail fold.
- A topical broad-spectrum antifungal agent, such as clotrimazole, ketoconazole, econazole, or miconazole, is often combined with a potent topical corticosteroid to provide antifungal as well as antiinflammatory effects.
- If topical therapy is ineffective, systemic broad-spectrum antiyeast therapy such as itraconazole (Sporanox) may be tried if clinically indicated and there are no contraindications to its use.

 POINTS TO REMEMBER

- Chronic paronychia is frequently misdiagnosed—and treated—as an acute staphylococcal paronychia.
- Chronic paronychia is distinct from onychomycosis, which is a fungal infection of the nail itself.

ONYCHOMYCOSIS

For a complete discussion, see Chapter 7, "Superficial Fungal infections."

NAIL PROBLEMS: MISCELLANEOUS DISORDERS

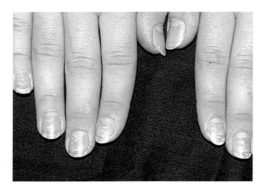

FIGURE 13.11   Leukonychia striata.

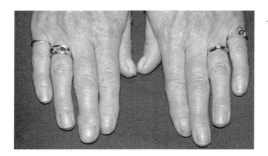

FIGURE 13.12   Yellow nail syndrome.

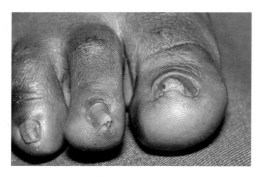

FIGURE 13.13   Pincer nails.

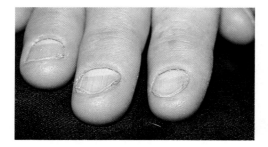

FIGURE 13.14   Koilonychia.

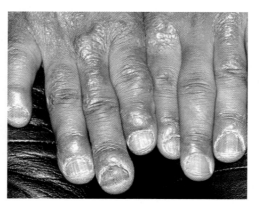

FIGURE 13.15   Sarcoidosis.

BASICS

In addition to the disorders already described, various other conditions can affect the nails. Some of these disorders produce characteristic nail findings that may serve as clues to unrecognized systemic disease.

Leukonychia Striata (Figure 13.11)

These white lines result from an injury to the nail matrix that occurred about 2 to 3 months earlier. The underlying injury is often an antecedent illness or the repeated trauma of manicuring; occasionally, it develops after liquid nitrogen therapy for warts. Leukonychia striata, which is also called *transverse striate leukonychia,* is often mistaken for a fungal nail infection.

Yellow Nail Syndrome (Figure 13.12)

The nails are yellow, curved, and grow slowly. This syndrome is associated with certain respiratory disorders (e.g., bronchiectasis, chronic respiratory infections, lymphedema, pleural effusion, ascites). Yellow nail discoloration also has been reported in patients with acquired immunodeficiency syndrome.

Pincer Nails (Figure 13.13)

This overcurvature of the nail produces lateral compression on the surrounding skin. It may result in ingrown, painful nails, particularly when there is additional compression from footwear. Pincer nails, also known as *trumpet nails,* are often congenital and may be seen in persons with the yellow nail syndrome or as a normal variant.

Koilonychia (Figure 13.14)

Acquired koilonychia, also known as *spoon nails,* may be seen in association with trauma to the cuticle and proximal nail folds, iron deficiency anemia, hemochromatosis, or endocrine or cardiac disease. Spoon-shaped or concave nails may also be seen in early infancy and may be self-limited. The koilonychia shown in Figure 13.14 is limited to those fingers that were subjected to trauma to the cuticle and proximal nail fold.

Sarcoidosis (Figure 13.15)

Dystrophic, thickened nail plates result from infiltration of the proximal nail folds by sarcoidal plaques. Only those nail folds with plaque are associated with nail plate dystrophy.

Dermatomyositis (Figure 13.16)

The proximal nail fold demonstrates periungual erythema, telangiectasias, thickening of the cuticles ("ragged cuticles"), and distal nail plate thinning.

Subungual Verruca (Figure 13.17)

A wart lifting the nail plate is seen in Figure 13.17. A solitary wart of the nail bed is often mistaken for a fungal infection. The possibility of subungual squamous cell carcinoma, basal cell carcinoma, or other neoplasm should always be considered.

Junctional Nevus (Figure 13.18)

An evenly pigmented linear nevus that emanates from nests of nevus cells in the nail matrix. These lesions are quite common in blacks and may be multiple. They are much less common in whites. Any smudging or leaching of pigment or variation from the original black band should undergo biopsy immediately, to rule out malignant melanoma (see Figure 22.38).

Terry's Nails (Figure 13.19)

The patient shown in Figure 13.19 had a liver transplant for cirrhosis. His nail beds are white with a narrow zone of pink under the distal end of the plate. Terry's nails are associated with cirrhosis, congestive heart failure, and adult-onset diabetes mellitus. This condition also may be seen as a normal finding associated with age.

Half-and-Half Nails (Figure 13.20)

The color changes in Figure 13.20 are seen in chronic renal failure. The proximal half of the nail is white and the distal portion retains the normal pink color.

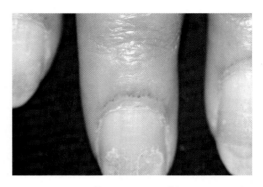

FIGURE 13.16   Dermatomyositis.

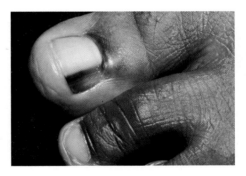

FIGURE 13.17   Subungual verruca.

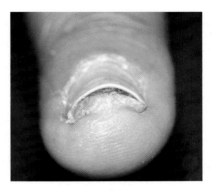

FIGURE 13.18   Junctional nevus.

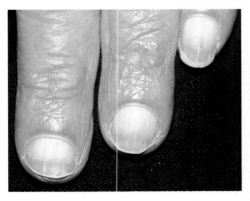

FIGURE 13.20   Half-and-half nails. Note proximal half is white and distal half is pink.

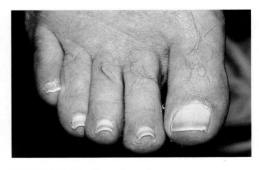

FIGURE 13.19   Terry's nails.

CHAPTER 14

Pigmentary Disorders

VITILIGO VULGARIS

BASICS

An acquired disorder of skin depigmentation, vitiligo vulgaris (common vitiligo) affects 1% to 2% of the world's population. Thirty percent of patients with vitiligo report a positive family history of the disorder. A distinct form of vitiligo occurs in children, and this form is often segmental or dermatomal in its distribution.

Pathogenesis

Although the cause of vitiligo vulgaris is still unknown, the condition is thought to result from an autoimmune process that prompts the loss of melanocytes. Vitiligo may develop in patients with other diseases that are believed to have an autoimmune basis (e.g., **thyroid dysfunction, Addison's disease, alopecia areata, diabetes mellitus, and pernicious anemia**), and this finding supports the hypothesis that an immune mechanism may be involved in its pathogenesis. However, another theory proposes that vitiligo is caused by an abnormality of nerve endings adjacent to skin pigment cells.

DESCRIPTION OF LESIONS

- Physical examination of a patient with vitiligo reveals hypopigmented (Figure 14.1) or depigmented, chalk-white macules.
- Occasionally, the lesions may have various shades of color and may include islands of repigmentation (Figure 14.2).
- In dark-skinned people, pigmentary loss may be observed at any time of year, whereas in light-skinned people, the lesions may be most obvious in the summer, because the tanning effects of the summer sun can accentuate the contrast between the light and dark skin.

DISTRIBUTION OF LESIONS

- Vitiliginous lesions tend to have a bilateral, symmetric distribution.
- They frequently occur on acral areas (e.g., the hands and feet), body folds, bony prominences, and external genitals.
- Lesions characteristically appear around orifices (e.g., the mouth, eyes, nose, and anus), but they may also involve the eyebrows, eyelashes, and scalp hair, resulting in white hairs *(leukotrichia)*.
- In severe cases, vitiligo may be more widespread (Figure 14.3) or even total *(vitiligo universalis)*.

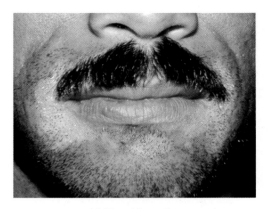

FIGURE 14.1 Vitiligo. Hypopigmented macules are characteristic of vitiligo vulgaris. Note white hairs.

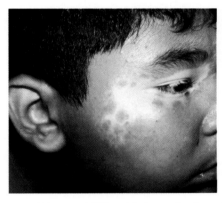

FIGURE 14.2 Vitiligo. Various shades of hypopigmentation, depigmentation, and islands of spontaneous repigmentation can be seen in this patient with vitiligo. Note the white eyelashes.

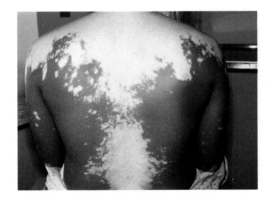

FIGURE 14.3 Vitiligo. Extensive depigmentation.

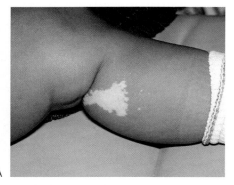

A

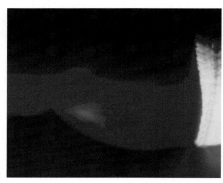

B

FIGURE 14.4 *B:* Wood's lamp examination reveals fluorescence in areas depigmented by vitiligo *(A).*

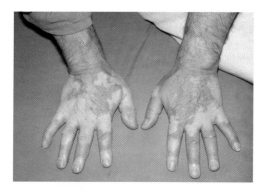

FIGURE 14.5 Vitiligo. Chemically induced depigmentation is limited to this patient's hands. Exposure to a cleaning product containing phenol caused the areas of hypopigmentation shown here.

CLINICAL MANIFESTATIONS

- Clinical manifestations often develop cyclically. A rapid loss of pigment is followed by a stable period (during which some repigmentation may occur), and then generally by recurrence.
- Some patients spontaneously experience partial repigmentation; total repigmentation is unusual.
- Patients with severe vitiligo may experience embarrassment and lowered self-esteem.

DIAGNOSIS

- A clinical diagnosis of vitiligo is usually based on the characteristic appearance of the skin lesions.
- The diagnosis can be aided by **Wood's lamp examination;** this should reveal a milk-white fluorescence. Wood's lamp is a handheld black light that makes hypopigmented areas appear lighter and depigmented areas (e.g., those produced by vitiligo) appear as a pure white or bluish white fluorescence (Figure 14.4).

 DIFFERENTIAL DIAGNOSIS

Postinflammatory Hypopigmentation (see later)
- Because the lesions of this disorder are not totally depigmented, they are generally off-white. Often, patients who have postinflammatory hypopigmentation reveal a history of preexisting inflammatory dermatitis, such as eczema or tinea versicolor. When there is no such history and no plausible explanation for the hypopigmentation (as is often the case), the condition is then considered idiopathic.

Hypopigmented Tinea Versicolor
- This disorder is frequently mistaken for vitiligo vulgaris. Patients with active, untreated tinea versicolor have a whitish scale. In addition, under Wood's lamp examination, the lesions may appear as a yellow-orange fluorescence, and skin scrapings tested with potassium hydroxide will be positive for the hyphae and spores of the responsible yeast. Inactive, or postinflammatory, spots of tinea versicolor lack scale and are hypopigmented (see Chapter 7, "Superficial fungal Infections").

Chemically Induced Vitiligo
- This develops on the hands of persons who work with germicidal detergents or with certain rubber-containing compounds that destroy melanocytes. The diagnosis is established based on the location of the lesions (e.g., only on the hands) and a history of exposure (Figure 14.5).

Leprosy
- Cutaneous leprosy often manifest with areas of hypopigmentation. Leprosy is extremely rare in the United States, but occasionally it may be seen in patients who emigrate from endemic areas, such as India or parts of South and Central America. The lesions of leprosy may appear as hypopigmented macules, plaques, or nodules that become insensitive to touch.

MANAGEMENT

- Treatment options for vitiligo include repigmentation therapies for the macules and depigmentation of the remaining healthy skin in patients with extensive disease.
- If administered early to patients with limited disease, potent and superpotent topical corticosteroids are occasionally helpful in promoting repigmentation. The hands and feet respond poorly to this approach.
- Reports of repigmentation have been noted in some patients who applied tacrolimus (Protopic) 0.1% ointment twice daily.
- Photochemotherapy, using psoralens and natural sunlight or psoralens and ultraviolet A light (PUVA) in a phototherapy light box, is sometimes tried. However, this treatment is time-consuming and often ineffective. It should generally not be used for children younger than 9 years. The treatments are 50% to 70% successful in restoring some color on the face, trunk, and upper arms and legs. Again, the hands and feet respond poorly to this method.
- Minigrafting of normal skin to areas of vitiligo may be helpful for some patients. However, it does not result in total return of normal pigment.
- An approach under study involves the application to vitiligo patches of a synthetic enzyme, pseudocatalase, that results in repigmentation after exposure to narrow-band ultraviolet B.
- Aspirin and vitamins B_6, B_{12}, C, and E have been reported to be of some value in treating vitiligo. However, none of these approaches has been studied rigorously.
- Special cosmetic makeup that is formulated to match the patient's normal skin color (e.g., Dermablend or Covermark) or self-tanning compounds that contain dihydroxyacetone may effectively hide the white patches.
- Sunscreens can be used to avoid exacerbating the contrast between normal skin and lesions and to protect the lesions, which are sensitive to the sun.
- Some patients with extensive vitiligo (more than 50% loss of pigment) may elect to have the remaining skin "bleached" with Benoquin (20% monobenzyl ether of hydroquinone). The results are permanent (Figure 14.6).

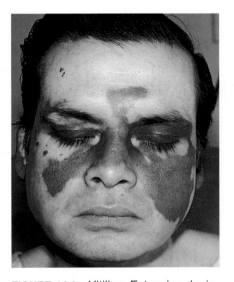

FIGURE 14.6 Vitiligo. Extensive depigmentation. The residual normal pigmentation was treated with Benoquin.

POINTS TO REMEMBER

- Health care professionals should resist the tendency to trivialize vitiligo by referring to it as only a cosmetic disorder.
- Clinicians should urge patients to use sunscreens whenever they are out in the sun. By minimizing tanning, sunscreens lessen the contrast between healthy skin and lesions; they also protect the vitiliginous skin, which is sensitive to the sun.
- If indicated by positive findings in the patient's history or physical examination, screening for autoimmune diseases should be done.
- Response rates to treatments for vitiligo often are disappointing.

HELPFUL HINT

Health care professionals should be sensitive to patients who have emigrated from countries in which leprosy is endemic—and generally dreaded. Such patients may feel particularly embarrassed and stigmatized by focal areas of lightened skin color, regardless of the cause of the hypopigmentation.

SEE PATIENT HANDOUT, PAGE 473

NONVITILIGINOUS FORMS OF HYPOPIGMENTATION

BASICS

Hypopigmentation and depigmentation are more obvious in dark-skinned persons; however, they can cause problems even in light-skinned persons, particularly those who tan. Postinflammatory reactions are the most common cause of hypopigmentation. In addition, neonates and toddlers may exhibit congenital areas of hypopigmentation such as congenital nevi; older children may develop halo nevi, which are melanocytic nevi encircled by a white halo of depigmentation (see Chapter 21, "Benign Skin Neoplasms"). In middle-aged and older persons, idiopathic white spots may also develop.

Localized alterations in skin color are not uncommon after many cutaneous inflammatory conditions. Affected areas may become lighter *(postinflammatory hypopigmentation)* or darker *(postinflammatory hyperpigmentation)* than the surrounding normal skin. Occasionally, a combination of light and dark patches may develop. Persons with dark complexions appear to be at increased risk for developing these pigmentary changes.

Often, the pigmentary changes are self-limited; they require only time for resolution. Nevertheless, they can be a source of embarrassment for many patients. Providing reassurance and practical advice on how best to conceal the areas of altered skin color can help patients to cope better with these disorders.

Postinflammatory Hypopigmentation

Lightening of the skin may follow nearly any inflammatory cutaneous eruption (e.g., eczema or psoriasis; Figure 14.7). In **pityriasis alba,** hypopigmented round spots are commonly seen on the faces in children with atopic dermatitis. Occasionally, the slightly scaly patches that precede the hypopigmentation may be seen (Figure 14.8). **Postinflammatory hypopigmentation** may also develop after an injury to the skin, such as a burn or surgical scar. The areas of hypopigmentation roughly correspond to the location and shape of the antecedent eruption ("footprints").

In general, the pigmentary changes that follow mild inflammatory dermatoses slowly revert to normal over several months. However, those that follow more severe inflammation or injury may be permanent.

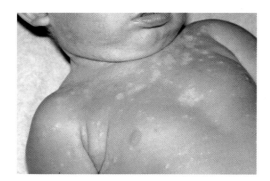

FIGURE 14.7 Atopic dermatitis. Postinflammatory hypopigmented macules can be seen in this infant who has atopic dermatitis. Note active areas of inflammation on the neck and axillary areas.

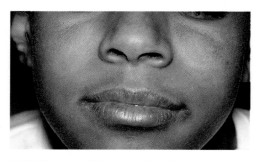

FIGURE 14.8 Pityriasis alba. Hypopigmented round spots are commonly seen on the faces in children who have atopic dermatitis. Also note postinflammatory hyperpigmentation in the center of the lesion.

MANAGEMENT

- The passage of time often improves the cosmetic abnormality.
- In the interim, makeup products such as Covermark and Dermablend can be used to conceal the areas of hypopigmentation.
- Artificial tanning lotions can also help.

IDIOPATHIC GUTTATE HYPOMELANOSIS

Idiopathic guttate hypomelanosis is the formal name for the idiopathic white spots that often appear on the arms and lower legs of middle-aged and elderly people. This condition occurs in all races, but as with vitiligo, it is more apparent in persons with darker skin.

- These spots tend to develop more commonly in areas of chronic sun damage, particularly on the anterior lower legs.
- They produce no symptoms other than skin discoloration.
- There is no effective treatment.

HELPFUL HINT

- Patients should be reassured that this is not vitiligo.

OTHER TYPES OF HYPOMELANOSIS

Numerous systemic and congenital conditions may cause hypopigmentation. They include the following:

- Endocrine diseases, such as Addison's disease and hypothyroidism, may cause hypopigmentation.
- Genetic conditions, such as congenital vitiligo, tuberous sclerosis, and albinism, may also cause this condition.
- Neonates and toddlers may exhibit congenital areas of hypopigmentation such as congenital nevi (Figure 14.9).
- Infectious diseases, such as leprosy, pinta, and yaws, may be causes.
- In addition, hypomelanosis may result from the use of topical therapeutic agents, such as corticosteroids, hydroquinone, and retinoids. Chemicals that contain phenol may also depigment the skin (Figure 14.5). Nutritional deficiencies (especially vitamin B_{12} deficiency and kwashiorkor) may also cause a loss of pigmentation. These disorders should be considered in the appropriate clinical or environmental context.

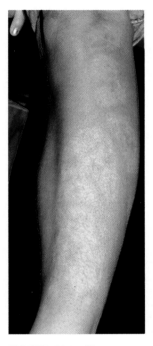

FIGURE 14.9 Nevus depigmentosus. This off-white linear hypomelanosis has been present since birth. It has enlarged commensurate with the patient's growth.

POINTS TO REMEMBER

- Both postinflammatory hypopigmentation and hyperpigmentation result from inflammation or injury to the skin.
- The likelihood that normal pigmentation will return depends on the degree and type of injury.

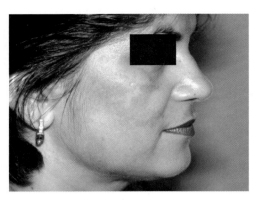

FIGURE 14.10 Melasma of cheeks. Melasma may result from pregnancy, oral contraceptive use, or menopause, or it may arise *de novo* for no apparent reason.

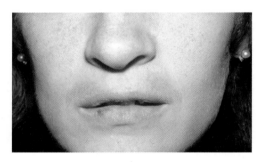

FIGURE 14.11 Melasma of the "moustache" area. Note the darkening above the patient's upper lip.

MELASMA

BASICS

Formerly known as *chloasma,* melasma, or the "mask of pregnancy," is an acquired form of hyperpigmentation that is seen most commonly on the face. It may result from pregnancy, oral contraceptive use, or menopause, or it may arise *de novo* for no apparent reason. It is exacerbated by exposure to sunlight.

Melasma is seen most frequently in young women of childbearing age, particularly those who have darker complexions and live in sunny climates. It is seen in Asia, the Middle East, South America, Africa, and the Indian subcontinent. In North America, melasma is most prevalent among Hispanics, African-Americans, and immigrants from countries in which it is common.

CLINICAL MANIFESTATIONS AND DESCRIPTION OF LESIONS

- Clinically, melasma is primarily a cosmetic problem.
- It consists of asymptomatic, blotchy darkening of the facial skin.
- Lesions are tan to brown, hyperpigmented macules that may coalesce into symmetric, well-demarcated patches (Figure 14.10).
- During pregnancy, the darkening of the skin often occurs in the second and third trimesters and spontaneously fades after termination of pregnancy.
- Melasma also tends to fade on discontinuance of oral contraceptives or avoidance of sunlight; however, it may persist indefinitely.

DISTRIBUTION OF LESIONS

- Lesions are found mainly on the cheeks, angles of the jaw, forehead, nose, chin, and above the upper lip (Figure 14.11).

DIFFERENTIAL DIAGNOSIS

The differential diagnosis of melasma includes postinflammatory hyperpigmentation and solar lentigines.

Postinflammatory Hyperpigmentation (see later)
- This may often be explained by a previous inflammatory eruption or injury. In general, lesions roughly correspond to the location of inflammation or injury, and they have less clearly defined margins than seen in melasma.

Solar Lentigines (Singular, Lentigo), or "Liver Spots"
- These lesions have uniform coloration and are acquired during middle age on sun-exposed areas, such as the face and backs of the hands (see also Chapter 21, "Benign Skin Neoplasms").

MANAGEMENT

- Treatment of melasma involves a combination approach using one or more bleaching agents and cosmetic camouflage. In addition, sun avoidance and the use of sun blocks are essential.
- Bleaching creams that contain the tyrosinase inhibitor hydroquinone are readily available. Over-the-counter preparations such as Ambi and Esoterica contain 2% hydroquinone.
- Preparations of 3% hydroquinone (Melanex) and 4% hydroquinone (Eldoquin-Forte) are available by prescription only. Some products such as Eldopaque contain a sun block; Lustra, a 4% hydroquinone agent, also contains vitamins C and E and glycolic acid.
- Hydroquinone preparations are applied twice daily to areas of darkening only.
- Other lightening agents include the tyrosinase inhibitor, azelaic acid (Azelex 20% cream), which may be used in addition to hydroquinone.
- Topical tretinoin can also be used in combination with both hydroquinone and a topical steroid (Tri-Luma cream).
- Alpha-hydroxy acid products, such as mild glycolic acid peels, may also be used to hasten the effect of other topical lightening agents. They should be used cautiously in darkly pigmented Hispanics, Asians, and blacks because of the risk for postinflammatory pigmentary hyperpigmentation (see later).
- Kojic acid, a tyrosinase inhibitor, is used in Japan and the Middle East, and it seems to have an efficacy similar to that of hydroquinone.

POINTS TO REMEMBER

- A patient's concern regarding melasma should not be dismissed as frivolous.
- Treatment requires patience during the many months in which lightening agents must be applied.
- Without the strict avoidance of sunlight, potentially successful treatments for melasma are doomed to failure.

HELPFUL HINTS

- Patients receiving treatment should be cautioned to expect slow but gradual lightening.
- Destructive modalities (e.g., cryotherapy, medium-depth chemical peels, lasers) yield unpredictable results and are associated with numerous potential adverse effects.
- Sunscreens containing *opaque* physical blockers such as titanium dioxide and zinc oxide are preferred over chemical sunscreens because of their broader protection.
- Melasma is a chronic condition, and patients are best kept on maintenance therapy.

POSTINFLAMMATORY HYPERPIGMENTATION

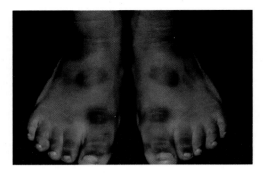

FIGURE 14.12 Postinflammatory hyperpigmentation. In this patient, the cause was contact dermatitis from wearing sandals. Note how the lesions conform to the shape of the sandals.

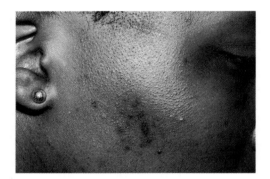

FIGURE 14.13 Postinflammatory hyperpigmentation. In this patient, the cause was healing acne lesions.

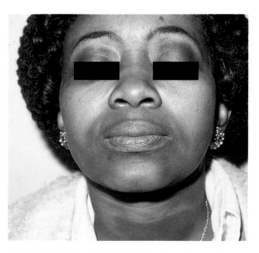

FIGURE 14.14 Postinflammatory hyperpigmentation. This patient has atopic dermatitis that has resolved with hyperpigmentation.

BASICS

Darkening of the skin may occur after nearly any inflammatory eruption, including eczema or acne, or after an injury such as a burn. Elective skin treatments (e.g., chemical peels, laser resurfacing, or dermabrasion) may also precipitate it.

The hyperpigmentation stems from the melanocytes' exaggerated response to cutaneous insult, which results in an increased or abnormal distribution of the pigment melanin. Like melasma, postinflammatory hyperpigmentation tends to develop more often in people with dark complexions.

DESCRIPTION AND DISTRIBUTION OF LESIONS

Lesions tend to conform in location and shape to the preceding eruption or injury. On occasion, lesions may mimic the exact shape of the inciting insult (Figures 14.12 to 14.14).

MANAGEMENT

- Often, the passage of time, coupled with sun protection, affords a gradual lightening of darkened areas.
- Avoidance of the inciting event may prevent future lesions. Treatment of acne, for example, prevents the formation of new inflammatory lesions and allows old pigmented lesions to fade.
- When lesions persist, many of the measures used to treat melasma (see earlier) may be tried. However, persistent postinflammatory hyperpigmentation tends to be much more recalcitrant than is melasma to therapeutic measures, and cosmetic coverups may be used.

ACANTHOSIS NIGRICANS

BASICS

- A characteristic hyperpigmented skin pattern, acanthosis nigricans occurs primarily in flexural folds. The skin is thought to darken and thicken in reaction to circulating growth factors.
- Most cases of acanthosis nigricans, including idiopathic cases and those associated with obesity, are referred to as *benign acanthosis nigricans*. Other benign forms of acanthosis nigricans are associated with endocrine disorders, such as insulin-resistant diabetes, polycystic ovary syndrome, Cushing's disease, Addison's disease, pituitary tumors, pinealomas, and hyperandrogenic syndromes with insulin resistance. Acanthosis nigricans is sometimes related to drug use, most commonly secondary to glucocorticoid, nicotinic acid, diethylstilbestrol, or growth hormone therapy. Acanthosis nigricans may also be inherited without any disease associations.

- The rare, so-called "malignant" acanthosis nigricans is associated with an internal malignant disease, usually an intraabdominal adenocarcinoma. Affected patients generally have a poor prognosis. The skin condition is sometimes seen before the cancer is recognized; it can also be associated with recurrences and metastases.

DESCRIPTION OF LESIONS

- Acanthosis nigricans generally presents with a gradual evolution of symmetric, asymptomatic, tan or brown to black, leathery or velvety plaques. The plaques are sometimes "warty" (papillomatous) and studded with skin tags. They have linear, alternating, dark-and-light pigmentation that becomes more apparent when the skin is stretched (Figure 14.15).

DISTRIBUTION OF LESIONS

- The most common sites of involvement are the axilla, the base of the neck, the inframammary folds, the inguinal areas, and the antecubital fossa.
- The dorsum of the hands (especially on the knuckles), the elbows, and the knees are also common locations.
- Less commonly, mucous membranes, the vermilion border of the lips, and the eyelids are involved.

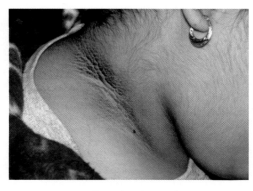

FIGURE 14.15 Acanthosis nigricans. Linear, alternating dark and light pigmentation becomes more apparent when the skin is stretched.

MANAGEMENT

- Acanthosis nigricans is primarily a cosmetic concern.
- Treatment is generally not effective.

POINTS TO REMEMBER

- Malignant acanthosis nigricans generally has a sudden onset, but otherwise it clinically resembles the benign form of the disorder.
- Concern is greatest when acanthosis nigricans suddenly arises in a nonobese adult who has no family history of the condition.

Pruritus: The "Itchy" Patient

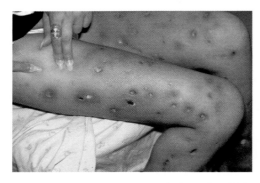

FIGURE 15.1 Neurotic excoriations (factitia). The self-induced ulcers are seen in a patient convinced that she was infested with lice.

Overview

Pruritus is the most common symptom of all skin diseases. It can be simply defined as an unpleasant sensation that elicits the urge to scratch.

The source of pruritus may result from the following:

- Primary skin disorders such as eczema, xerosis (dry skin), and dermatitis herpetiformis
- Exogenous causes such as drugs, scabies, lice, fiberglass, and aquagenic pruritus
- Internal disorders such as chronic renal disease, acquired immunodeficiency syndrome, polycythemia vera, cholestasis, pregnancy related disorders, primary biliary cirrhosis, diabetes mellitus, thyroid disease, and carcinoid syndrome
- Psychogenic causes such as delusions of parasitosis, neurotic excoriations, and obsessive—compulsive disorder
- Associated malignant diseases such as Hodgkin's disease, leukemia, and multiple myeloma
- Pruritus of unknown origin, or itching for more than 2 to 6 weeks with no determined cause

DESCRIPTION OF LESIONS

- Linear excoriations, crusts, lichenified plaques, and wheals may be present.
- Pruritus with no lesions is also quite common.
- The lesions may have a bizarre appearance with deep ulcers and scars (factitia or "neurotic excoriations") (Figure 15.1) (see also Chapter 2, "Eczema").

DISTRIBUTION OF LESIONS

- Symptoms or clinical lesions may be localized (Figure 15.2) or widespread.

DIAGNOSIS

A search for the cause of the pruritis is based on the following:

- A careful history
- Physical evidence (linear excoriations, crusts)

The workup for pruritus of unknown origin includes the following:

- Rectal and pelvic examinations, if indicated
- Complete blood count
- Stool examination for parasites and occult blood
- Chest radiograph
- Thyroid, renal, and liver function tests
- Follow-up of the patient for as long as necessary to make a diagnosis

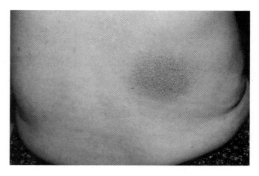

FIGURE 15.2 Notalgia paraesthetica. Note the typical location on the lower scapula. The postinflammatory hyperpigmentation resulted from the chronic rubbing and scratching of this itchy area.

CLINICAL VARIANTS

- A patient may complain of itching caused by reasons that seem totally inexplicable or bizarre. Many histories have various twists and turns, such as the following:
  - The person with *aquagenic pruritus* experiences intense itching *only* after exposure to water.
  - A patient may insist that driving with the car window open makes the wind blow on his or her forehead and causes it to itch intensely; the itch instantly disappears when the window is closed.
  - Some localized itching is described as *notalgia paraesthetica*. This not uncommon condition most often consists of a localized, very focal, often unilateral area of recurrent itching that characteristically occurs on the lower or middle of the scapula. The postinflammatory hyperpigmentation that sometimes results from the chronic rubbing and scratching reveals the diagnosis (Figure 15.2).

MANAGEMENT

- Whenever possible, treatment of the underlying systemic disease that causes the pruritus may bring relief.
- Antihistamines are of more benefit in the treatment of allergic conditions, urticaria, and drug reactions than they are for the treatment of itching and may be no more effective than placebo. Despite this finding, the powerful effect of antihistamines as placebos should not be overlooked.
- Topical therapy that can be soothing and helpful in some patients includes the following:
  - Menthol, phenol, camphor, calamine lotions (e.g., Sarna, Prax, PrameGel) may be used. Topical steroids are generally not very helpful when no lesions are apparent.
  - Cold applications of frozen vegetable packets may be useful.

For Pruritus of Chronic Renal Disease
- Ultraviolet B therapy is used.
- Oral ingestion of activated charcoal may be helpful.
- Cholestyramine is given.

For Pruritus Caused by Liver Disease
- Cholestyramine is used.

For Pruritus Resulting from Xerosis
- Moisturizers may be helpful.
- Topical steroids are used only when there are inflammatory skin lesions.

 POINTS TO REMEMBER

- Antihistamines often exert their antipruritic action by inducing sleep (soporific effect).
- Topical emollients are an essential component of the therapy of pruritus when xerosis is present.

 HELPFUL HINTS

- The dosage of antihistamines should be titrated gradually upward using nonsedating agents during the daytime and sedating agents at bedtime.
- Scabies should be considered if more than one family member itches.
- Hodgkin's disease may present with pruritus that precedes the diagnosis by up to 5 years.

CHAPTER 16

Xerosis: The "Dry" Patient

Overview

Xerosis, or dry skin, is a common occurrence in winter climates, particularly in conditions of cold air, low relative humidity, and indoor heating. Xerosis can affect anyone, but it tends to be more severe in certain persons, especially those with an hereditary predisposition.

Modern lifestyles are also contributing factors. In Western societies, people tend to overbathe, and they often live and work in overheated spaces.

The word "dry" is sometimes misapplied. Skin that appears to be dry (i.e., that shows a buildup of scale) may not always be suffering from a lack of water, but from an overadherence or hyperproliferation of scale. Overadherence of scale may occur in patients with ichthyosis (see Chapter 2). Hyperproliferation of scale is noted in atopic dermatitis, psoriasis, seborrheic dermatitis, and common dandruff.

Xerosis In Elderly Persons

Dry skin tends to be most apparent on the hands and lower legs. It becomes especially common in persons who are older than 65 years (Figure 16.1).

Pathogenesis

The reasons why the skin becomes—or appears to become—dry are not well understood. It has been proposed that xerosis may be secondary to diminished production of sebum *(asteatosis)*, as well as to reduced eccrine sweat activity. However, other biochemical factors related to aging skin have also been implicated.

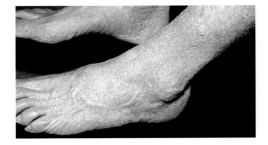

FIGURE 16.1 Xerosis. Dry skin tends to be most apparent on the hands and lower legs. This elderly patient's legs are dry and scaly.

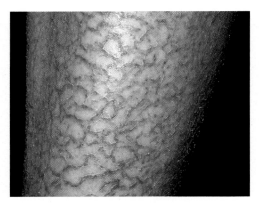

FIGURE 16.2 Asteatotic eczema. This condition often develops on the shins, arms, hands, and trunk. The skin resembles a cracked porcelain vase *(erythema craquelé)*.

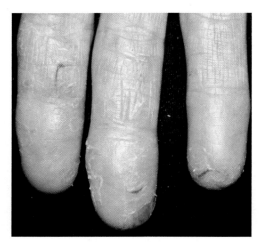

FIGURE 16.3 Atopic dermatitis. Dry, sensitive, itchy, lichenified skin is characteristic of this condition. This patient has painful fissures of distal fingers.

Asteatotic Eczema

Occurring exclusively in adults, asteatotic eczema *(winter eczema)* most commonly appears on the shins, arms, hands, and trunk (see Chapter 2, "Eczema"). Because the eruption often resembles the surface of a cracked porcelain vase, it is often referred to as *erythema craquelé*. It is also likened to the appearance of a dry river bed (Figure 16.2).

Asteatotic eczema is a common, sometimes pruritic, dermatitis that appears in dry, cold winter months. It is caused by a relative loss of water from the skin through evaporation, a lack of normal desquamation, and, possibly, a decline in the production of sebum (the skin's natural lubricant and sealant).

Atopic Dermatitis

Dry, exquisitely sensitive, itchy skin is the major feature of atopic dermatitis (eczema) (see Chapter 2, "Eczema"). Atopic skin is often characterized by decreased water content, increased water loss, and reduced water-binding capacity, as well as epidermal hyperproliferation resulting in lichenification (an exaggeration of normal skin markings) and buildup of scale.

Patients with atopic dermatitis usually have a personal or family history of allergies, asthma, or hay fever. In addition to scaly eczematous plaques, such patients may develop painful linear cracks or fissures from xerosis, particularly on the palms, soles, and fingertips (Figure 16.3).

 DIFFERENTIAL DIAGNOSIS

Ichthyosis Vulgaris (see Figure 2.18)
- Ichthyosis vulgaris (the most commonly seen variant of ichthyosis) resembles dry skin; however, it is actually caused by overadherence of scale.
- It is frequently associated with atopy.
- Skin with ichthyosis vulgaris resembles fine fish scales and tends to be most clinically obvious on the shins.
- Ichthyosis vulgaris is inherited in an autosomal dominant fashion and tends to improve with age.

Scabies
For a full discussion of this condition, see Chapter 20, "Bites, Stings, and Infestations."

- Scabies usually appears in a characteristic distribution of lesions, particularly in the finger webs, wrists, feet, penis, scrotum, and buttocks.
- Occasionally, epidemics occur in nursing homes and similar extended-care institutions. Under these circumstances, scabies may present uncharacteristically as "dry," minimally, itchy, or eczematous skin. Scabies may also be seen with crusted, keratotic plaques—so-called "Norwegian scabies" (see Figure 24.19).

MANAGEMENT

Moisturizers

Moisturizers do not add water to the skin, but they help to retain or "lock in" water that is absorbed while bathing. Therefore, moisturizers should be applied while the skin is still damp. There are numerous over-the-counter preparations in ointment bases, cream bases, and lotions. Some moisturizers contain alpha-hydroxy acids. The choice of product is based on personal preference, ease of application, cost, and effectiveness.

Ammonium lactate 12% (Lac-Hydrin) lotion or cream is a prescription alpha-hydroxy acid preparation that may be applied after bathing. It is very effective and is used for more severe cases of xerosis.

The 12% ammonium lactate preparation may be purchased over the counter as AmLactin. Carmol 40 (40% urea) lotion is useful for moderate to severe dryness. It is available by prescription only.

Other Strategies

- Low- to medium-potency topical corticosteroids are valuable for treating itching and erythema. In severe cases, more potent topical corticosteroids may be applied.
- Showers and baths that are less frequent and shorter may be helpful. Only tepid water should be used.
- Mild soaps (e.g., Dove, Basis) or a soap substitute (e.g., Cetaphil lotion) may be tried. However, excessive use of any soap or substitute should be avoided, especially on affected areas.
- Adhesive dressings (Band-Aids) are effective in promoting healing of fissures.
- Lined gloves worn while washing dishes can keep hands dry.
- Scarves, gloves, and other apparel can help to provide adequate protection from outdoor cold exposure.

The use of room humidifiers and the ingestion of copious amounts of water are of questionable value.

POINTS TO REMEMBER

- Dry skin and persistent pruritus—especially in elderly patients— may be evidence of a systemic condition (e.g., hypothyroidism or hypoparathyroidism), renal disease, or an underlying malignant disease.
- Dry or scaly skin may be associated with the use of cholesterol-lowering agents, in particular nicotinic acid.

HELPFUL HINTS

- Cocoa butter, petroleum jelly, or even vegetable shortening (e.g., Crisco) can be used as inexpensive moisturizers when cost is a consideration. They are very effective and do not contain many additives that may be sensitizing.
- For fissures, Krazy Glue, a cyanoacrylate glue, carefully applied to "seal the cracks," is a nontoxic dressing that is reported to promote healing.

SEE PATIENT HANDOUT, PAGE 475

CHAPTER 17

Drug Eruptions

Overview

- An adverse drug reaction is any nontherapeutic deleterious effect of a prescribed or over-the-counter medication.
- Drug eruptions can mimic almost any inflammatory dermatosis.
- Drug reactions may be allergic (immunologic) or nonallergic (toxic).

Allergic-type drug reactions are not dose dependent. They are classified as the four following types of immunologic reactions:

- Type I: Classic immediate hypersensitivity (urticaria, angioedema, anaphylaxis)
- Type II: Cytotoxic (hemolysis, purpura)
- Type III: Immune complex (vasculitis, serum sickness, urticaria, angioedema)
- Type IV: Delayed hypersensitivity (contact dermatitis, exanthematous reactions, photoallergic reactions)

Nonallergic drug eruptions are more common than allergic-type eruptions; they may be dose related or idiosyncratic. Vertigo due to high dose minocycline, demethylchlortetracycline photosensitive reactions, and irritant reactions from topical retinoids are examples.

BASICS

- Most drug eruptions are exanthematous (red rashes) and usually fade in a few days.
- More serious reactions include erythema multiforme major (Stevens–Johnson syndrome), toxic epidermal necrolysis, and serum sickness.

The presence of urticaria, mucosal involvement, extensive or palpable purpura, or blisters almost always requires discontinuation of the responsible drug. Certain classes of systemic medications, such as antimicrobial agents, nonsteroidal antiinflammatory drugs (NSAIDs), cytokines, chemotherapeutic agents, and psychotropic agents, are associated with a high rate of cutaneous reactions. Risk factors include the following:

- Age is a factor. Drug eruptions are more commonly seen in elderly persons because they often take more drugs than younger people, they often take more than one drug at a time, and they are more likely to have been previously sensitized.
- A history of previous drug reactions is a risk factor.
- A family history of drug eruptions is another factor.
- Prolonged use of the drug can predispose patients to drug eruptions.
- Paradoxically, although human immunodeficiency virus (HIV) infection causes profound anergy to other immune stimuli, the frequency of drug hypersensitivity reactions is increased markedly compared with both immunocompetent and HIV-negative immunocompromised populations.

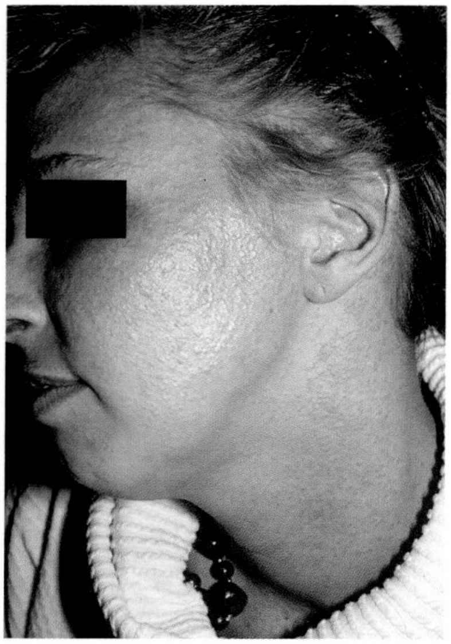

Characteristic Skin Reactions Produced by Drugs

Adverse cutaneous drug reactions can mimic many common non–drug-related skin eruptions, and certain drugs are more likely to cause characteristic reactions in the skin, as follows:

- **Exanthems and urticarial reactions:** Sulfonamides, penicillins, hydantoins, allopurinol, quinidine, angiotensin-converting enzyme inhibitors, barbiturates, carbamazepine, isoniazid, NSAIDs, and phenothiazine, as well as thiazide diuretics, aspirin, blood products, cephalosporins, dextran, opiates, radiocontrast dye, ranitidine, and vaccines
- **Acneiform eruptions:** systemic steroids, topical steroids, lithium, oral contraceptives, and androgenic hormones
- **Photo-induced:** tetracyclines, particularly demethylchlortetracycline and doxycycline, griseofulvin, sulfonamide diuretics, sulfonylurea agents used to treat diabetes, NSAIDs (Figure 17.1), and phenothiazines
- **Erythema nodosum:** iodides, oral contraceptives, penicillin, gold, amiodarone, sulfonamides, and opiates
- **Bullous eruptions:** penicillin, sulfonamides, captopril, iodides, gold, and furosemide
- **Purpura:** anticoagulants and thiazides
- **Vasculitic eruptions:** Allopurinol, aspirin or other NSAIDs, cimetidine, gold, hydralazine, penicillin, phenytoin, propylthiouracil, quinolones, sulfonamide, tetracycline, and thiazides
- **Erythema multiforme major (Stevens–Johnson syndrome)** and **erythema multiforme minor:** sulfonamides, penicillins, tetracyclines, hydantoins, and barbiturates
- **Fixed drug eruptions:** tetracyclines, sulfonamides, griseofulvin, barbiturates, phenolphthalein, and NSAIDs
- **Contact dermatitis:** neomycin and preservatives in topical medications

DESCRIPTION OF LESIONS

The morphology of a drug eruption can often provide clues to the most likely responsible agent.

Exanthematous Drug Eruption (Figure 17.2)

- Lesions are morbilliform (resembling measles).
- There may be areas of confluence.
- Lesions are pink, "drug red," or purple.

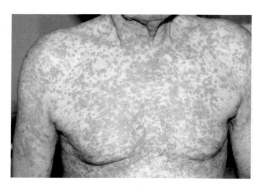

FIGURE 17.1 Photosensitivity versus phototoxic eruption, due to Feldene (piroxicam). Two days after this patient began taking Feldene, a nonsteroidal antiinflammatory drug, she went to the beach and developed an eruption in a photo distribution. Note the sparing under her sun-protected jaw.

FIGURE 17.2 Drug eruption. Exanthematous ampicillin reaction.

Urticarial Drug Eruption (Figure 17.3)

- Urticarial drug eruptions usually occur as wheals that may coalesce or take cyclic or gyrate forms.

Vasculitic Drug Eruption

- This may present as palpable purpura (see Figure 18.13).

Drug Photosensitive or Phototoxic Eruption

- This may appear as erythematous (an exaggerated sunburn) (Figure 17.4), eczematous, or lichenoid (resembling lichen planus).

Fixed Drug Eruption

This is a reaction of red plaques or blisters that recur at the same cutaneous site each time the drug is ingested. In other words, a rechallenge of the drug results in an identical eruption at the same site or sites.

- Lesions may be round or oval, single (Figures 17.5 and 17.6) or multiple.
- Lesions initially are erythematous; later they become violaceous.
- Lesions often blister and erode.
- The eruption often heals with postinflammatory hyperpigmentation.

DISTRIBUTION OF LESIONS

Drug eruptions tend to be symmetric and occasionally generalized in distribution; however, certain eruptions have specific regional predilections.

- Exanthems are noted particularly on the trunk, thighs, upper arms, and face. The rash is often symmetric and typically spares the palms and soles.
- In contact dermatitis, the distribution most often corresponds the area of initial insult to the skin.
- A fixed drug eruption may present as a solitary isolated lesion occurring most often on the extremities, glans penis (Figure 17.6), or trunk; multiple lesions may also occur.
- A photo-induced drug eruption occurs on the face, dorsal forearms, and "V" of the neck and upper sternum.
- Erythema nodosum occurs characteristically in the pretibial area.
- Purpura and vasculitic drug eruptions also tend to occur on the lower extremities.
- Steroid rosacea occurs on the face.
- Steroid atrophy most often occurs in body folds (axillae and inguinal creases).
- Urticaria can be seen anywhere on the body.
- Angioedema occurs in a periorbital, labial, and perioral distribution.
- Erythema multiforme lesions commonly manifests on mucous membrane as well as on the palms and soles; they can also be widespread (see Chapter 18, "Diseases of the Vasculature").

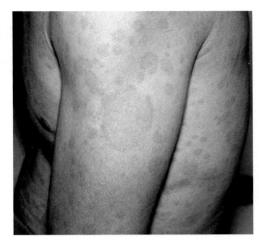

FIGURE 17.3 Urticarial drug eruption. Note the bizarre shapes of the urticarial plaques.

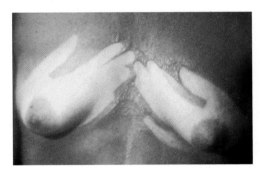

FIGURE 17.4 Drug photosensitivity eruption. Erythematous (exaggerated sunburn) reaction in a person who was taking demeclocycline (Declomycin) and fell asleep on the beach. (Courtesy of the Albert Einstein College of Medicine, Division of Dermatology, Bronx, New York.)

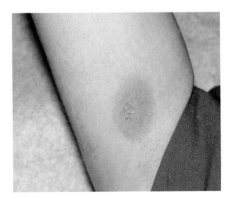

FIGURE 17.5 Fixed drug eruption. An oval lesion occurred at the identical site where it had occurred previously. In both episodes, the rash emerged after this patient ingested a sulfonamide antibiotic. Note the eroded blister in the center of the lesion.

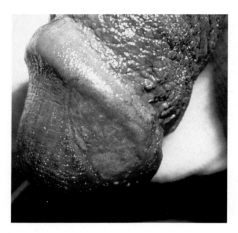

FIGURE 17.6 Fixed drug eruption. An oval erosion on the glans penis occurred in this patient who was taking minocycline. According to the patient, an identical lesion appeared when he was given minocycline previously.

CLINICAL MANIFESTATIONS

- Pruritus is a common complaint; however, adverse drug reactions also can cause pruritus unaccompanied by a rash.
- Acute urticarial lesions usually appear shortly after onset of drug therapy and resolve rapidly when the drug is withdrawn.
- Mucous membrane lesions are often painful (e.g., erosions, ulcers).
- Drug eruptions may be associated with systemic anaphylaxis or with extensive mucocutaneous exfoliation and multisystemic involvement; however, most drug eruptions are mild and self-limited, resolving after the offending agent is discontinued.
- In drug eruptions with vasculitis, fever, myalgias and arthritis, and abdominal pain may be present. Vasculitis typically begins 7 to 21 days after onset of drug therapy. The vasculitic process also may include other organ systems.

DIAGNOSIS

- Obtaining a detailed, careful history from the patient or family is paramount.
- A handy reference to drug eruptions and interactions should be always available.
- Patients occasionally have eosinophilia.
- Skin biopsy of an exanthem showing perivascular lymphocytes and eosinophils may be helpful, but it is not diagnostic. Characteristic histopathologic changes may occur in some cases, such as leukocytoclastic vasculitis in palpable purpura and panniculitis in erythema nodosum; however, these findings are not necessarily diagnostic of a drug-related origin.

 DIFFERENTIAL DIAGNOSIS

- Viral or bacterial exanthems generally occur with fever and other symptoms; however, they are often indistinguishable from a drug eruption.
- Pityriasis rosea should be considered.
- Acute urticaria (not drug-induced) is another possible diagnosis.
- Chronic urticaria (not drug-induced) should be considered.

 MANAGEMENT

- The drug should be discontinued, if feasible. However, the decision to discontinue a potentially vital drug presents a dilemma.
- If the patient is taking multiple medications and it is not possible to isolate which drug is the cause, the number of medications should be reduced to an absolute minimum, and the remaining drugs switched to alternative agents when possible.
- Oral antihistamines, such as diphenhydramine (Benadryl), hydroxyzine (Atarax), or the nonsedating agents cetirizine (Zyrtec) and loratadine (Claritin), may be helpful.
- Systemic steroids are given only in severe cases in which an infectious cause has been excluded.

POINTS TO REMEMBER

- Prompt recognition and withdrawal of an offending drug are important, particularly in patients with severe reactions.
- If a patient is taking multiple medications, it is often impossible to identify the agent responsible for an adverse reaction. In these instances, the drug that is most likely to cause the reaction should be suspected.
- If it is necessary to continue the drug (i.e., there is no alternative medication) and the adverse reaction is mild or tolerable, the difficulty may be minimized by decreasing the dosage or treating the adverse reaction.
- Persons who are immunocompromised have a greater risk for developing a drug eruption than the general population.

 HELPFUL HINTS

- Drug reactions can occur even after years of continuous therapy with the same drug.
- Drug reactions can occur days after a drug has been discontinued.
- A drug eruption may easily be confused with a feature of the condition that it is intended to treat (e.g., a viral exanthem treated with an antibiotic).
- Patients with infectious mononucleosis are likely to develop a morbilliform rash when they are given ampicillin.

CHAPTER 18

Diseases of Vasculature

BASICS

- Urticaria, commonly known as hives, is a reaction of cutaneous blood vessels that produces a transient dermal edema consisting of papules or plaques of different shapes and sizes (wheals).
- Angioedema refers to edema that is deeper than urticaria and involves the dermis and subcutaneous tissue.
- By definition, an individual urticarial lesion lasts less than 24 hours.
- A total of 10% to 20% of the population has at least one episode of urticaria or angioedema at some point in his or her lifetime.

Pathophysiology

Release of histamine and other compounds by mast cells and basophils causes the appearance of urticaria. Mast cell activation causes degranulation of intracellular vesicles that contain histamine, leukotriene C_4, prostaglandin D_2, and other chemotactic mediators that recruit eosinophils and neutrophils into the dermis. Histamine and chemokine release lead to extravasation of fluid into the dermis (edema). Histamine effects account for many of the clinical and histologic findings of urticaria. As with drug reactions, urticaria may be immune mediated or nonimmune mediated (see Chapter 17, "Drug Eruptions").

Causes of urticaria and angioedema include the following:

- Immunologic causes, mediated by immunoglobulin E (IgE), include food, drugs, and parasites.
- Complement-mediated causes include serum sickness and whole blood transfusions.
- Physical stimuli include cold, sunlight, and pressure (e.g., dermatographism).
- Occult infections include sinusitis, dental abscesses, and tinea pedis. However, such problems are rarely associated with chronic urticaria.

In 85% to 90% of patients with chronic urticaria, the origin is unknown (i.e., chronic idiopathic urticaria).

CLASSIFICATION

Urticaria may be classified as acute or chronic urticaria, physical urticaria, urticarial vasculitis, and hereditary angioedema (rare).

Acute Urticaria

Acute urticaria, by definition, lasts less than 30 days.

- Outbreaks are often IgE mediated.
- Many patients have an atopic history.
- There may be an obvious precipitant such as an acute upper respiratory infection, drug, parasitic infection, or bee sting.
- The most common drugs that may cause acute hives are antibiotics (especially penicillin and sulfonamides), pain medications such as aspirin, nonsteroidal antiinflammatory drugs (NSAIDs), narcotics, radiocontrast dyes, diuretics, and opiates such as codeine.

- The most common foods associated with acute urticaria are: milk, wheat, eggs, chocolate, shellfish, nuts, fish, and strawberries. Food additives and preservatives such as salicylates and benzoates may also be responsible.
- Acute urticaria also may be caused by physical stimuli such as pressure, cold, sunlight, or exercise. Such hives are called physical urticarias (see later).
- Anaphylaxis or an anaphylactoid reaction can occur.

Chronic Urticaria
Chronic urticaria is, by definition, urticaria that lasts longer than 4 to 6 weeks.

- There is a 2:1 female-to-male ratio of occurrence.
- The cause is usually unknown; however, chronic urticaria may, very infrequently, be a sign of one of the following systemic diseases: systemic lupus erythematosus, serum hepatitis, lymphoma, polycythemia, macroglobulinemia, or thyroid disease.

DESCRIPTION OF LESIONS

- Papules and plaques are of varying sizes.
- Wheals are the color of the patient's skin or pale red; a halo may be noted at the periphery of the lesions (Figure 18.1).
- Lesions have various shapes; they can be annular, linear, arciform, or polycyclic, and frequently they are multiple, with bizarre shapes (Figures 18.2 and 18.3).
- Individual lesions disappear within 24 hours (evanescent wheals).
- Lesions may be accompanied by a deep swelling (angioedema) around the eyes, lips, and tongue that often looks frightening. Fortunately, angioedema usually lasts less than 24 hours.

DISTRIBUTION OF LESIONS

- Angioedema is noted primarily in the periorbital area (Figure 18.4), lips, and tongue.
- Urticarial lesions may occur anywhere on the body and may be localized or generalized.

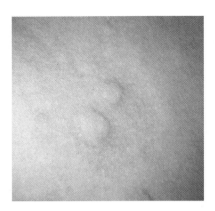

FIGURE 18.1 Urticaria. Skin-colored wheals are present.

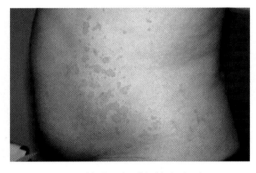

FIGURE 18.2 Urticaria. Multiple lesions have various shapes and sizes. Note whitish halos.

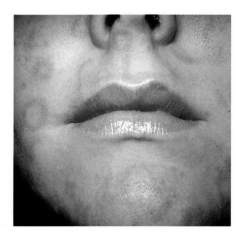

FIGURE 18.3 Acute urticaria. Lesions are annular, arciform, and polycyclic, with bizarre shapes.

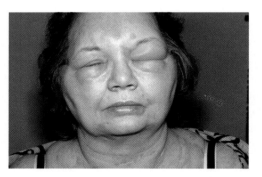

FIGURE 18.4 Urticaria. Marked angioedema is noted.

CLINICAL MANIFESTATIONS

- Lesions generally itch.
- Arthralgia, fever, malaise, and other symptoms may accompany urticaria when it is the result of hepatitis or serum sickness, for example.
- Scratching and rubbing of lesions generally do not produce scabs or crusts similar to those seen in atopic dermatitis.
- Acute urticaria lasts for hours to days (generally less than 30 days).
- Approximately 50% of patients with chronic urticaria are free of lesions in 1 year; in other patients, lesions may recur for many years.
- Emotional stress may trigger recurrences.

CLINICAL VARIANTS

Physical Urticarias

Physical factors are the most commonly identified causes of chronic urticaria. Physical urticarias are diagnosed by challenge testing. The following is a list of some physical urticarias and their causes:

- Dermatographism results from firm stroking or scratching.
- Cold urticaria is caused by cold exposure.
- Aquagenic urticaria results from contact with water.
- Cholinergic urticaria is caused by heat or exercise.
- Solar urticaria results from sun exposure.

Dermatographism ("Skin Writing") (Figure 18.5)

- Dermatographism affects more than 4% of the general population, in whom it is physiologic and asymptomatic.
- Linear erythematous wheals occur 3 to 4 minutes after firmly stroking the skin with the wooden handle of a cotton swab; they fade within 30 minutes.
- Lesions are seen under constrictive garments, such as belts and bras, or after a person scratches.
- In some persons, itching is the primary symptom.
- Episodes of dermatographism may persist for years.

Cold Urticaria (Figure 18.6)
- Cold urticaria occurs in young adults and children.
- Itchy hives occur at sites of cold exposure, such as areas exposed to cold winds or immersion in cold water.
- In the "ice cube test," a wheal arises on the skin after application of an ice cube.

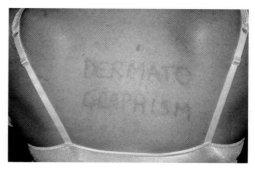

FIGURE 18.5 Dermatographism ("skin writing"). These lesions occurred 3 minutes after stroking with the wooden tip of a cotton swab.

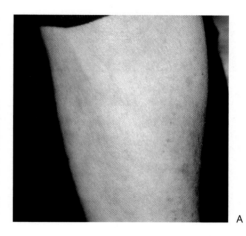

A

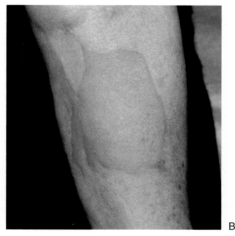

B

FIGURE 18.6 Cold urticaria. The "ice cube test." Before *(A)* and 5 minutes after *(B)* application of an ice cube. A large wheal and surrounding erythema have appeared.

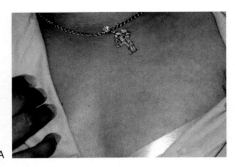

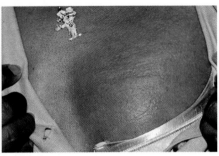

FIGURE 18.7 Solar urticaria induced by ultraviolet A light. Before sun exposure *(A)* and after 15 minutes of sun exposure through a glass window *(B)*. The glass window filters out ultraviolet B light.

Light-Induced (Solar) Urticaria (Figure 18.7)

- Urticaria that occurs in sun-exposed areas of the skin and is triggered by different wavelengths of light.

Cholinergic Urticaria

- This type of urticaria is induced by exercise.
- The patient exercises to the point of sweating, which provokes lesions and establishes the diagnosis.
- Typical lesions are multiple small monomorphic wheals.

Other Physical Urticarias

These include those induced by pressure, vibration, and water *(aquagenic urticaria)*.

DIAGNOSIS

The diagnosis of acute and chronic urticaria is usually made on **clinical observation** and **history.** If a complete review of systems is normal, and a physical urticaria is ruled out, it is often futile to perform multiple laboratory tests to determine a cause for chronic urticaria. Nonetheless, a positive **symptom-directed search** for underlying illness (e.g., systemic lupus erythematosus, thyroid disease, lymphoma, and necrotizing vasculitis) may warrant evaluations such as:

- Complete blood count
- Erythrocyte sedimentation rate
- Fluorescent antinuclear antibody test
- Thyroid function studies
- Hepatitis-associated antigen test
- Assessment of the complement system
- Radioallergosorbent test for IgE antibodies
- In the presence of eosinophilia, stool examination for ova and parasites

 DIFFERENTIAL DIAGNOSIS

Insect Bite Reactions

These reactions are also known as **papular urticaria.** For a full discussion of insect bite reactions, see Chapter 20, "Bites, Stings, and Infestations."

- Reactions to insect bites may be indistinguishable from ordinary hives.
- Bites are generally seen on exposed areas.
- They may have a central punctum and crust; they also may blister.
- Individual lesions may last more than 24 hours.

Erythema Multiforme Minor (see later)

- Lesions are targetoid.
- Lesions last more than 24 hours.
- Lesions are generally nonpruritic.

Erythema Migrans (Acute Lyme Disease)

For a full discussion of this condition, see Chapter 20, "Bites, Stings, and Infestations."

- Erythema migrans may be indistinguishable from urticaria.
- Lesions are usually solitary.
- A lesion may last more than 24 hours.
- Lesions are generally nonpruritic.

Urticarial Vasculitis

This condition is rare.

- Persistent hivelike lesions last more than 24 hours.
- Evidence of vasculitis (e.g., purpura) is occasionally seen in the lesions.
- The diagnosis is confirmed by skin biopsy.
- Patients may have hypocomplementemia and an elevated erythrocyte sedimentation rate.
- Urticarial vasculitis may be associated with collagen vascular diseases.

MANAGEMENT

- If possible, the cause of the hives should be eliminated, and tight clothing and hot baths and showers should be avoided, particularly in people who have physical urticaria.
- Histamine H_1 blockers include hydroxyzine (Atarax), diphenhydramine (Benadryl), and cyproheptadine (Periactin); H_1 and H_2 blockers may be used in combination, such as cimetidine (Tagamet) plus hydroxyzine. These first-generation antihistamines compete with histamine at the tissue receptor level.
- Newer, nonsedating antihistamines, such as loratadine (Claritin), desloratadine (Clarinex), and cetirizine (Zyrtec), may be used during the day, and a more sedating H_1 blocker or a tricyclic antidepressant drug, such as doxepin (Sinequan, Zonalon), may be tried at bedtime. Doxepin can be given at bedtime at a much lower dosage than when it is used as an antidepressant; it has antihistaminic properties and is several hundred times more potent than diphenhydramine. In addition, doxepin has both H_1 and H_2 antihistaminic properties.
- Oral doxepin alone, at doses ranging from 5 mg twice daily to 50 mg three times daily, has successfully suppressed chronic urticaria.
- Systemic steroids are sometimes used for short periods to break the cycle of chronic urticaria; however, they are not indicated for long-term use in the treatment of chronic idiopathic urticaria.
- Salicylates, NSAIDs, and narcotics, which are all histamine-releasing agents, may aggravate both acute and chronic urticaria and should be avoided.
- If all else fails, a diary of daily foods eaten may be kept, with subsequent food elimination. However, this approach is rarely successful.

POINTS TO REMEMBER

- Except for the physical urticarias and urticaria that is obviously associated with drugs and systemic disease, determining the cause of chronic urticaria is generally a fruitless task.
- Routine blood tests are of little or no value in determining the cause of acute or chronic urticaria.
- Allergy testing is expensive, and often tests are positive for allergies that have no relation to the patient's urticaria.
- When individual wheals persist for more than 24 hours, the process is unlikely to be urticaria.

HELPFUL HINTS

- Epinephrine, which is often administered by intramuscular or subcutaneous injection for acute urticaria, **should not be used** for routine cases of hives. It should be reserved for cases of acute anaphylaxis.
- Patients with documented cold urticaria should be advised not to immerse themselves abruptly in cold water.
- Patients with severe reactions should consider wearing a Medic Alert bracelet that describes their problem.
- Montelukast (Singulair), a leukotriene receptor antagonist used to treat asthma, has been found to be effective in some cases of chronic idiopathic urticaria that are refractory to antihistamines.
- The mainstay of treatment of chronic urticaria is the use of antihistamines; however, immunotherapies using plasmapheresis, intravenous immunoglobulin, and cyclosporine have been used in severe, recalcitrant cases.

SEE PATIENT HANDOUT, PAGE 477

BASICS

- Erythema multiforme is a confusing condition for many health care providers. The classic description of erythema multiforme made by Ferdinand von Hebra in the late 19th century was very specific and is still currently used: "a self-limited eruption characterized by symmetrically distributed erythematous papules, which develop into characteristic target-like lesions consisting of concentric color changes with a dusky central zone that may become bullous." This classic form of erythema multiforme is currently defined as **erythema multiforme minor.**
- The more serious variant, with extensive mucous membrane involvement, systemic symptoms, and more widespread lesions, is called **erythema multiforme major (Stevens–Johnson syndrome).**
- Erythema multiforme is a reaction pattern of dermal blood vessels with secondary changes noted in the epidermis that results clinically in curious targetlike shapes.
- Erythema multiforme is most commonly seen in late adolescence and in young adulthood. Affected persons are generally in good health.

Causes

The list of causes of erythema multiforme is long and is, in many cases, a duplication of the list of causes of urticaria (see earlier). Most cases of both erythema multiforme major and minor are idiopathic, however, the following are the most well-documented associations:

- The most common precipitating cause of erythema multiforme minor is recurrent labial herpes simplex virus infection (Figure 18.8); recurrences of herpes progenitalis also have been reported to precede or sometimes occur simultaneously with episodes of recurrent erythema multiforme minor. Erythema multiforme minor is unlikely related to drugs.
- Precipitating factors in erythema multiforme major are drugs (sulfonamides, penicillin, hydantoins, barbiturates, allopurinol, NSAIDs), *Mycoplasma* infection, pregnancy, *Streptococcus* infection, hepatitis A and B, coccidioidomycosis, and Epstein–Barr virus infection.

DESCRIPTION OF LESIONS

- Lesions begin as round, erythematous macules.
- Some lesions evolve to form targetoid plaques *(iris lesions)* with a dark center that may become vesicobullous.
- Lesions persist (are "fixed") for at least 1 week.
- Erosions and crusts form.

DISTRIBUTION OF LESIONS

- Lesions are bilateral and symmetric.
- The palms and soles, dorsa of hands and feet, extensor forearms and legs, face, and genitalia are affected.
- Mucous membrane lesions are limited to the mouth in erythema multiforme minor.
- Extensive mucous membrane lesions in erythema multiforme major may be located in multiple sites, including the mouth, pharynx, eyes, and genitalia (Figure 18.9).

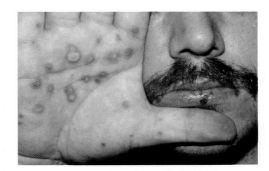

FIGURE 18.8 Erythema multiforme minor. This patient has a recurrent herpes simplex virus infection. Note the drying crust of the herpetic "cold sore" on his lower lip and the target-like lesions on his palm.

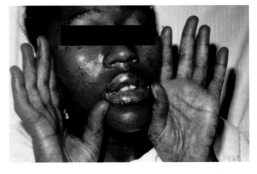

FIGURE 18.9 Erythema multiforme major. Extensive hemorrhagic crusting on mucous membranes is noted in a patient with fever and extensive erythematous lesions.

CLINICAL MANIFESTATIONS

Erythema Multiforme Minor
- The eruption is acute, self-limited, and often recurrent.
- Evidence of herpes labialis may be present.
- Little or no mucous membrane involvement is noted.

Erythema Multiforme Major
- This is often accompanied by symptoms of fever, malaise, and myalgias.
- Severe, painful mucous membrane involvement occurs.
- Possible complications include keratitis, corneal ulcers, upper airway damage, and pneumonia.

DIAGNOSIS

- Typical target lesions are present.
- Skin biopsy is performed, if necessary.

 DIFFERENTIAL DIAGNOSIS

Urticaria
- Lesions are transient, not "fixed."
- Lesions are pruritic.
- The center of annular lesions is not dusky in color.

Primary Herpes Gingivostomatitis and Primary Bullous Diseases of the Oral Cavity
- In the absence of nonmucous membrane skin lesions, other diseases of the mucous membranes may be clinically indistinguishable from those of erythema multiforme.
- Mucous membrane biopsy may be necessary to distinguish oral bullous erythema multiforme from primary bullous diseases such as pemphigus vulgaris or bullous pemphigoid.

MANAGEMENT

- If known, the precipitating cause should be eliminated or treated.
- Suspected etiologic drugs should be discontinued.
- Empiric treatment with oral acyclovir, famciclovir, or valacyclovir may prevent or mitigate recurrences if erythema multiforme is due to herpes simplex virus infection.
- Wet dressings (e.g., Burow's solution) and topical steroids may be applied.
- In life-threatening situations, such as may be seen in erythema multiforme major, hospitalization is often essential. The use of systemic steroids in such severe cases is controversial, and their effectiveness has not been established.

POINTS TO REMEMBER

- Erythema multiforme is not a disease but a syndrome with multiple causes and various degrees of severity.
- Even in the clinical absence of herpes simplex virus infection, recurrent erythema multiforme may be suppressed with oral acyclovir, famciclovir, or valacyclovir.

BASICS

Purpura is a hemorrhage of blood into the skin. Purpura may be seen after the following:

- Minor trauma to the skin may precipitate purpura, particularly when a patient is taking drugs such as aspirin or other NSAIDs and warfarin (Coumadin), agents that increase clotting time.
- Long-term application of potent topical steroids on the skin of elderly patients may also produce purpura.

It also may be seen in association with the following:

- Blood dyscrasias and coagulopathies, such as thrombocytopenia, leukemia, and disseminated intravascular coagulopathy, may result in purpura.
- Actinic purpura (formerly known as *senile purpura*) is a prevalent finding on the dorsal forearms in elderly persons. Such ecchymoses are believed to result from minor trauma to an area of chronic sun exposure. Thinning of skin and "fragile capillaries" are considered the cause (Figure 18.10).
- Chronic venous insufficiency of the lower extremities may result in purpuric changes in the skin.

There are also the so-called "benign" variants of purpura such as:

- **The benign pigmented purpuras,** of which there are several varieties, are caused by capillaritis, which allows blood to exit small vessels (extravasation), and create petechiae.

As their name implies, these benign purpuras are not associated with any systemic disease.

    Schamberg's purpura is the most common of the benign pigmented purpuras. It is characterized by so-called "cayenne pepper" purpura (Figure 18.11).

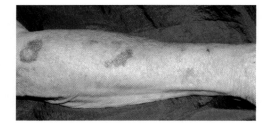

FIGURE 18.10 Senile, or actinic, purpura. Ecchymoses are present on the dorsal forearms in an elderly person.

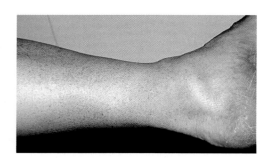

FIGURE 18.11 Schamberg's purpura. "Cayenne pepper" petechiae are seen on the lower extremities.

DESCRIPTION OF LESIONS

- Lesions begin as nonblanching, red, pinpoint macules *(petechiae),* or bruises *(ecchymoses)* that may coalesce.
- Older lesions become purple, then brown as hemosiderin forms.

DISTRIBUTION OF LESIONS

- **Purpura due to blood dyscrasias and coagulopathies** are noted more commonly on dependent areas (i.e., lower legs and ankles; buttocks in bedridden patients).
- **Actinic purpura** is seen on the dorsa of forearms.
- **Schamberg's purpura** and other variants of benign pigmented purpura are most commonly seen on the lower extremities.
- **Chronic venous insufficiency** (often with secondary stasis dermatitis) is also seen on the lower legs (Figure 18.12) (see the discussion of stasis dermatitis in Chapter 2, "Eczema").

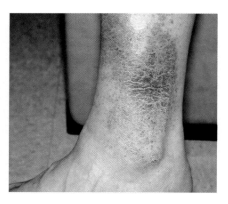

FIGURE 18.12 Stasis dermatitis. Purpura and lichenification are noted.

CLINICAL MANIFESTATIONS

- Lesions are generally asymptomatic, but they may be mildly pruritic.
- Pruritus is more severe when stasis dermatitis complicates chronic venous insufficiency (see Chapter 2, "Eczema").
- Purpuric lesions may be of cosmetic concern to patients; other patients wish to be reassured that purpura is not a sign of a serious disease.
- Lesions may persist for months to years or indefinitely.

DIAGNOSIS

- The diagnosis is made on clinical presentation.
- Lesions are not palpable and are nonblanching on diascopy (direct pressure).
- A coagulopathy or blood dyscrasia should be ruled out if it is clinically suspected.

 DIFFERENTIAL DIAGNOSIS

- Biopsy may be necessary at times to distinguish benign purpura from leukocytoclastic vasculitis (see later).

 MANAGEMENT

- Benign pigmented purpura generally requires no workup; however, if a blood dyscrasia or coagulopathy is suspected, appropriate laboratory tests should be ordered.
- Possible offending drugs should be evaluated regarding their risk-to-benefit ratio.

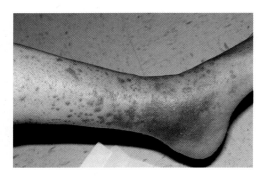

FIGURE 18.13 Leukocytoclastic vasculitis. Palpable purpura and ecchymoses are present.

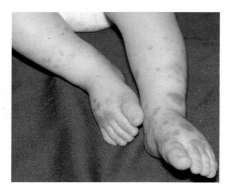

FIGURE 18.14 Henoch-Schönlein purpura. Resolving palpable purpura is shown in an infant.

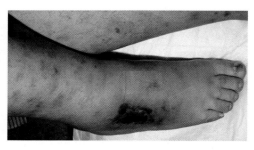

FIGURE 18.15 Leukocytoclastic vasculitis. Ulceration has occurred in this patient who has vasculitis.

BASICS

- **Hypersensitivity vasculitis** refers to a group of vasculitic conditions involving the vessels that lie within the middle to upper dermis.
- Clinically, hypersensitivity vasculitis is manifested in the skin as **palpable purpura.** It is caused by deposition of circulating immune complexes in the postcapillary venules, primarily in the legs (Figure 18.13).
- The circulating immune complexes may also deposit in organs and may cause systemic vasculitis with resultant gastrointestinal bleeding, hematuria, and arthralgias.
- **Henoch-Schönlein purpura (HSP)** is a type of hypersensitivity vasculitis caused by group A streptococci that demonstrates an IgA immunofluorescent pattern. This term, HSP, should be reserved for disease that follows an upper respiratory infection, generally in children (Figure 18.14).
- Vasculitis may also be associated with a hypersensitivity to antigens from drugs, infectious agents, neoplasms, or other underlying diseases such as collagen vascular disease and cryoglobulinemias, or it may be idiopathic. (Hypersensitivity vasculitis is idiopathic in more than 50% of cases.)
- **Leukocytoclastic vasculitis** is the histopathologic hallmark of hypersensitivity vasculitis.

DESCRIPTION OF LESIONS

- Lesions are frequently palpable and do not blanche *(palpable purpura).*
- Ulceration may develop (Figure 18.15).

DISTRIBUTION OF LESIONS

- Lesions are most often seen in dependent areas such as the lower legs and ankles and on the buttocks in bedridden patients.
- In severe forms, lesions can be generalized.

CLINICAL MANIFESTATIONS

- Lesions may be asymptomatic, slightly painful, or mildly pruritic.
- Lesions sometimes recur.
- There may be associated malaise and possible fever.
- In Henoch-Schönlein purpura, abdominal pain, arthralgia, hematuria, and proteinuria may be present.
- In systemic vasculitis, symptoms are referable to the organ involved.

DIAGNOSIS

- Laboratory investigation is made for underlying disease: complete blood count, erythrocyte sedimentation rate, urinalysis, and stool examination for occult blood. Further studies (e.g., serum complement, anti-nuclear antibodies) should be directed by the patient's symptoms.
- Biopsy of lesions shows characteristic leukocytoclastic vasculitis ("nuclear dust").
- Patients with Henoch-Schönlein purpura caused by group A streptococci have a perivascular IgA immunofluorescent deposition in the skin and kidneys.

  DIFFERENTIAL DIAGNOSIS

- Palpable and nonpalpable purpura may also be seen in **septic vasculitis,** in which lesions are generally acral and tend to be few (e.g., gonococcemia) (Figure 18.16).
- Patients who have septic vasculitis may also be febrile and show other signs and symptoms of the underlying infection.

 MANAGEMENT

- If known, the precipitating cause (e.g., drug) should be eliminated or treated.
- In general, no treatment is necessary for mild, self-limited episodes.
- Systemic steroids and appropriate antibiotics are administered, if indicated.
- Nonsteroidal medications may include dapsone or colchicine.
- Immunosuppressants are sometimes used in conjunction with systemic steroids as steroid-sparing agents.

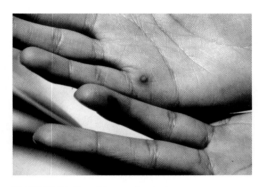

FIGURE 18.16 Disseminated gonococcemia. This is an example of septic vasculitis. Note the two palpable purpuric hemorrhagic vesicles.

 POINT TO REMEMBER

- Palpable purpura may be a sign of systemic vasculitis, sepsis, drug allergy, underlying disease, or an idiopathic benign reaction pattern.

CHAPTER 19

Sexually Transmitted Diseases

Mary Ruth Buchness and Herbert P. Goodheart

BASICS

Anogenital warts are sexually transmitted viral warts caused by infection with specific types of human papillomavirus (HPV). It is estimated that 1% of the population of the United States has clinically evident lesions, and 15% has latent HPV infection.

- The incubation period is variable, ranging from 3 weeks to 8 months, with an average of 2.8 months reported in one study.
- HPV has been identified in the skin of infected persons at a distance of up to 1 cm from the actual lesion; this feature may explain the high recurrence rate. HPV types 16, 18, 31 to 35, 39, 42, 48, and 51 to 54 have been identified in cervical and anogenital cancers.
- Lesions tend to be more extensive and recalcitrant to treatment in immunocompromised persons; they also tend to grow larger and more numerous during pregnancy. Women with HPV infection who are pregnant or who are considering pregnancy pose specific challenges. In addition to the potential for rapid proliferation of external genital warts during pregnancy, the mere presence of HPV infection raises concerns regarding mode of delivery and the risk for oropharyngeal or genital HPV infections in the newborn. Although neonates are at greater risk for exposure to HPV after vaginal delivery than they are after cesarean section, the significance of such exposure remains controversial. Moreover, cesarean section does not confer complete protection.

Risk Factors
- Transmission of anogenital HPV infection occurs largely by sexual intercourse.
- Other risk factors for infection include cigarette smoking, participating in sexual activity at an early age, having a high number of sexual partners, having another sexually transmitted disease, immunosuppression, and having an abnormal Pap smear result.

DESCRIPTION OF LESIONS

There are five morphologic types, and a patient may manifest more than one type. The appearance of warts depends on its location; for example, the condyloma acuminatum type tends to occur on moist surfaces:

1. Condyloma acuminatum may resemble small cauliflowers (Figure 19.1).
2. Warts may appear as smooth, dome-shaped papular lesions (Figure 19.2).
3. They can look like typical verrucous papules or plaques that resemble common warts (Figure 19.3).
4. Occasionally, they present as flat papules that may be hyperpigmented.
5. Mucous membrane lesions often appear white from maceration.

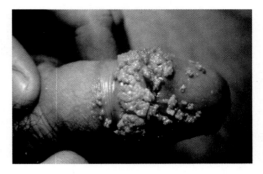

FIGURE 19.1 Condyloma acuminatum. Lesions resemble small cauliflowers.

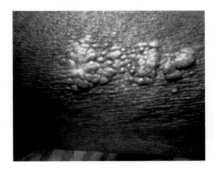

FIGURE 19.2 Penile warts. Smooth, dome-shaped papular lesions are present.

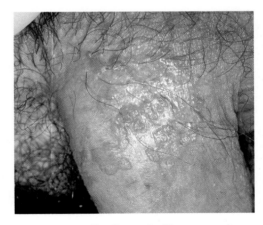

FIGURE 19.3 Penile warts. These papules have the appearance of common warts.

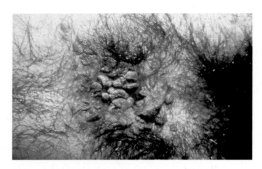

FIGURE 19.4 Condyloma acuminatum. Perianal warts are noted.

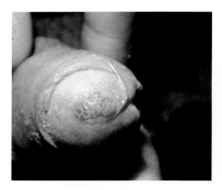

FIGURE 19.5 Condyloma acuminatum. Periurethral warts are seen.

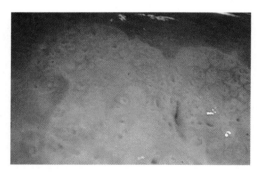

FIGURE 19.6 Cervical warts. Acetowhitening of subclinical lesions on the cervical mucosa is shown here.

DISTRIBUTION OF LESIONS

Anogenital Lesions
- In men, lesions occur on the penis, scrotum, mons pubis, inguinal crease, and perianal area (Figure 19.4).
- In women, the vagina, labia, mons pubis, perianal area, and uterine cervix are the most common locations.
- Intraanal warts are seen predominantly in patients who have engaged in receptive anal intercourse.
- Warts may also be found in the peri- and intraurethral areas (Figure 19.5).

Outside the Genital Area
- HPV has been associated with conjunctival, nasal, oral, and laryngeal warts.

CLINICAL MANIFESTATIONS

- Genital warts are usually asymptomatic.
- Lesions may become pruritic, particularly perianal and inguinal lesions.
- They may be painful or bleed if traumatized.
- Genital warts may resolve spontaneously or, rarely, progress to invasive squamous cell carcinoma.

DIAGNOSIS

- The diagnosis of anogenital warts is generally straightforward when the patient presents with the typical cauliflowerlike lesions of condyloma acuminatum or with characteristic verrucous or filiform warts. However, when lesions are papular, planar (flat-topped), pigmented, moist, or erosive, the diagnosis may not be as clinically obvious.
- Normal anatomic structures found on mucous membranes, such as vestibular papillae and sebaceous glands **(Fordyce spots)** in women and **pearly penile papules** in men, are frequently mistaken for—and treated as—warts by overzealous clinicians misled by a high index of suspicion for HPV (see later).
- On non–mucous membrane skin, further potential diagnostic pitfalls are presented by the dome-shaped, waxy papules of **molluscum contagiosum** (see Figure 19.10) and by the smooth, skin-colored or pigmented lesions known as **skin tags** (acrochordons).

Acetowhite Test on Mucous Membranes
- In women, colposcopy is performed using 35% acetic acid, which produces an acetowhitening of subclinical lesions on the vaginal and cervical mucosa (Figure 19.6).
- Atypia or koilocytosis found on Pap smears may represent early changes resulting from HPV infection.

Acetowhite Test on Non–Mucous Membrane Areas
- A 5% concentration of acetic acid applied for 15 to 20 minutes makes subclinical lesions turn white.
- This method results in the overdiagnosis of warts because of false-positive results and is no longer recommended for routine screening.

Biopsy

A biopsy may be needed to identify confusing anogenital lesions.

- After local anesthesia with lidocaine, curved iris scissors are used to obtain a small specimen (snip biopsy) from the labia minora or perianal area. A punch biopsy or, more simply, a shave biopsy may be obtained from non–mucous membrane skin (see Chapter 26, "Basic Dermatologic Procedures"). If an ulcer or an indurated nodule is present—particularly if carcinoma is suspected—a punch or excisional biopsy should be performed.
- A biopsy is used to rule out anogenital bowenoid papulosis or frank squamous cell carcinoma in atypical or recalcitrant lesions.

 DIFFERENTIAL DIAGNOSIS

Normal Variants

- In women, **vestibular papillae** are normal anatomic structures. Unlike warts, vestibular papillae *(vulvar papillomatosis)* occur near the vaginal vestibule in symmetric clusters or in a linear pattern. They often appear as monotonous, small, smooth projections that resemble cobblestones (Figure 19.7).
- In men, **pearly penile papules** are frequently mistaken for warts. They are small, skin-colored to shiny, pearly papules that are located around the rim of the corona of the glans penis (Figures 19.8 and 19.9).
- Fordyce spots are angiokeratomas. They occur on the medial labia minora in many women (see Figure 21.34).

Benign Lesions

- Common benign skin lesions, such as skin tags, seborrheic keratoses, and melanocytic nevi, may also be easily mistaken for warts.
- Skin tags are smooth and may be pigmented or skin-colored.
- Seborrheic keratoses and melanocytic nevi often have a verrucous (keratotic) appearance and may be pigmented.

Other Conditions

- **Hemorrhoids.** Not infrequently, anal hemorrhoids are mistaken for warts. Hemorrhoids are bluish, smooth, and compressible.
- **Molluscum contagiosum.** When found in the pubic area, vulvae, or medial thighs (Figure 19.10), molluscum contagiosum can easily be confused with, and may coexist with, genital warts. Molluscum contagiosum is a common superficial viral infection of the epidermis. It is seen most often in young children and in patients with human immunodeficiency virus (HIV) infection and in sexually active young adults (see Chapter 6, "Superficial Viral Infections," and Chapter 24, "Cutaneous Manifestations of HIV Infection"). The lesions are dome-shaped, waxy or pearly white papules with a central white core, which is often revealed by inspection with a handheld magnifier. Lesions are generally 1 to 3 mm in diameter. Frequently, the lesions are grouped. A short application of liquid nitrogen accentuates the central core. A smear or a shave biopsy of a lesion demonstrates characteristic "molluscum bodies" (see Figure 6.18).
- **Condyloma latum of secondary syphilis.** Lesions are moist, smooth-surfaced, and, usually, whitish and flat-topped. Serologic tests for syphilis are positive (see Figure 19.20).

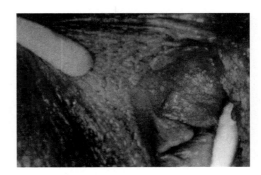

FIGURE 19.7 Vestibular papillae (vulvar papillomatosis). These lesions occur near the vaginal vestibule in symmetric clusters or in a linear pattern. They are frequently mistaken for warts.

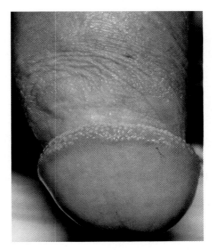

FIGURE 19.8 Pearly penile papules. Shiny papules are present around the corona of the glans penis.

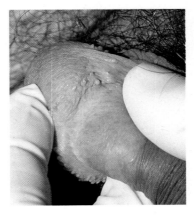

FIGURE 19.9 Pearly penile papules. These hairlike papules are sometimes referred to as "hirsutoid papules." They are also frequently misdiagnosed and treated as warts.

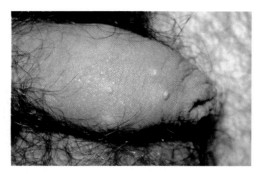

FIGURE 19.10 Molluscum contagiosum. Dome-shaped papules have central white core.

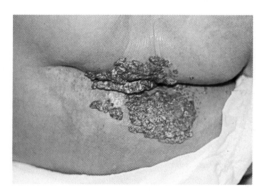

FIGURE 19.11 Giant condyloma acuminatum. This lesion is a low-grade, locally invasive malignant tumor that can arise from and appear as a fungating condyloma.

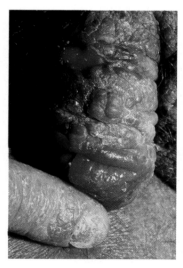

FIGURE 19.12 Squamous cell carcinoma. These lesions are beefy red and eroded.

Neoplasms

- Other neoplasms that should be considered in the differential diagnosis include bowenoid papulosis, giant condyloma acuminatum, and squamous cell carcinoma. When any of these conditions are suspected, a biopsy should be performed.
- **Bowenoid papulosis.** These lesions are clinically similar to, and often indistinguishable from, flat or dome-shaped genital warts. They are associated with HPV type 16 or 18. Histologically, bowenoid papulosis demonstrates squamous cell carcinoma *in situ;* however, it follows a largely benign clinical course.
- **Giant condyloma acuminatum.** Also known as a Buschke-Löwenstein tumor, this lesion is a low-grade, locally invasive squamous cell carcinoma that can arise from and appear as a fungating condyloma (Figure 19.11).
- **Squamous cell carcinoma.** These lesions are rapidly growing nodules or tumors, or they may be erosive or ulcerative (Figure 19.12).

MANAGEMENT

Counseling

- Patients should be advised about the long latency period of HPV; thus, a patient may not have contracted condyloma from his or her current partner.
- Sexual transmission. Male patients should use condoms at least 1 year after clinical infection is treated; however, condoms are not perfect protection because warts can occur on genital areas other than the penis or vagina.
- In affected women, there is a risk for malignant degeneration to cervical intraepithelial neoplasia or squamous cell carcinoma. If cervical warts are found during examination or if vulvar neoplasia is confirmed by biopsy, referral for colposcopic evaluation is indicated.
- Once a woman is diagnosed with condyloma acuminatum, she should have Pap smears every 6 months.
- The United States Centers for Disease Control and Prevention (CDC) recommends cesarian section only when the vaginal outlet is obstructed by extensive condylomata or if vaginal delivery would cause excessive bleeding.
- Patients who have internal anal or rectal warts tend to have continual recurrences of external warts and should be referred to a rectal surgeon.

Surgical Therapy

- Liquid nitrogen cryosurgery
- Electrodesiccation and curettage
- Carbon dioxide laser treatment (more expensive)
- Surgical excision

Intralesional Therapy

- Interferon-α2b (11.5 units three times weekly for 3 weeks [not recommended by the CDC because of high expense and no increased efficacy over other treatments])

Topical Therapy

- Various topical treatments are available.

TOPICAL THERAPY		
	TREATMENT	**APPLICATION**
PATIENT-APPLIED THERAPIES	Imiquimod 5% (Aldara) cream	It is used three times weekly for up to 16 weeks. It is believed to act by enhancing a patient's immunity to human papillomavirus by increasing local production of interferon. Efficacy in immunocompromised patients is unknown. Safety for use in pregnancy is not known.
	Podofilox (Condylox) 0.5% solution or gel	It is used twice daily, morning and evening, for 3 days, then followed by 4 days without therapy. This 1-week cycle of treatment may be repeated up to four times until no wart remains. Safety for use in pregnancy is not known.
PROVIDER-APPLIED THERAPIES	Podophyllin resin 10% to 25% in tincture of benzoin	It is carefully applied to the wart surface. The patient is instructed to wash the area in 4 to 6 hours, and the interval is increased on subsequent treatments. It is most effective on mucosal warts. Podophyllin is an antimitotic agent that causes local tissue destruction.
	Tricholoracetic or bichloroacetic acid 80% to 90%	First, the surrounding normal epithelium is coated with a protective substance, such as 2% lidocaine jelly or Vaseline Petroleum Jelly, and then a small, cotton-tipped applicator is used to apply the medication carefully to the wart surface. These agents can cause intense burning of mucosal surfaces. They are most effective on small warts and on nonmucosal surfaces. They may be followed by the use of podophyllin on nonmucosal surfaces.

Treatments during pregnancy: In the ambulatory setting, appropriate treatment choices for pregnant women include trichloroacetic or bichloracetic acid and ablative procedures, such as cryosurgery.

POINTS TO REMEMBER

- Affected women should have Pap smears every 6 months.
- Immunosuppressed patients, such as those with acquired immunodeficiency syndrome (AIDS) and those taking immunosuppressive therapy (e.g., renal transplant recipients), are more likely than others to develop persistent HPV infection and subsequent dysplasia and malignant disease.
- Malignant degeneration may be indicated by increasing size, pain, or bleeding.
- Pearly penile papules and normal findings on the penis are often mistaken for condyloma acuminatum.

HELPFUL HINT

- Although skin warts are common in the general pediatric population, genital warts are uncommon in children. Consequently, the diagnosis of genital warts in children should alert the health care provider to the possibility of sexual abuse.
- A vaccine that prevents infection with human papillomavirus type 16 (HPV-16), one of the viruses linked to cervical cancer, has been shown to be safe and effective.

SEE PATIENT HANDOUT, PAGE 479

BASICS

Herpes simplex genitalis is a genital disease caused most commonly by herpes simplex virus type 2 (HSV-2), although HSV-1 also can infect genital skin. It is most commonly, but not invariably, sexually transmitted. HSV is the most common cause of ulcerative genital lesions. The disease is highly contagious during the prodrome and while the lesions are active it establishes latency in the dorsal root ganglia and will reappear after different triggers in individual patients. Triggers include psychological or physiologic stress, physical trauma such as from sexual intercourse, menses, and immunosuppression. Affected patients may have recurrences that are infrequent or as common as once monthly. Patients who have six or more episodes per year are candidates for long-term suppressive therapy.

Risk Factors
- Women have higher acquisition rates and more recurrences than do men.
- People between the ages of 15 and 35 years have a greater chance to contract HSV.
- As with HPV infection, those who have a greater number of sexual partners are also more likely to develop HIV.

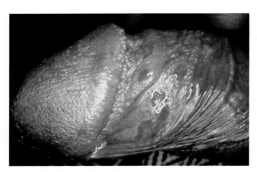

FIGURE 19.13 Herpes simplex virus. Multiple grouped erosions are seen on an erythematous base.

DESCRIPTION OF LESIONS

- Initially, lesions appear as grouped vesicles on an erythematous base.
- Lesions may then become pustular, crusted, and eroded (Figure 19.13).
- Crusting of the lesions occurs over 15 to 20 days, before reepithelialization begins.
- Chronic ulcerations or crusted or verrucous papules may develop in immunocompromised patients.

DISTRIBUTION OF LESIONS

- In women, the vulva, perineum, inner thighs, buttocks, and sacral area are the most common sites of involvement.
- In men, the penis, scrotum, thigh, and buttocks are the typical locations.

CLINICAL MANIFESTATIONS

Primary Herpes Simplex
- This may be more severe than recurrent infections.
- The duration is generally from 10 to 14 days.

- Regional adenopathy may be present.
- Fever, dysuria, and constipation may also occur.

Alternatively,

- The patient may be asymptomatic, so the initial outbreak looks like recurrent HSV.

Recurrent Herpes Simplex
- There is often a prodrome of itching, burning, numbness, tingling, or pain 1 to 2 days before a clinical outbreak.
- Lesions are localized and recur at the same site or in close proximity each time.
- Regional adenopathy may be present.
- Vulvar involvement may cause dysuria.
- The duration is generally from 3 to 5 days.
- Chronic ulcerative lesions are indicative of immunosuppression.
- The risk for neonatal transmission is less than 3% and is greatest in patients with primary HSV at the time of delivery.

DIAGNOSIS

- Most often, the diagnosis is based on the clinical appearance.
- The Tzanck preparation (see Chapter 6, "Superficial Viral Infections") may be helpful.
- Viral culture is the current standard of diagnosis.
- Diagnosis in tissue culture using monoclonal antibodies or polymerase chain reaction is sensitive; however, it is very expensive.
- Serologic testing is of little value.

 DIFFERENTIAL DIAGNOSIS

Herpes Zoster (see Figure 6.31)
- Herpes simplex may be dermatomal and may clinically be identical to herpes zoster.
- A history of recurrences suggests HSV.

Primary Syphilis (Chancre) (see Figures 19.15 and 19.16)
- Classically, the lesion is painless (this is not always true).
- The border is indurated.

Chancroid
- Multiple painful ulcers (Figure 19.14).

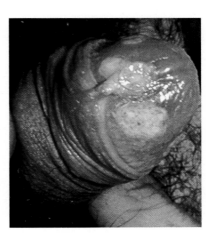

FIGURE 19.14 Chancroid. This patient has multiple painful ulcers on the glans penis.

MANAGEMENT

Patient Education
- The patient should be given written educational materials and clear instructions regarding safe sexual practices.
- The use of condoms should be encouraged.
- The patient should be advised about asymptomatic viral shedding.
- The risk for neonatal infection should be emphasized to both female *and* male patients.

Topical Therapy
- Topical antivirals are of limited effectiveness.
- Symptomatic relief may be achieved with cold compresses, viscous lidocaine (Xylocaine), EMLA (lidocaine and prilocaine), or oral analgesics.

Systemic Antiviral Therapy
Primary Herpes Simplex
- Acyclovir (200 mg five times per day or 400 mg three times daily for 10 days) *or*
- Famciclovir (250 mg three times daily for 10 days) *or*
- Valacyclovir (1 g twice daily for 7 to10 days)

Episodic Therapy for Recurrent Herpes Simplex
Treat at the first sign of the prodrome.

- Acyclovir (200 mg five times per day or 400 mg three times daily for 5 days) *or*
- Famciclovir (125 mg twice daily for 5 days) *or*
- Valacyclovir (500 mg twice daily for 3 days)

Daily Suppressive Therapy for Recurrent Herpes Simplex with More than Six Recurrences per Year or Chronic Recurrent Erythema Multiforme
- Treat as for recurrent HSV for 5 days, then continue therapy with acyclovir (200 mg three times daily or 400 mg twice daily) *or*
- Famciclovir (250 mg twice daily) *or*
- Valacyclovir (250 mg twice daily, 500 mg once per day, or 1,000 mg once per day)

After one year of treatment with these agents, the medication should be discontinued to determine the recurrence, and the dosage can be adjusted as needed.

Acyclovir-Resistant Herpes Simplex
- This is seen in patients with AIDS.
- Coresistance to famciclovir and valacyclovir has been reported.
- Foscarnet can be given (40 mg/kg intravenously two to three times daily for 14 to 21 days).
- Recurrent HSV after foscarnet treatment is often acyclovir sensitive.

(continued)

Herpes Simplex in Pregnant Women

- The safety and efficacy of oral antiviral therapy during pregnancy are being investigated.
- Although acyclovir readily crosses the placenta, several studies did not reveal any increased risk to the developing fetus.
- Antiviral therapy is recommended for pregnant women who are experiencing a primary HSV infection.
- If vaginal delivery occurs through an infected birth canal, the neonate should be observed, and any suspicious lesions should be cultured.
- If no symptoms or signs are present during labor, vaginal delivery is recommended.
- Although the risk for neonatal infection is lower in women with recurrent HSV than it is in women with primary infection, the presence of active herpetic lesions or symptoms of vulvar pain or burning may call for cesarean delivery, regardless of the type of maternal herpetic infection.

 POINTS TO REMEMBER

- Oral antiviral treatment should be initiated during the prodromal phase.
- Asymptomatic infections are common and contribute significantly to HSV transmission because of subclinical viral shedding.
- Condoms are clearly not foolproof, because the virus spreads by contact with herpes sores and condoms may not cover all of them.

 HELPFUL HINT

- A recent study found that 500 mg Valtrex taken once daily by people with HSV-2, decreased by 50% the risk for transmitting the infection to uninfected partners. This suggests that Valtrex can be prescribed in so-called discordant couples—those in which one partner is infected and the other is not.

BASICS

Syphilis is a sexually transmitted systemic disease caused by the spirochetal bacterium *Treponema pallidum*. It is divided into primary, secondary, early latent, late latent, and tertiary stages. Tertiary syphilis is exceedingly rare in the modern era, presumably because most infected patients have had exposure to multiple courses of antibiotics during the course of their lives, and this treatment prevents the infection from progressing.

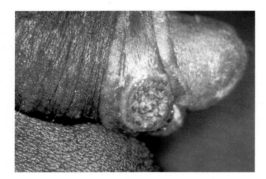

FIGURE 19.15 Chancre of primary syphilis. This ulcer has a rolled, indurated border (chancre) and a "clean" base.

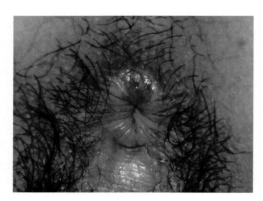

FIGURE 19.16 Chancre of primary syphilis. Note the lesion on the anus.

PRIMARY SYPHILIS

DESCRIPTION OF LESIONS

- A painless ulceration is seen, with a rolled, indurated border *(chancre)* (Figure 19.15).
- Lesions are usually single, but they may be multiple.
- The base of the ulcer is "clean" unless it is superinfected.
- There are no vesicles.

DISTRIBUTION OF LESIONS

- The primary chancre most often presents on or near the glans penis in men; it appears less commonly on shaft of the penis.
- The chancre may occur at base of the penis in condom wearers.
- A visible chancre is less common in women.
- In women, lesions may occur on the labia majora or minora, the clitoris, or the posterior commissure.
- Anal lesions may occur after receptive anal intercourse (Figure 19.16).
- Less frequently, extragenital chancres can occur.

CLINICAL MANIFESTATIONS

- The primary chancre is usually asymptomatic.
- Regional adenopathy may be present.
- An untreated chancre heals within 3 months.

DIAGNOSIS

The following diagnostic methods are used:

- Dark-field examination of the ulceration
- Skin biopsy
- Nontreponemal serologic tests VDRL (Venereal Disease Research Laboratory), RPR (rapid plasma reagent), automated reagin test, which become positive at a rate of 25% of patients per week of infection

DIFFERENTIAL DIAGNOSIS

Herpes Simplex
- Lesions are generally painful.
- Vesicles precede the ulceration.

Chancroid
- Chancroid is unusual in the United States.
- In Africa, chancroid is often present as a coinfection.
- Lesions are painful.

 MANAGEMENT

- Test for HIV infection.

Non–Penicillin-Allergic Patients
- Benzathine penicillin G (2.4 million units intramuscularly in a single dose)

Penicillin-Allergic Nonpregnant Patients
- Doxycycline (100 mg orally twice daily for 2 weeks) *or*
- Tetracycline (500 mg four times daily for 2 weeks)

Penicillin-Allergic Pregnant Patients
- Desensitization to penicillin
- Subsequent treatment with benzathine penicillin G (2.4 million units intramuscularly, with a second dose 1 week later)

HIV-Infected Patients
- Benzathine penicillin G (2.4 million units intramuscularly in one dose)
- Some experts recommend repeated treatment

 POINTS TO REMEMBER

- Patients should be evaluated at 3 and 6 months after treatment. Nontreponemal tests should be negative or have decreased fourfold in titer.
- If the antibody titer does not drop fourfold, suspect treatment failure, reinfection, or HIV infection.

SECONDARY SYPHILIS

DESCRIPTION OF LESIONS

- Scaly, erythematous oval papules appear (Figure 19.17) and are usually asymptomatic.

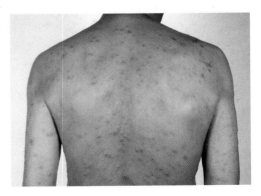

FIGURE 19.17 Secondary syphilis. Scaly, erythematous oval patches and papules are noted.

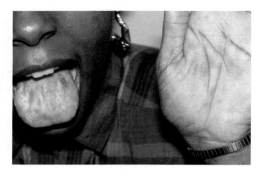

FIGURE 19.18 Secondary syphilis. Mucous patches are present and characteristic copper colored palmar lesions are seen.

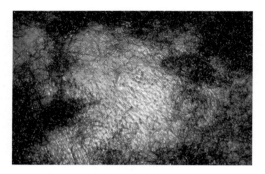

FIGURE 19.19 Secondary syphilis. "Moth-eaten" alopecia is evident.

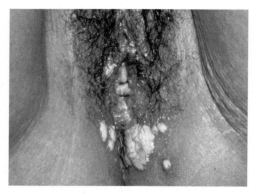

FIGURE 19.20 Secondary syphilis. Condyloma latum is noted. These moist, wartlike papules are highly infectious.

- **Mucous patches** may be noted (Figure 19.18).
- "Moth-eaten" alopecia (Figure 19.19) and **condyloma latum** (Figure 19.20) are also seen in secondary syphilis.

DISTRIBUTION OF LESIONS

- Lesions are widespread and include the palms, soles (Figure 19.21), scalp, and mucous membranes.

CLINICAL MANIFESTATIONS

- Generalized adenopathy and mild systemic symptoms are often present.

DIAGNOSIS

- The diagnosis is often suggested by the clinical presentation.
- If available, a dark-field examination of serum expressed from lesions can confirm the diagnosis. *or*
- Positive treponemal (fluorescein treponemal antibody) and nontreponemal serologic tests (100% of non–HIV infected patients, usually at titer greater than 1:16 for the nontreponemal test) confirm the diagnosis. *or*
- A skin biopsy with silver or immunoperoxidase stain may confirm the diagnosis.
- Serologic titers may be negative in HIV-infected persons.

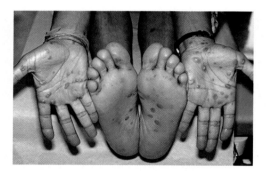

FIGURE 19.21 Secondary syphilis. Characteristic copper or "ham" colored, palmo-plantar papulosquamous lesions seen on this patient's palms and soles.

DIFFERENTIAL DIAGNOSIS

Pityriasis Rosea (see Figures 4.1 to 4.4)
- Usually, pityriasis rosea is confined to the skin above the knees, and it spares the face, palms, and soles. It is prudent to check syphilis serologic tests in patients with pityriasis rosea.

Other Diagnoses
- Other papulosquamous eruptions such as psoriasis, lichen planus, and drug eruptions should be considered.

 MANAGEMENT

This is the same as for primary syphilis.

LATENT SYPHILIS

- Latent syphilis is manifested by positive serologic tests for nontreponemal and treponemal antibodies in the absence of clinical manifestations. It is divided into early latent syphilis and late latent syphilis.
- Early latent syphilis is syphilis documented to be of less than 1 year's duration and is treated with the same regimen as primary and secondary infections.
- The duration of late latent syphilis is more than 1 year or is unknown. Patients are treated with the same regimen as those with tertiary syphilis. HIV-infected patients with latent syphilis of any duration should have a cerebrospinal fluid examination to rule out neurosyphilis before treatment.

TERTIARY SYPHILIS

- Tertiary syphilis occurs about 20 years after the onset of untreated syphilis, and it is rare in the antibiotic era.
- Congenital syphilis can affect babies born to mothers with untreated syphilis, with syphilis treated during pregnancy with erythromycin, with syphilis treated less than 1 month before delivery, and with syphilis treated with penicillin without a fourfold decrease in serologic titer. The CDC recommends testing all pregnant women for syphilis at least once during pregnancy and at the time of delivery in at-risk populations.

CHANCROID

BASICS

Chancroid is an ulcerative sexually transmitted disease that is most common in developing countries and is rare in the United States and Western Europe. In the United States, it is associated with the use of crack cocaine. The causative organism, *Haemophilus ducreyi*, a gram-negative rod, is fastidious and requires specific conditions for culture. Chancroid occurs as a mixed infection with syphilis or herpes simplex in 10% of cases. Clinical infection is more common in men than in women.

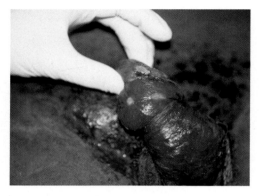

FIGURE 19.22 Chancroid. Multiple painful ulcers and a bubo are present.

DESCRIPTION OF LESIONS

- The earliest manifestation is a papule, which becomes a pustule and ulcerates.
- Fully developed lesions are painful, with undermined borders and peripheral erythema (Figure 19.22).
- Borders are not indurated.
- There may be satellite ulcers.

DISTRIBUTION OF LESIONS

- The location of lesions depends on the site(s) of inoculation.
- In **men,** the prepuce, balanopreputial fold, and the shaft of the penis are the typical sites.
- In **women,** lesions are noted on the labia majora, posterior commissure, or perianal area.
- Extragenital lesions have been described.

CLINICAL MANIFESTATIONS

- The incubation period is 25 days.
- Tenderness and pain are common.
- Unilateral or bilateral inguinal adenopathy (buboes) may be present.

DIAGNOSIS

- The diagnosis is often made based on the clinical appearance.
- A negative dark-field examination, syphilis serologic testing, and HSV cultures help to exclude syphilis.
- Obtaining a culture is difficult.
- A Gram stain shows characteristic "schools of fish" or "Chinese characters."
- Polymerase chain reaction may help in making a diagnosis.

DIFFERENTIAL DIAGNOSIS

- Herpes simplex is preceded by blisters, and the borders are not undermined.
- Chronic HSV in patients with AIDS may resemble chancroid.
- In primary syphilis, the borders are indurated, not undermined, and the lesion is generally painless.

 MANAGEMENT

Drug Therapy
- Azithromycin (1 g orally in a single dose) *or*
- Ceftriaxone (250 mg intramuscularly in a single dose) *or*
- Erythromycin (500 mg orally four times daily for 7 days)

HIV Testing
Pregnant women and HIV-infected patients should be treated with erythromycin.

- Symptomatic improvement usually occurs in 3 days; objective improvement is seen in 7 days.
- Complete healing may take more than 2 weeks.

 POINTS TO REMEMBER

- Chancroid is rare in the United States, but epidemics have been described in crack cocaine users.
- Chancroid predisposes to HIV infection because of recruitment of CD4 cells into the ulcer.
- Always test for coinfection with HIV, syphilis, and HSV.

BASICS

Lymphogranuloma venereum (LGV) is caused by *Chlamydia trachomatis* types L1, L2, and L3. It is most often sexually transmitted. It is rarely seen in the United States and is most common in tropical countries. An inconspicuous cutaneous ulceration occurs at the site of inoculation, and it often heals without being noticed.

DESCRIPTION OF LESIONS

- Evanescent papulopustule or ulceration occurs.
- Regional lymphadenitis is characteristic. The groin fold divides lymph nodes into upper and lower groups ("the groove sign") (Figure 19.23). Sometimes, the adenopathy is bilateral.
- Fluctuance and sinus tracts may develop.

DISTRIBUTION OF LESIONS

- The primary lesion, if present, is found on the penis, vaginal wall, cervix, or perirectally. It is rarely seen in women.

CLINICAL MANIFESTATIONS

- LGV may be associated with malaise and joint stiffness.
- Scarring may result in genital lymphedema.
- Erythema nodosum occurs in 10% of women with LGV.

DIAGNOSIS

- The diagnosis of LGV depends mainly on the exclusion of other causes of suppurative adenopathy and serologic testing: a complement fixation test, and two immunofluorescent tests.
- Culture of the organism is also available.

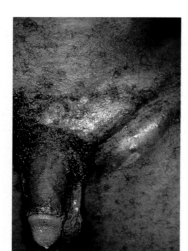

FIGURE 19.23 Lymphogranuloma venereum. Regional lymphadenitis ("the groove sign") is present.

DIFFERENTIAL DIAGNOSIS

Catscratch Disease
- Usually, there is a history of traumatic contact with cats at a site proximal to involved lymph nodes.

Pyogenic Adenitis
- A positive Gram stain and bacterial cultures may be found.

Tuberculous Adenitis
- A positive acid-fast bacillus stain and cultures and a positive purified protein derivative test (PPD) are obtained.

 MANAGEMENT

- Doxycycline (100 mg orally twice daily for 3 weeks minimum) *or*
- Alternative regimen: sulfisoxazole (500 mg orally four times daily for 3 weeks minimum)
- In pregnancy, erythromycin (500 mg orally four times daily for 3 weeks minimum)

 POINTS TO REMEMBER

- Infection is rare in the United States.
- Cutaneous manifestations are usually inapparent.

BASICS

- Granuloma inguinale is a chronic granulomatous ulcerative disease of the genitalia caused by the gram-negative bacillus *Calymmatobacterium granulomatis*. It is thought to be sexually transmitted, with low infectivity.
- It is rare in the United States and is widespread in the tropics and subtropics. The frequency of the disease in homosexuals suggests that the causative organism may reside in the gastrointestinal tract.

DESCRIPTION OF LESIONS

- The initial lesion is a papule or a nodule that ulcerates.
- The ulcer is painless and has an undermined border.
- There is no regional adenitis.

DISTRIBUTION OF LESIONS

- Granuloma inguinale appears in the genital, pubic, perineal, groin, or perianal areas.
- Extragenital lesions occur in 3% to 6% of cases.

CLINICAL MANIFESTATIONS

- The presence of pain or adenitis suggests superinfection.

DIAGNOSIS

- Smears from the edge of the lesion may show characteristic Donovan bodies (organisms within macrophages).
- The biopsy specimen should be taken from the edge of lesion.

 DIFFERENTIAL DIAGNOSIS

Syphilis
- Syphilis must be excluded by dark-field and serologic examinations.
- The borders of the ulcers are indurated, not undermined.

MANAGEMENT
- Tetracycline (500 mg four times daily for 10 to 20 days) *or*
- Trimethoprim-sulfamethoxazole (one double-strength tablet twice daily for 3 weeks minimum) *or*
- Doxycycline (100 mg twice daily for 3 weeks minimum) *or*
- Gentamicin for treatment failures

CHAPTER 20

Bites, Stings, and Infestations

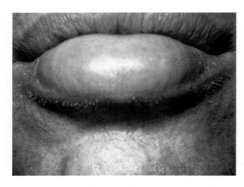

FIGURE 20.1 Angioedema due to a bee sting. This patient developed an immediate hypersensitivity reaction after being bitten on the lip.

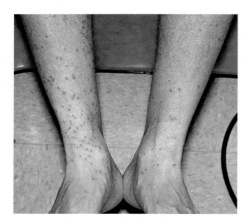

FIGURE 20.2 Chigger bites. This person was bitten while walking barefoot in tall grass. These lesions are intensely pruritic. Chiggers are nonscabetic harvest mites.

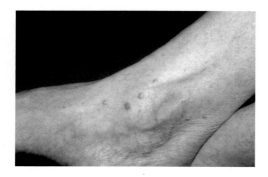

FIGURE 20.3 Flea bites. Note the arrangement of lesions in groups of three ("breakfast, lunch, and dinner"); the fourth lesion probably represents a "midnight snack."

BASICS

In much of the world, insect bites commonly serve as vectors that transport diseases such as malaria, leishmaniasis, filariasis, and rickettsial diseases. In modern industrial societies, insect bites are more of a nuisance than a potential carrier of a life-threatening illness. In the East Coast and Midwest of the United States, mosquitoes and biting flies as well as ticks account for most bites. In arid areas, including much of the Southwest and parts of California, flying insects are less common, and crawling arthropods are the primary cause of bites and stings.

There is individual variability in the attraction of insects, possibly related to pheromones. Furthermore, reactions to bites and stings are probably related to individual hypersensitivity.

Pathogenesis

The physical insult of an insect bite or sting causes little injury; instead, lesions occur as a result of the body's immune response to injected foreign chemicals and proteins introduced by the bite or sting. The time it takes for reactions reflects the immune mechanism involved.

- **Immediate** hivelike skin lesions reflect hypersensitivity to the bite or sting. It is mediated by immunoglobulin E (Figure 20.1).
- **Delayed** pruritic papules, nodules, and vesicles usually become symptomatic within 48 hours after the insult. They are manifestations of delayed hypersensitivity (type IV cell-mediated immunity).
- Less commonly, tissue necrosis occurs as a result of toxins introduced by the bite or sting (e.g., brown recluse spider bites).
- Insects that bite include mosquitoes, fleas, flies, ticks, chiggers (Figure 20.2), and lice. Mosquito and fly bites occur most often from outdoor exposures, particularly in the summer. Flea bites are most often acquired indoors from pets.
- Insects that sting include bees, wasps, hornets, and fire ants.

DESCRIPTION OF LESIONS

- Bite reactions typically present as intensely pruritic erythematous papules that commonly are excoriated.
- Bite reactions may be indistinguishable from ordinary hives.
- Lesions may have a central punctum and crust and also may blister.
- Grouping of lesions often occurs, particularly after flea bites ("breakfast, lunch, and dinner") (Figures 20.1 through 20.3).
- Insect bite reactions are also known as *papular urticaria* when lesions persist for longer than 48 hours.

DISTRIBUTION OF LESIONS

- Lesions are found on exposed areas, more often on nonclothed body parts: distal lower extremities, forearms, and hands. These regions correspond to areas exposed while handling infested animals.
- The papules of flea bites are typically asymmetric in distribution.
- Lesions are most likely seen on the lower legs, forearms, lower trunk and waist; the axillary and anogenital areas are usually spared.

CLINICAL MANIFESTATIONS

- Insect bites may be a chronic, recurrent problem or simply a nuisance.
- Itching may be intense and may persist for weeks.
- Secondary bacterial infection may occur.
- Stings generally cause immediate pain and are therefore usually remembered.
- Bites often go unnoticed, and the lesions that arise from them may not appear for days after the bite because of what is often a delayed immune-mediated hypersensitivity reaction. Consequently, a patient may seek medical advice for unexplained itchy bumps or blisters.

DIAGNOSIS

- The diagnosis is usually made on clinical appearance and history.
- Inquiry about household pets currently and formerly residing in the house may be a clue to the diagnosis. If the residence was formerly host to a dog or cat infested with fleas, the fleas left behind may have found new human hosts.
- A skin biopsy is not diagnostic, but it may show suggestive findings consisting of a dense lymphocytic infiltrate (resembling lymphoma) with many eosinophils. The responsible agent is rarely found in a biopsy specimen (Figure 20.4A and B).

 DIFFERENTIAL DIAGNOSIS

Urticaria Unrelated to Insect Bites (see Chapter 17, "Drug Eruptions")
- It lacks a central punctum.
- It is often indistinguishable from insect bites.

Fiberglass Dermatitis
- Nonspecific itching is noted.
- The patient has a history of exposure (e.g., patient works with roofing materials).

Scabies
See the discussion later in this chapter.

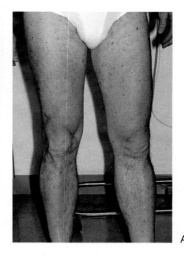

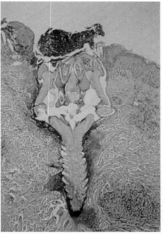

FIGURE 20.4 Tick bites. *A:* This patient developed pruritic papular lesions after spreading manure. *B:* A mouth part—a rare finding—with barblike "teeth" (hypostome) was fortuitously found in this skin biopsy specimen. The "teeth" face backward and enable the organism to be lodged securely in the skin during feeding.

MANAGEMENT

- Insect repellents help to prevent against bites and stings.
- Acute reactions to stings are treated symptomatically with topical or intralesional steroids and oral antihistamines; people with severe reactions from stings may profit from desensitization therapy.
- Anaphylactic reactions require epinephrine, systemic steroids, and antihistamines.
- If flea infestation is suspected, pets should be evaluated by a veterinarian. If fleas are present in the home, thorough vacuuming and shampooing of flea-infested areas and sometimes even fumigation may be necessary.

POINTS TO REMEMBER

- A careful history and knowledge of the patient's environment and possible exposures should be sought.
- Symptoms may persist for weeks after the original bites.
- Other causes should be diligently sought if symptoms persist for more than 4 to 6 weeks.

HELPFUL HINTS

- Patients who seek medical help generally do not consider "mundane" insect bites to be the cause of their dermatosis or itching; rather, they seek attention because they assume that other factors cause their problem.
- Avoiding perfumes and bright clothing can reduce the risk of bee stings.

LYME DISEASE (LYME BORRELIOSIS)

BASICS

- Lyme disease, or Lyme borreliosis (LB), is a systemic infection caused by the spirochete, *Borrelia burgdorferi*. Bacteria are introduced into the skin by a bite from an infected *Ixodes* tick.
- Successful transmission of the spirochete seems to require 48 to 72 hours, thus affording the tick (usually the larva or nymph) enough time to embed in the skin.
- Once in the skin, the spirochete may stay localized at the site of inoculation, or it may disseminate via the blood and lymphatics. Hematogenous dissemination can occur within days or weeks of the initial infection. The organism can travel to other parts of the skin, the heart, the joints, the central nervous system, and other parts of the body.
- The tick vector of LB, *I. dammini,* is found in the northeastern and midwestern United States, where most cases are reported. *I. scapularis* in the southeastern United States, *I. pacificus* on the Pacific coast, and *I. ricinus,* the sheep tick, in Europe are also vectors. Because the disease depends on deer, mice, ticks, and bacteria, it is limited geographically to the areas where these organisms are present. Eight states, from Maryland north to Massachusetts, account for about 90% of reported cases in the United States.
- LB can occur in any season, although it is most prevalent during the warmer months from May through September during the nymphal stage of the tick. The ticks cling to vegetation (not trees) in grassland, marshland, and woodland habitats. They transfer to animals and humans brushing against the vegetation.

DESCRIPTION OF LESIONS

- Initially, the LB lesion is a red macule or papule at the site of a tick bite. The bite itself usually goes unnoticed (only 15% of patients report a tick bite). Approximately 2 to 30 days after infection, the rash appears.
- The lesion expands to form an annular erythematous lesion, erythema migrans (EM), which is the classic lesion of LB (Figure 20.5). The lesion measures from 4 to 70 cm in diameter, generally with central clearing.
- The center of the lesion, which corresponds to the putative site of the tick bite, may become darker, vesicular, hemorrhagic, or necrotic.

DISTRIBUTION OF LESIONS

- Initially, there may be multiple lesions, presumably arising at the sites of multiple tick bites or, more likely, resulting from bacteremia (Figures 20.6 and 20.7).
- Lesions may be confluent (not annular), and concentric rings may form (Figure 20.8).
- Only 50% to 80% of patients with LB exhibit EM. Multiple lesions occur in approximately 50% of patients.
- Common sites are the thigh, groin, trunk, and axillae.

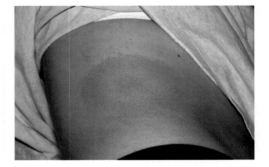

FIGURE 20.5 Lyme disease. A solitary annular, targetlike, erythematous plaque of erythema migrans is seen.

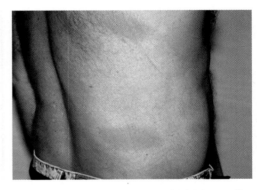

FIGURE 20.6 Lyme disease. Multiple confluent lesions of erythema migrans are noted.

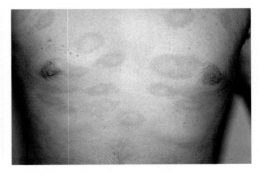

FIGURE 20.7 Lyme disease. Multiple annular lesions of erythema migrans are seen here.

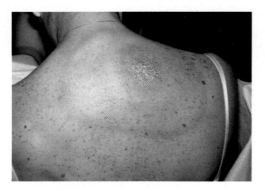

FIGURE 20.8 Lyme disease. In this patient, erythema migrans is manifested by concentric rings with drying central vesicles.

CLINICAL MANIFESTATIONS

Early Lyme Disease
- At the early stage of disease, flulike symptoms, such as malaise, arthralgias, headaches, fever, and chills, may occur, as can stiffness of the neck and muscles, difficulty in concentrating, and fatigue.
- The EM rash itself is usually asymptomatic.

Intermediate and Chronic Lyme Disease
Some of the signs and symptoms of LB may not appear for weeks, months, or even years after the initial tick bite and are probably driven by immunopathogenetic mechanisms. These include the following:

- Patients may have **arthritis** in one or more large joints, nervous system problems that may include **pain, paresthesias, Bell's palsy, headaches,** and **memory loss,** and **cardiac dysrhythmias.**
- Rarely, a lesion of **lymphocytoma cutis** may develop, usually occurring on the earlobe or nipple. These lesions are bluish red nodules.
- **Acrodermatitis chronica atrophicans** is a manifestation of chronic LB that begins as an inflammatory phase marked by edema and erythema, usually on the distal extremities.

Later, atrophy occurs, and thin "cigarette-paper" skin is seen. Because of the loss of subcutaneous fat, underlying venous structures are more visible, and the skin becomes thin, atrophic, and dry.

- Both lymphocytoma cutis and acrodermatitis chronica atrophicans are very rare findings in the United States and are seen primarily in European patients. The clinical differences probably result from the different antigenic strains of *Borrelia*.

DIAGNOSIS

- The diagnosis of LB is often difficult because the disease mimics many other conditions. Viral infections, such as influenza and mononucleosis, also may manifest with rash, aches, fever, and fatigue. Drug eruptions and insect bite reactions other than those caused by the *Ixodes* tick closely match the rash of early LB.

Early Diagnosis
To diagnose early LB, the following are important:

- There is a history of tick exposure or bite in an area endemic for LB.
- The specific tick is identified as a potential vector of LB.
- The various presentations of EM are recognized.

Laboratory Testing
- Serologic testing, using enzyme-linked immunosorbent assay (ELISA) and Western blot analyses for *B. burgdorferi*, are notoriously unreliable. At the early presenting stage of LB, serologic testing has been reported to be positive in only 25% of infected patients. After 4 to 6 weeks, approximately 75% of these patients test positive, even after antibiotic therapy.

- The poor reputation of serologic testing is derived somewhat from the many false-negative test results of patients treated very early in the course of the disease and from the many misdiagnosed cases of supposed LB.
- The United States Centers for Disease Control and Prevention currently recommends a two-step testing procedure consisting of a screening ELISA or immunofluorescent assay followed by a confirmatory Western immunoblot test on any samples with positive or equivocal results on ELISA.

Other Tests

Other diagnostic measures, such as polymerase chain reaction and cultures for *B. burgdorferi*, have met with some success; however, these techniques are time-consuming and expensive. Skin biopsies may give both false-positive and false-negative results.

 DIFFERENTIAL DIAGNOSIS

Tinea Corporis (Figure 20.9)
See Chapter 7, "Superficial Fungal Infections."

- There may be a history of exposure to fungus.
- Lesions are also annular (ringlike) and clear in the center; however, tinea corporis has an "active" scaly border (epidermal involvement).
- Lesions are potassium hydroxide positive, or the fungal culture grows dermatophytes.
- Tinea corporis generally itches.

Acute Urticaria
See Chapter 18, "Diseases of Vasculature."

- This may be indistinguishable from LB.
- Individual lesions disappear within 24 hours.
- It generally itches.

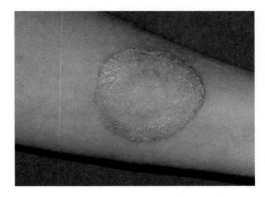

FIGURE 20.9 Tinea corporis. The scaly border is potassium hydroxide positive.

Granuloma Annulare
For a full discussion of this condition, see Chapter 4, "Inflammatory Eruptions of Unknown Cause."

Erythema Multiforme
For a full discussion of this condition, see Chapter 25, "Cutaneous Manifestations of Systemic Disease."

Erythema Annulare Centrifugum
This condition is less common.

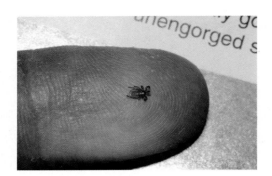

FIGURE 20.10 *Ixodes* tick. An adult tick is the size of the head of a match.

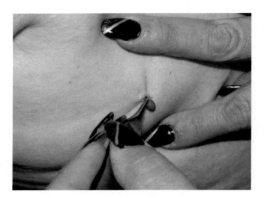

FIGURE 20.11 Dog tick. An intact engorged adult dog tick being removed by the head.

MANAGEMENT

Tick Recognition
- *Ixodes* ticks are much smaller than dog ticks. In their larval and nymphal stages, they are no bigger than a pinhead; unengorged adult ticks are the size of the head of a match (Figure 20.10).

Tick Removal
- An attached tick should be removed carefully by using a pair of tweezers. The tick should be grasped by the head (not the body) as close as possible to the skin, to avoid force that may crush it. It is then gently pulled straight out of the patient's skin (Figure 20.11).

Treatment of Erythema Migrans (Early Lyme Borreliosis)
- Doxycycline (100 mg twice per day for 21 days [do not use in children younger than 10 years or in pregnant women]) *or*
- Amoxicillin (500 mg three times per day for 21 days) *or*
- Ceftriaxone or cefuroxime (500 mg twice per day for 21 days [expensive; use if patient is unable to tolerate the other antibiotics])
- Azithromycin (Zithromax) and erythromycin: second-line drugs that should be considered in pregnant patients who are allergic to beta-lactam antibiotics

Prevention
People who are outdoors in endemic areas in the summer should wear long pants and socks, use insect repellents, and frequently look for ticks on themselves and their clothing.

Lyme Disease Vaccine (LYMErix)
A vaccine directed against the outer surface protein A of *B. burgdorferi* was removed from the United States market in 2002.

POINTS TO REMEMBER
- Serologic testing is usually negative early in the course of infection.
- Serologic testing should not be used to make a diagnosis, only to help confirm it.

HELPFUL HINTS
- Patients can be reinfected. There is no lasting immunity to LB.
- Coinfection by *Ehrlichia* species and *Babesia microti* are reported with increased frequency, in as many as 10% to 15% of patients with LB in some studies.
- Antibiotic prophylaxis after tick bites is controversial. Clearly, prevention of bites is a better means of preventing disease.

BASICS

- Scabies is a skin infestation caused by the mite, *Sarcoptes scabiei*, var. *hominis*. It is usually spread by skin-to-skin contact, most frequently among family members and by sexual contact in young adults. Occasionally, epidemics occur in nursing homes and similar extended-care institutions, where scabies is spread by person-to-person contact and possibly by mite-infested clothing and bed linen. The diagnosis can be easily overlooked, and treatment is often delayed for long periods.
- The diagnosis of scabies should be considered when an individual complains of intractable, persistent pruritus, especially when other family members, consorts, or fellow inhabitants of an institution, such as a nursing home or school, have similar symptoms.
- Although scabies is found more commonly in poor, crowded living conditions, it occurs worldwide and is not limited to the impoverished or those who practice poor personal hygiene. Blacks infrequently acquire scabies; the reason is unknown.

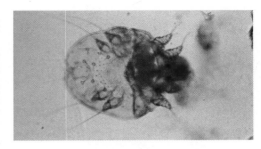

FIGURE 20.12 Scabies. A fertilized female mite is visible.

Etiology

A fertilized female mite (Figure 20.12) excavates a burrow in the stratum corneum, lays her eggs, and deposits fecal pellets (scybala) behind her as she advances. The egg laying, scybala, or other secretions act as irritants or allergens, which may account for the itching and subsequent delayed type IV hypersensitivity reaction that occurs approximately 30 days after infestation.

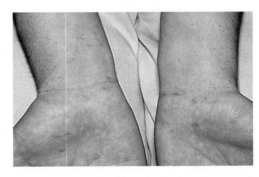

FIGURE 20.13 Scabies. Lesions are present on the flexor wrists.

DESCRIPTION OF LESIONS

- The initial lesions of scabies include tiny pinpoint vesicles and erythematous papules, some of which evolve into burrows, the classic telltale lesions of scabies (Figures 20.13 and 20.14).

The Burrow

- The burrow is a linear or S-shaped excavation that is pinkish white and slightly scaly and ends in the pinpoint vesicle or papule. This is where the mites may be found.
- Burrows are easiest to find on the hands, particularly in the finger webs and wrists in adults and on the palms and soles in infants.
- Sometimes burrows can be highlighted by applying black ink with a felt-tipped pen to the suspected areas.

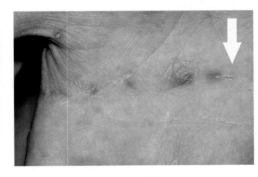

FIGURE 20.14 Scabies. This close-up view shows a burrow *(arrow)* on the palm.

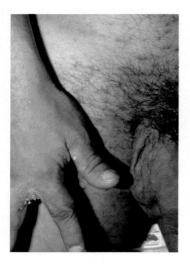

FIGURE 20.15   Scabies. Finger web and groin lesions are noted.

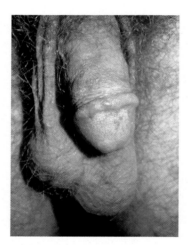

FIGURE 20.16   Scabies. Pruritic papules and nodules are present on the penis and scrotum.

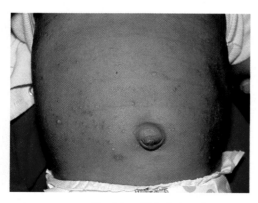

FIGURE 20.17   Scabies. This infant has papular and vesicular lesions on the trunk.

DISTRIBUTION OF LESIONS

- Lesions are most often located on the interdigital finger webs (Figure 20.15), sides of the hands and feet, flexor wrists, umbilicus, waistband area, axillae, ankles, buttocks, and groin.
- An important diagnostic sign is that children and adults rarely have lesions above the neck.
- Infants tend to have more widespread involvement including the face and scalp and especially the palms and soles.
- Immunocompromised patients also tend to have a widespread distribution of lesions.

CLINICAL MANIFESTATIONS

- Because the incubation period from initial infestation to the onset of pruritus is usually approximately 1 month, it is not uncommon for contacts to be asymptomatic, especially if they have been recently infested.
- Itching (**nocturnal pruritus**) has traditionally been considered a symptom that is characteristic of scabies; however, it should be kept in mind that pruritis that occurs in many other skin conditions also tends to be more severe during the night time hours when people are inclined to be less distracted by their daytime routines.

Course and Secondary Lesions
- Initially, itching is rather mild and focal, but when lesions begin spreading rapidly, usually after 4 to 6 weeks, it can sometimes become intolerable.
- A generalized distribution of lesions is probably the result of a hypersensitivity reaction. In this case, a more pleomorphic array of lesions, such as juicy papules and nodules, may be seen.
- Hemorrhagic crusts and ulcerations may replace the primary lesions.
- In men, itchy papules and nodules, particularly on the penis and scrotum, are virtually pathognomonic for scabies (Figure 20.16).

CLINICAL VARIANTS

Scabies in Infants
- Frequently, intact vesicles are seen on the palms and soles. A typical clinical picture of an infant with scabies is one who doggedly pinches his or her skin (Figure 20.17).

Scabies in the Elderly
- Patients, particularly in an institutional setting, can have intense pruritus and few papular lesions, excoriations, or simply have dry, scaly skin.

Norwegian or Crusted Scabies

- Norwegian, or crusted scabies (Figure 20.18) (see also Chapter 24, "Cutaneous Manifestations of HIV Infection," Figure 24.13) occurs in people with varying degrees of immune deficiency such as that seen in Down's syndrome, leukemia, nutritional disorders, and acquired immunodeficiency syndrome (AIDS).
- The lesions tend to involve large areas of the body.
- The hands and feet may be scaly and crusted with a thick keratotic material that can also be seen under the nails.
- There may be wartlike vegetations on the skin, which are host to thousands of mites and their eggs.

DIAGNOSIS

A conclusive diagnosis is made by finding scabies mites, eggs, or feces.

- A drop of mineral oil is applied to the most likely lesion (usually a vesicle on the finger web or wrist is chosen). The site is then scraped with a No. 15 blade (Figure 20.19); the scrapings are placed on a slide, and a cover slip is then applied (see also Figures 24.14 and 24.15).
- Adults, who are more efficient scratchers than children, tend to remove the definitive evidence of scabies, (i.e., mite) with their fingernails. Because mites are few and are particularly hard to find in adults, the time and effort spent searching for the mite may be better used by taking a thorough history and counseling the patient and his or her contacts. Thus, if scabies is strongly suspected on clinical grounds, scabicidal treatment should be initiated.

 DIFFERENTIAL DIAGNOSIS

- Insect bites, such as fleas, generally spare areas that are covered (e.g., the groin and axillae).
- Pruritus associated with systemic diseases, such as renal disease, hepatic disease, lymphomas, AIDS, leukemias, and Hodgkin's disease, should be excluded.

Other Diagnoses
- **Atopic dermatitis** or **dyshidrotic eczema** should be considered.
- **Drug eruptions** and **other itchy rashes,** including urticaria, tinea, xerosis, and contact dermatitis, are possible diagnoses.

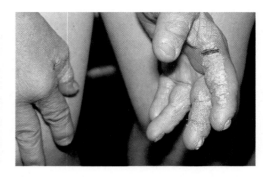

FIGURE 20.18 Norwegian scabies. This child with Down's syndrome has verrucous plaques on his hands and thickened dystrophic nails. The lesions are teeming with mites.

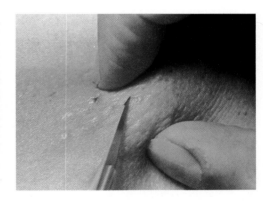

FIGURE 20.19 Scabies. Scraping for scabies is performed.

MANAGEMENT

- Treatment is directed at killing the mites with a scabicide. It is also aimed at affording rapid symptomatic relief using appropriate oral antihistamines and topical corticosteroids, if necessary.

Permethrin (Elimite and Acticin)

The prescription drugs Elimite and Acticin both contain permethrin cream 5%. They are safe and effective scabicides that are currently considered the treatment of choice for scabies. A prescription is required. They have not been proven to be safe in infants younger than 2 months or in pregnant and nursing women.

Instructions for Use

- After a warm bath, the cream is applied to all skin surfaces "from head to toe" (including the palms and soles and scalp in small children) and is left on for 8 to 12 hours, usually overnight. It is washed off the next morning.
- If indicated, other family members and contacts should be treated simultaneously. All bed linen and intimate undergarments should be washed in hot water after treatment is completed.
- Generally, only one treatment is necessary; however, a second treatment is often recommended in 4 to 5 days, especially in long-standing cases and for infants with scabies of the palms and soles.
- Patients should be advised that it is normal to continue itching for days or weeks after treatment, albeit less intensely. The medication should not be applied repeatedly. Systemic antihistamines and a topical corticosteroid can be used for these symptoms.

Lindane (Kwell Lotion, Scabene)

This is the generic name for gamma benzene hexachloride. Until recently, it was the mainstay of scabies treatment; now it is recommended as an alternative agent. It is available in a 1% formulation and also requires a prescription. It is also safe and effective, but controversy arose about its safety after several reports of neurotoxicity in infants. Ultimately, it was concluded that the drug was overused in these cases and led to systemic absorption. In addition, there have been reports of resistance to lindane.

Instructions for Use

- Used as an overnight treatment, it is applied from the neck to toes, and the patient is instructed to wash it off in 8 to 12 hours.
- Treatment may be repeated in 4 to 5 days, if there is little symptomatic improvement.
- Lindane is to be avoided in infants, in pregnant or nursing women, or in people with a history of seizure disorders.

Precipitated Sulfur Ointment (6%)

- This is used in pregnant or lactating women and in infants younger than 2 months. It is applied nightly for 3 nights. It is messy and malodorous, but it is effective and safe.

Ivermectin

- Ivermectin is an antihelmintic that can be administered in a single oral dose. It can be used when topical therapy is difficult or impractical (e.g., widespread infestations in nursing homes).
- It has been used safely and effectively in patients who are seropositive for human immunodeficiency virus and in some patients with Norwegian scabies.
- This agent is used adjunctively with a topical scabicide.
- It is available as Stromectol, in 3- and 6-mg tablets.
  - Dosage: 0.2 mg/kg in a single oral dose; repeat in 10 days
- This drug is not currently approved by the United States Food and Drug Administration for the treatment of scabies in humans, and there are no studies to establish its safety for use in pregnancy or in children.

Crotamiton (Eurax Lotion and Cream)

- This preparation is not very effective against scabies.

Management of Institutional Scabies

- Treatment must be conducted in an organized, cooperative fashion.
- A scabicide is applied to all patients, staff, family members, and frequent visitors.
- Laundering of all bed linen and clothes is necessary shortly after treatment.

POINTS TO REMEMBER

- Scabies mimics other skin diseases.
- Scabies rarely occurs above the neck in immune-competent adults.
- Treat contacts simultaneously to avoid "ping-ponging" (reinfection).
- Treatment failure may result from noncompliance (i.e., treating lesions only) or reinfection.
- Symptoms may persist after appropriate treatment.
- Lesions that resemble insect bites, an eczematous dermatitis, and so-called neurotic excoriations may confuse an unsuspecting diagnostician.
- Because the mite can survive away from the skin for 2 to 5 days on inanimate objects such as clothing of an affected person, it is believed that indirect contact with such personal items can transmit the organism. This is most applicable in immuno-compromised and institutionalized elderly patients.

HELPFUL HINTS

Think scabies when you see:

- An infant with palmar or plantar vesicles or pustules
- More than one family member, roommate, or sexual partner who is itching
- Pruritic scrotal or penile nodules
- Vesicles in the finger webs

SEE PATIENT HANDOUT, PAGE 481

BASICS

There are two species of sucking lice: *Pediculosis humanus* and *Phthirus pubis* (pubic lice, sometimes called "crabs"). *P. humanus* is further divided into two subspecies: *P. humanus capitis* (the head louse) and *P. humanus corporis* (the body louse).

Head Lice (Pediculosis Capitis)
- Head lice spread from human to human; epidemics of head lice are most commonly seen in schoolchildren.
- Head lice occur more often in girls and women than in boys and men; they are unusual in African-Americans, but not in African blacks.

Body Lice (Pediculosis Corporis)
- Body lice are most often found in situations of poor personal hygiene, such as in homeless people.
- They are historically prevalent in war conditions.

Pubic Lice
- Pubic lice are generally transmitted by sexual contact.

DESCRIPTION OF LESIONS

Head Lice
- There are no primary lesions; however, secondary crusts and eczematous dermatitis resulting from scratching may be present.
- Nits (louse eggs) are cemented to the hairs (Figure 20.20).
- It is difficult to find living lice.

Body Lice
- Lesions begin as small papules.
- Later, secondary lesions develop from scratching and may produce crusted papules, infected papules, and ulcerations.

Pubic Lice
- Small brown lice may be seen at the base of hairs (Figure 20.21).
- Blue macules *(maculae ceruleae)* may occur on nearby skin.

DISTRIBUTION OF LESIONS

Head Lice
- Only the scalp is involved.

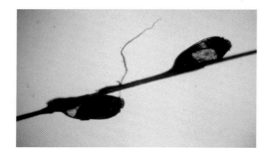

FIGURE 20.20 Head lice. The nits are attached to the hair shaft.

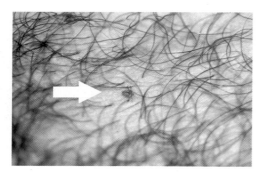

FIGURE 20.21 Pubic lice. A small brown living crab louse is seen at the base of hairs *(arrow).*

Body Lice
- Covered areas (under infested clothing) of the body may be affected.

Pubic Lice
- Pubic hair, eyebrows, eyelashes, and axillary hair may be infested.

CLINICAL MANIFESTATIONS

Head, Pubic, and Body Lice
- Itching is the predominant symptom.
- Affected children with head lice may be asymptomatic.
- There is a possibility of secondary infection from scratching.
- With the exception of body lice, which have historically been known to carry epidemic typhus, trench fever, and relapsing fever, lice are not known to transmit any disease.

DIAGNOSIS

Head Lice
- Knowledge of an epidemic at school generally alerts parents or school nurses to look for evidence of lice.
- White nits may be very obvious on a background of darker hair.
- A hair may be plucked and examined for nits using the low power of a microscope.
- A nit is attached to the base of a hair shaft when the egg is first laid and remains cemented to the growing hair (Figure 20.20).

Body Lice
- The diagnosis is not made from examining the patient, but from the seams of his or her clothing where the lice are found.

Pubic Lice
- Lice are present (Figure 20.21).
- Pruritus is noted.
- Blue macules may be seen.
- Often, a sexual partner has "crabs."

 DIFFERENTIAL DIAGNOSIS

Head Lice
- Atopic dermatitis of the scalp should be considered.

Body Lice and Pubic Lice
- Atopic dermatitis or another type of eczematous dermatitis should be considered.
- Scabies should be excluded.

MANAGEMENT

Head Lice

Remove nits with a fine-tooth comb after soaking the hair in a vinegar solution; this helps to soften the cementing substance that attaches the nit to the hair.

First-Line Treatment
Over-the-Counter Nix Creme Rinse, RID, and Acticin

These products all contain low concentrations of permethrin; they are very effective in killing adult lice and nymphs, but not as effective in killing nits (eggs). There has been a growing resistance of head lice to these agents.

How to use:

- The hair is washed with a nonmedicated shampoo and is towel dried; the agent is applied as a cream rinse, is allowed to remain in place for 10 minutes, and then is rinsed off thoroughly.
- Because these agents do not destroy nits effectively, a second application (using the same technique) often is recommended 7 to 10 days after the initial therapy.

Strategies for Resistant Cases
Ovide (Malathion Lotion 0.5%)

This agent is considered the most effective treatment for head lice. It is both a pediculicide and an ovicide.

Caution: Ovide Lotion is flammable. Treated areas that are wet with this product should be kept away from open flames and electric heat sources such as hairdryers.

How to use:

- The lotion is applied to **dry** hair in a quantity sufficient to wet hair and scalp.
- It is then massaged into the scalp and is left on for 8 to 12 hours. Heat (e.g., hairdryers, hot curlers) should not be used to dry the lotion.

- The hair is then rinsed, and the nits are removed with a fine-tooth (nit) comb.
- Treatment should be repeated in 7 to 10 days if lice are still present (using the same technique).

Elimite Cream (5% Permethrin Cream)

This is available by prescription. It is left on overnight under an occlusive shower cap; and the application is repeated in 1 week to destroy any remaining eggs.

Other Treatment Options

Oral Ivermectin, which has not yet been approved for the treatment of head lice. The dosage is 0.2 mg/kg in a single dose. A second treatment may be required.

There have been reports of therapeutically recalcitrant cases of head lice responding to **trimethoprim-sulfamethoxazole,** which presumably destroys essential bacteria in the louse's gut and causes it to starve to death.

Petrolatum such as Vaseline Petroleum Jelly is quite messy and hard to remove, but is an inexpensive and sometimes effective method that asphyxiates the lice and nits. It is applied to the entire scalp and is left on under a shower cap overnight.

Pubic Lice
- Kwell shampoo is lathered and is left on for 10 minutes.
- Kwell, RID, and Nix lotions are also effective.
- Treatment should include contacts of infested patients, especially sexual partners.

Body Lice
- A shower and clean clothing will generally cure body lice.
- Clothing should be washed at hot temperatures to kill the lice.

HELPFUL HINTS

- Shaving of pubic, scalp, or body hair is not necessary to treat lice.
- In resistant cases, particularly after repeated treatment failures, **delusions of parasitosis** should be considered in the differential diagnosis in adult patients.

SEE PATIENT HANDOUT, PAGE 483

BASICS

- There are two types of stinging jellyfish seen floating in the coastal waters of North America: the smaller sea nettle and the more dangerous Portuguese man-of-war, whose poison may be fatal.
- The tentacles of jellyfish have many stinging nematocysts, which contain a hollow poisonous tip and hooks. The hooks hold the victim while the nematocysts discharge the toxic venom into their aquatic prey.

DESCRIPTION OF LESIONS

- The shape of the lesions, which are like linear welts that develop at the site of contact, often give the victim the appearance of having been whipped (Figure 20.22).
- Lesions may fade or blister and become necrotic, depending on the amount of injected venom and individual sensitivity.

DISTRIBUTION OF LESIONS

- The distribution is unilateral.

CLINICAL MANIFESTATIONS

- Victims usually describe a stinging or burning sensation.
- The sting of the Portuguese man-of-war is more painful than a common jellyfish sting. It has been described as feeling like being struck by a lightning bolt, and some victims dread it more than a shark bite (Figure 20.23).
- There have been reported cases of anaphylactic reactions and fatalities.

DIAGNOSIS

- The diagnosis is based on the reported sting occurring in an endemic area and its characteristic eruption.

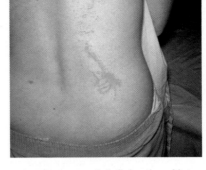

FIGURE 20.22 Jellyfish sting. Note the curvilinear, whiplike shape of the lesions.

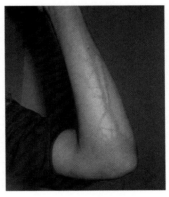

FIGURE 20.23 Portuguese man-of-war sting. Note the linear shape of the lesions. The sting of the Portuguese man-of-war is more painful than a common jellyfish sting.

DIFFERENTIAL DIAGNOSIS

- Other bites or stings should be considered.

 MANAGEMENT

- Mild stings may be treated symptomatically with cool soaks and topical steroids.
- For more severe reactions, the affected area should be washed with sea water, alcohol, or vinegar to remove nematocysts and to inactivate any remaining toxins.

→ POINT TO REMEMBER

- Severe stings that result in systemic reactions may require life-support measures.

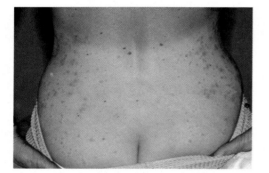

FIGURE 20.24 Seabather's eruption. This patient has just returned from bathing off the coast of Florida. The lesions are confined to the bathing suit area.

SEABATHER'S ERUPTION

- An intensely pruritic eruption develops **under** swimwear minutes to 12 hours after exposure to the larvae of the thimble jellyfish *(Linuche unguiculata)* in the salt waters off the coast of Florida and in the Caribbean.
- Itching is worse at night and tends to prevent the patient from sleeping.
- Erythematous macules and papules last for 2 to 14 days and resolve spontaneously (Figure 20.24).
- Treatment is symptomatic.

 DIFFERENTIAL DIAGNOSIS

- "Swimmer's itch" (cercarial dermatitis) occurs on **exposed sites** after freshwater swimming.

CUTANEOUS LARVA MIGRANS ("CREEPING ERUPTION")

BASICS

- As the name suggests, cutaneous larva migrans is a cutaneous eruption that creeps or migrates in the skin. It results from the invasion and movement of various hookworm larvae that have penetrated the skin through the feet, lower legs, or buttocks.
- *Ancylostoma braziliense* and *A. caninum*, *A. ceylanicum*, *Uncinaria stenocephala* (dog hookworm), *Bunostomum phlebotomum* (cattle hookworm), *A. duodenale*, and *Necator americanus* are the primary hookworms that cause cutaneous larvae migrans in the United States.
- The adult hookworm (nematode) resides in the intestines of dogs, cats, cattle, and monkeys. The feces of these animals contain hookworm eggs that are deposited on sand or soil, hatch into larvae if conditions are favorable, and then penetrate human skin, which serves as a "dead-end" host.
- At greatest risk are gardeners, seabathers, plumbers, and farm workers.
- A distinct variant of cutaneous larvae migrans, known as **larvae currens,** caused by *Strongyloides stercoralis,* may produce visceral disease.

DESCRIPTION OF LESIONS

- Patients have a characteristic curvilinear inflammatory lesion (Figure 20.25).

DISTRIBUTION OF LESIONS

- Areas that come into contact with the sand; most commonly the feet or buttocks (nude beaches), are affected.

CLINICAL MANIFESTATIONS

- This benign eruption is usually pruritic and self-limited because the larvae usually die within 4 to 6 weeks.

DIAGNOSIS

- This is based on clinical appearance.

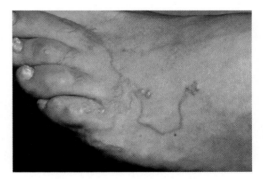

FIGURE 20.25 Cutaneous larva migrans. Note the serpiginous, erythematous, raised lesion that resembles a tunnel.

DIFFERENTIAL DIAGNOSIS

Granuloma Annulare
- Lesions are annular.
- It lacks scale and vesicles and does not itch.

Tinea Pedis
- The potassium hydroxide examination is positive.

Other Diagnoses
- Other bites or stings (e.g., jellyfish) should be considered.

 MANAGEMENT

- Superpotent topical steroids (e.g., clobetasol cream) for itching
- Topical thiabendazole suspension (500 mg/5 mL under occlusion three times per day for 1 week)
- Oral thiabendazole (Mintezol; 50 mg/kg per day in two daily doses for 2 to 5 days) *or*
- Albendazole (400 mg daily for 3 days [this drug has fewer side effects than thiabendazole])
- Liquid nitrogen, applied to the active, advancing end of the lesion

HELPFUL HINT

- If the patient has been vacationing on the beach in an endemic area, consider cutaneous larva migrans as a cause of a local itchy eruption on one foot.

CHAPTER 21

Benign Skin Neoplasms

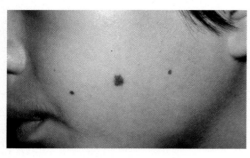

FIGURE 21.1 Junctional melanocytic nevi. These small, macular, frecklelike lesions may be brown to dark brown to black.

BASICS

- Nevi, commonly called moles or "beauty marks," are benign proliferations of normal skin components.
- Melanocytic nevi are composed of nevus cells that are derived from melanocytes. Melanocytic nevi may be congenital or acquired, and they are much more often seen in whites than in blacks or Asians.
- The acquisition of melanocytic nevi is greatest in childhood and adolescence. During adulthood, the development of new lesions tapers off, and many existing lesions gradually lose their capacity to form melanin and become skin-colored or disappear completely.

JUNCTIONAL MELANOCYTIC NEVI

- These small, macular, frecklelike lesions are uniform in color. Individual lesions may be brown to dark brown to black (Figure 21.1).
- Histologic examination reveals melanocytic nevus cells located at the dermoepidermal junction.
- Junctional nevi are most prevalent on the face, arms, legs, trunk, genitalia, palms, and soles.

 DIFFERENTIAL DIAGNOSIS

Freckles or Ephelides
- These small, tan macules appear on the sun-exposed skin of fair-skinned people (Figure 21.2). They darken after sun exposure and lighten when they are no longer exposed to the sun.

Lentigo (Plural: Lentigines) or "Liver Spot"
- These small, acquired tan macules occur on sun-exposed areas during middle age. They are uniform in color (Figures 21.3 and 21.4).

Lentigo Simplex
- This also has uniform coloration. It may be first noted in childhood and is not related to sun exposure.

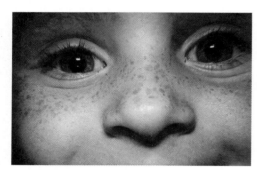

FIGURE 21.2 Freckles (ephelides). These lesions darken after sun exposure and lighten when they are no longer exposed to the sun.

DERMAL MELANOCYTIC NEVI

- Dermal melanocytic nevi may be elevated and dome-shaped, wartlike, or pedunculated. They are most often skin-colored, but may be tan or brown, or they may be dappled with pigmentation. Lesions tend to lose pigmentation with age and become skin-colored.
- They are most often seen on the face and neck (Figure 21.5).
- Microscopy reveals that dermal melanocytic nevus cells are located in the dermis.

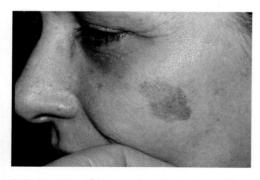

FIGURE 21.3 Solar lentigo. Note the uniformity in color (compare with Figures 22.33 and 22.34).

COMPOUND MELANOCYTIC NEVI

- Compound melanocytic nevi are elevated, dome-shaped papules or papillomatous nodules that are uniformly brown to dark brown, may contain hairs, and are seen most often on the face, arms, legs, and trunk (Figure 21.6).
- Their histologic structure combines features of junctional and dermal nevi.

CLINICAL MANIFESTATIONS

- Dermal nevi and compound nevi are asymptomatic unless they are irritated or inflamed.
- Rarely do they transform to malignant melanoma.

DIAGNOSIS

The diagnosis of melanocytic nevi is based on clinical appearance or, if necessary, on histopathologic evaluation after removal.

 DIFFERENTIAL DIAGNOSIS

Dermal nevi and compound nevi often resemble one another as well as the following:

- Atypical nevus
- Skin tags
- Seborrheic keratoses
- Dermatofibromas
- Neurofibromas
- Basal cell carcinomas
- Nodular melanoma
- Warts

When evaluating a junctional nevus, the following lesions should be considered in the differential diagnosis:

- Atypical nevus (see later)
- Early melanoma

CLINICAL VARIANTS

Blue Nevi

- These lesions are a benign variant of dermal melanocytic nevi. Blue nevi, which are blue-gray or blue-black macules, papules, or nodules, are rarely malignant (Figure 21.7).
- Like the more common dermal and compound melanocytic nevi, blue nevi usually begin to appear in adolescence or early adulthood.

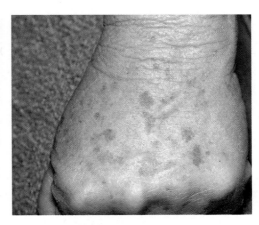

FIGURE 21.4 Solar lentigines. Tan macules arise on sun-exposed areas during middle age.

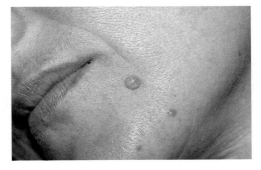

FIGURE 21.5 Dermal melanocytic nevi. Papules can be elevated and dome-shaped, wartlike, or pedunculated. These lesions tend to lose pigmentation as the patient ages.

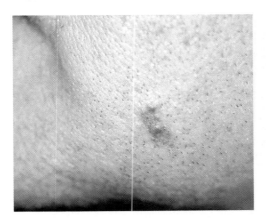

FIGURE 21.7 Blue nevus. This is a variant of melanocytic nevus. Note the blue–gray color.

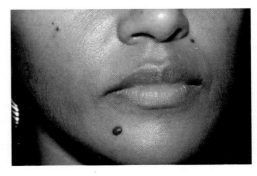

FIGURE 21.6 Compound melanocytic nevi. Elevated, dome-shaped papules or papillomatous nodules are uniformly brown to dark brown, may contain hairs, and are most often seen on the face, arms, legs, and trunk.

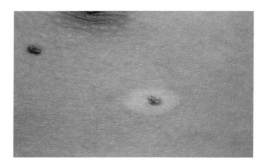

FIGURE 21.8 Halo nevus. An inflamed compound nevus is encircled by a white halo of depigmentation. Ultimately, the nevus may disappear, and the area will regain normal pigmentation.

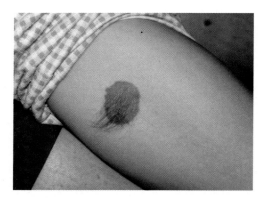

FIGURE 21.9 Small to medium-sized congenital hairy nevus. This lesion is evenly pigmented and symmetric and probably has little, if any, malignant potential.

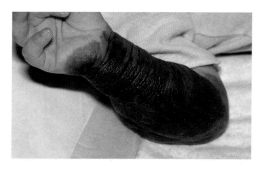

FIGURE 21.10 Giant pigmented hairy nevus. A patient with this lesion may have a greater than 6% lifetime risk for melanoma.

Halo Nevus

- A halo nevus is a melanocytic nevus that is encircled by a white halo of depigmentation. The halo represents a regression of a preexisting nevus caused by a lymphocytic infiltrate. Frequently, the entire nevus disappears, and the area regains normal pigmentation.
- Most often, halo nevi are initially seen on preadolescents; they usually appear on the trunk (Figure 21.8).
- If a halo nevus is seen on an adult, two rare possibilities should be considered: the lesion may be malignant, or a melanoma may be present elsewhere on the body. Biopsy and removal are indicated in this situation. Also bear in mind that in a patient of any age, a biopsy should be performed if the nevus has an atypical clinical appearance.

Congenital Melanocytic Nevi

- Melanocytic nevi that are present at birth or arise during the first year of life are known as congenital melanocytic nevi (Figures 21.9 and 21.10). Congenital nevi are of the greatest concern when they are 20 cm or larger in diameter. These nevi, which are often called *giant pigmented hairy nevi, garment nevi,* or *bathing trunk nevi,* may develop into melanoma—the lifetime risk is estimated to be greater than 6%. The malignant potential of small or medium-sized congenital melanocytic nevi is controversial. However, many experts believe that a small nevus does not significantly increase the lifetime risk for developing melanoma.
- All congenital nevi should be carefully examined and considered for biopsy, particularly if there is any suggestion of clinical atypia. They can also be removed for cosmetic purposes.

MANAGEMENT

For most melanocytic nevi, biopsy is not indicated. Persons with numerous melanocytic nevi, particularly atypical nevi (see later), are at greater risk for developing malignant melanoma.

Indications for Removal
- Atypical appearance
- Cosmetic reasons
- Repeated irritation by clothing, such as a bra strap
- Persistent discomfort (a lesion that itches, hurts, or bleeds)

Methods of Removal
Lesions can be removed by shave excision (which is often followed by electrodesiccation) or by elliptic excision (see Chapter 26, "Basic Dermatologic Procedures").

- *Shave excision*: This method is fast and economical, and it generally provides satisfactory cosmetic results. Its disadvantage is that it often results in only partial removal of the lesions, which infrequently necessitates a second excisional procedure.
- *Elliptic excision*: This technique is performed with the intent of removing lesions completely. Surgical margins can be identified. However, elliptic excision is slower than shave excision. It also requires suturing and suture removal, and it results in linear scars that may not be as cosmetically pleasing as scars that result from shave excisions.

ATYPICAL NEVUS (DYSPLASTIC NEVUS)

BASICS

- The atypical nevus, which is also called *dysplastic nevus,* an *atypical mole,* or *Clark's nevus,* is a controversial and confusing lesion. Even among dermatopathologists, there is no consensus regarding the histopathologic criteria for its diagnosis. This much is agreed on: when a patient has numerous atypical nevi and there is a positive family history of melanoma, the potential for melanoma in that patient and in his or her family is extremely high. Such dysplastic nevi may be inherited as an autosomal dominant trait (see the later discussion of **familial atypical mole syndrome**).
- Atypical nevi are rarely seen in black, Asian, or Middle Eastern populations.

DESCRIPTION OF LESIONS

Atypical nevi have some or all of the following features:

- They are usually larger than common moles and frequently measure 5 to 15 mm in diameter.
- Their borders are usually irregular, notched, and ill-defined.
- They have a macular appearance, but the centers may be raised (for this reason, they are sometimes called *sunny-side-up egg lesions*) (Figure 21.11).
- Their coloration (tan, brown, black, pink, or red) is irregular.

DISTRIBUTION OF LESIONS

- Atypical nevi are most often found on the trunk (Figure 21.12), legs, and arms; generally, the face is spared.

CLINICAL MANIFESTATIONS

- The exact risk for an individual atypical nevus developing into a melanoma is uncertain.
- Unlike dermal and compound nevi, these lesions often continue to appear into adulthood.

Sporadic Atypical Nevi
- A patient with an isolated atypical nevus and no family history of multiple atypical nevi or melanoma probably carries little risk for developing melanoma and should not necessarily be identified as prone to melanoma.

Multiple Atypical Nevi
- The exact risk for an individual nevus developing into a melanoma is uncertain.
- In certain situations, atypical nevi are considered possible precursors to, as well as potential markers for, the development of melanoma.

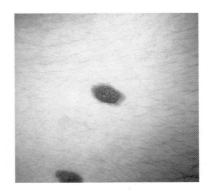

FIGURE 21.11 Atypical nevus (dysplastic nevus). Note the raised center and indistinct border; such a nevus is sometimes called a *sunny-side-up egg lesion*.

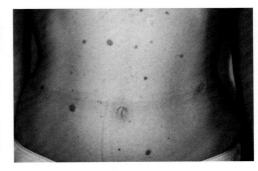

FIGURE 21.12 Multiple dysplastic nevi. Note the characteristic distribution on the trunk.

Familial Atypical Mole Syndrome

Those persons who meet the following criteria are considered to have an extremely high potential for developing malignant melanoma:

1. A first-degree (e.g., parent, sibling, or child) or second-degree (e.g., grandparent, grandchild, aunt, uncle) relative who has a history of malignant melanoma.
2. Many nevi—often more than 50—are present and some of them are atypical moles.
3. Moles show certain dysplastic features when examined under the microscope.

MANAGEMENT

- The method chosen for removing suspected atypical nevi depends on the purpose of treatment.
    - If melanoma is suspected, complete excision should be performed.
    - If melanoma is not suspected, the lesion can be removed and prepared for biopsy with a shave or punch biopsy technique.

Prevention

- Patients with many atypical nevi should avoid excessive sun exposure and should routinely use a sunscreen with a sun protective factor of 15 or greater.
- Patients who meet the criteria for familial atypical mole syndrome should examine their own skin every 2 to 3 months, in addition to having a full body examination and regular screening visits performed by a dermatologist.
- High-risk patients and their families should be taught self-examination to detect changes in existing moles and should be given printed material with photographs to help them recognize the features of malignant melanoma.

POINTS TO REMEMBER

- Any pigmented lesion that changes rapidly in size or color or that has an atypical appearance should be removed for biopsy.
- The risk for melanoma is greatly increased in patients who have multiple atypical nevi and a personal or family history of melanoma.
- Once a diagnosis of multiple atypical nevi is established, other family members should be examined.
- A person with an isolated atypical nevus probably carries little risk for developing melanoma and should not be identified as melanoma prone.
- Melanoma risk is greater for those persons who have one relative with melanoma than for those with no affected relative. The lifetime risk for melanoma may approach 100% in persons with atypical nevi who are from melanoma-prone families (i.e., individuals having two or more first-degree relatives with melanoma).

SEBORRHEIC KERATOSIS

BASICS

A seborrheic keratosis is an extremely common benign skin growth that becomes apparent in people after the age of 40 years. These lesions are the most common tumors in the elderly, and they have virtually no malignant potential. Patients often report a positive family history of seborrheic keratoses; men and women are equally affected. Seborrheic keratoses have been whimsically described as "barnacles in the sea of life," a metaphor intended to allay patients' anxieties.

DESCRIPTION OF LESIONS

- The typical seborrheic keratosis lesion has a warty, "stuck-on" appearance that ranges from tan to dark brown to black. The "dry," crumbly, keratotic surface of some lesions is sometimes rubbed or picked off, only to recur later. The use of the word "seborrheic," a misnomer, stems from the occasional "greasy" or shiny appearance of the lesions; seborrheic keratoses are actually epidermal in origin, with no sebaceous derivation.
- The appearance of individual lesions tends to vary considerably, even on the same person. Lesions may be warty, tortoise shell-like (Figure 21.13), scaly, flat or almost flat (Figure 21.14), or small pigmented papules similar to skin tags (discussed later) (Figure 21.15). The color, shape, and surface characteristics of seborrheic keratoses can change with the age and location of individual lesions. Lesions are often smooth and symmetric, uniformly pigmented, and small. To the untrained eye, however, these lesions may resemble melanomas (i.e., they may be asymmetric, have irregular or notched borders, and vary in color).

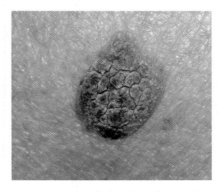

FIGURE 21.13 Seborrheic keratosis. This lesion has a warty, tortoise shell-like, "stuck-on" appearance.

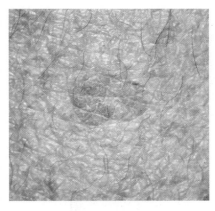

FIGURE 21.14 Seborrheic keratosis. This lesion is almost flat.

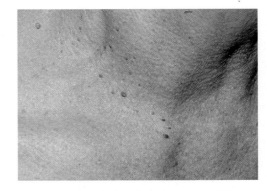

FIGURE 21.15 Seborrheic keratoses. These small seborrheic keratoses are clinically indistinguishable from pigmented skin tags.

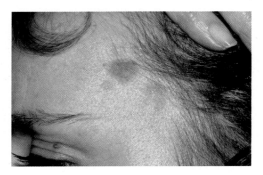

FIGURE 21.16 Seborrheic keratoses. The frontal hairline is a common location.

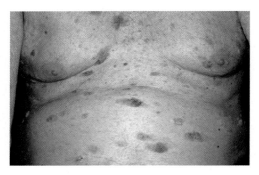

FIGURE 21.17 Seborrheic keratoses. Multiple lesions of various shapes, sizes, and colors are noted.

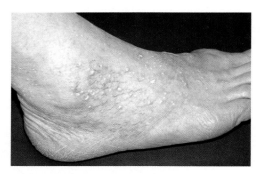

FIGURE 21.18 Stucco keratoses. These lesions have a whitish, "stuck-on" appearance.

DISTRIBUTION OF LESIONS

- Seborrheic keratoses most often are located on the back, chest, and face, particularly along the frontal hairline (Figure 21.16) and scalp. They are also frequently found on the arms, legs, and abdomen.
- Smaller lesions similar to skin tags can be seen around the neck, under the breast, or in the axillae.
- When many lesions are present, the distribution is usually bilateral and symmetric (Figure 21.17).

CLINICAL VARIANTS

Stucco Keratoses

These are a nonpigmented variant of seborrheic keratosis; they are seen most often in the elderly.

Description of Lesions

- Stucco keratoses are skin-colored or whitish papules that become whiter and scalier when they are scratched. They typify the "dry, stuck-on" type of seborrheic keratosis (Figure 21.18).

Distribution of Lesions

- They are commonly found on the distal lower leg, particularly around the ankles, and they may also be seen on the dorsal forearms.

Dermatosis Papulosa Nigra

This common manifestation is diagnosed primarily in African-Americans, Afro-Caribbeans, and sub-Saharan African blacks; however, it is also seen in darker-skinned persons of other races. Lesions start appearing in adolescence and increase in number as persons age. The lesions are histopathologically identical to seborrheic keratoses and are considered to be of autosomal dominant inheritance.

Description of Lesions

- The lesions are darkly pigmented and, in contrast to typical seborrheic keratoses, they have minimal, if any, scale.

Distribution of Lesions

- The lesions are generally seen on the face, especially the upper cheeks and lateral orbital areas (Figure 21.19).

Sign of Leser-Trélat

This refers to the sudden appearance of multiple seborrheic keratoses in a short period or a rapid increase in their size. It is a rare phenomenon and is presumed by some observers to be a cutaneous sign of leukemia or internal malignant disease, especially of the gastrointestinal tract, prostate, breast, ovary, uterus, liver, or lung. However, in light of the frequency of malignant disease in the elderly, and the ubiquitous presence of seborrheic keratoses in this age group, the relationship is believed by some observers to be fortuitous.

DIAGNOSIS

- With experience, seborrheic keratoses are easily recognized.
- If necessary, a shave biopsy (using a No. 15 scalpel blade) or curettage may be performed for histologic confirmation. An excisional biopsy is not necessary (see Chapter 26, "Basic Dermatologic Procedures").

 DIFFERENTIAL DIAGNOSIS

- Malignant melanoma (Figure 21.20)
- Pigmented basal cell carcinoma (see Figure 22.20)
- Verruca vulgaris (wart)
- Solar lentigo (especially early flat seborrheic keratoses)
- Pigmented solar keratosis (actinic keratosis)
- Melanocytic nevus
- Dysplastic nevus

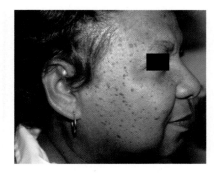

FIGURE 21.19 Dermatosis papulosa nigra. The lesions of this common inherited condition appear as small, pigmented papules on the face that resemble seborrheic keratoses.

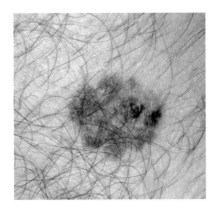

FIGURE 21.20 Malignant melanoma. Note the variegation in color and the irregular, notched border.

MANAGEMENT

- Patients with seborrheic keratoses are often referred to dermatologists with a presumptive diagnosis of warts or moles or to have these lesions evaluated for cancer, particularly melanoma.
- Learning to recognize seborrheic keratoses should obviate the need for many of these referrals. When a patient is referred, a biopsy (generally a shave biopsy) is performed if necessary to confirm the diagnosis or to distinguish seborrheic keratosis from a basal cell carcinoma, melanocytic nevus, wart, or melanoma.
- Because some patients have numerous lesions, it is an impractical expenditure of time and money to perform multiple biopsies of lesions, as long as the clinical appearance is typical. However, an excisional biopsy should be performed whenever malignant melanoma is suspected.

Treatment Methods
- Cryosurgery is performed with liquid nitrogen spray or cotton swab application or light electrocautery and curettage (treating the base of the lesion helps to prevent recurrence) (see Chapter 26, "Basic Dermatologic Procedures") *or*
- Excisional surgery, which results in scar formation, is unnecessary, unless a biopsy of a completely removed lesion is required to rule out malignant disease.

POINTS TO REMEMBER

- Seborrheic keratoses are mainly a cosmetic concern, except when they are inflamed or irritated and can be an annoyance. The challenge for primary care clinicians is to distinguish these lesions from skin cancer, particularly malignant melanoma.
- Lesions may be quite numerous on some persons. Because seborrheic keratoses may, at times, be confused with melanoma, careful visual examination of all lesions should be performed.

HELPFUL HINT

- Seborrheic keratoses present in many shapes, colors, and sizes. It is a good idea to become familiar with these lesions by consistently examining the skin of all adult patients.

BASICS

- These benign skin lesions are very common. They are sometimes referred to as *acrochordons, fibroepithelial polyps,* or, if large, *soft fibromas* or *pedunculated lipofibromas*. They are often seen in the body folds of obese persons.
- Skins tags were formerly suspected by several investigators to be markers for intestinal polyps or, possibly, internal malignant diseases, but current evidence suggests that this association is not justifiable.

DESCRIPTION OF LESIONS

- Skin tags are generally 1- to 10-mm fleshy papules.
- They may be skin-toned, tan, or darker than the patient's skin. They are sessile or pedunculated in shape.
- They are most often found on the neck (Figure 21.21), the axillae, the inframammary area, the groin (especially the inguinal creases), the upper thighs, and the eyelids. (Figure 21.22)

CLINICAL MANIFESTATIONS

- Skin tags are primarily of cosmetic concern; however, they may become a nuisance from the irritation of necklaces and underarm shaving, for example.
- In pregnant women, they tend to grow larger and more numerous over the course of the pregnancy.
- They are often seen in association with acanthosis nigricans.

DIAGNOSIS

- Skin tags are easy to recognize; a skin biopsy is rarely necessary.

 DIFFERENTIAL DIAGNOSIS

- Pedunculated seborrheic keratoses
- Compound or dermal nevi
- Neurofibromas

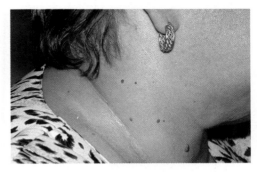

FIGURE 21.21 Skin tags. Pigmented papules are present around the neck.

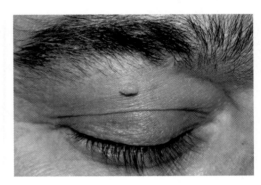

FIGURE 21.22 Skin tags. A solitary, skin-colored skin tag is present on the eyelid.

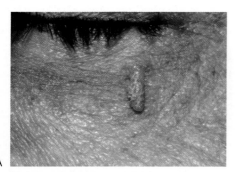

A

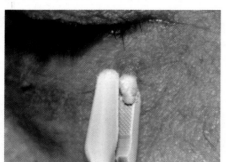

B

FIGURE 21.23 *A:* Skin tag. *B:* Treatment is performed with liquid nitrogen. Frost appears at the tip of the needle holder and on the skin tag. The frozen skin tag that will be shed in 7 to 10 days.

MANAGEMENT

- Small skin tags are easily removed by snipping them off at their base using iris scissors, with or without prior local anesthesia (see Chapter 26, "Basic Dermatologic Procedures"). The crushing action of the scissors results in little bleeding or pain.
- Skin tags, if disregarded, occasionally may spontaneously self-destruct. After torsion, they become necrotic and autoamputate.

HELPFUL HINTS

- A rapid and painless treatment for small skin tags is to dip a needle holder or nontoothed forceps into liquid nitrogen for 15 seconds and then gently grasp each skin tag for about 10 seconds. There is little or no collateral damage, just a narrow rim of erythema occurs. Multiple lesions can be treated by this method (Figure 21.23). The frozen skin tag will be shed in approximately 10 days.
- This is a good approach for skin tags hanging on the eyelids.

BASICS

- Sebaceous hyperplasia refers to small, benign papules on the face of adults representing hypertrophy of the sebaceous glands. They are fairly common lesions that are often confused with basal cell carcinomas.

DESCRIPTION OF LESIONS

- The yellow papules are often doughnut-shaped (with a dell in the center) (Figure 21.24).
- They are small in diameter (1 to 3 mm).
- Telangiectasias are present on the raised borders.

DISTRIBUTION OF LESIONS

- Lesions occur on the forehead and cheeks.

CLINICAL MANIFESTATIONS

- Lesions are asymptomatic.
- They may be of cosmetic concern.

DIAGNOSIS

- This is made by the lesion's typical clinical appearance ("little bagels").
- Biopsy is indicated, if basal cell carcinoma is suspected.

 DIFFERENTIAL DIAGNOSIS

- Basal cell carcinoma (see Chapter 22, "Premalignant and Malignant Neoplasms")

 MANAGEMENT

- The patient should be reassured about the benign nature of this condition.
- Light electrocautery may be performed to remove lesions, if desired.

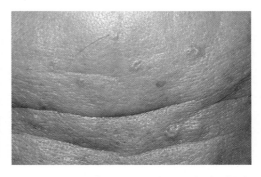

FIGURE 21.24 Sebaceous hyperplasia. Multiple yellowish papules are present. Note the central dell and telangiectasias.

BASICS

A cyst is a sac containing semisolid or liquid material. The sac contains keratin and lipid-rich debris. A cyst has an epithelial lining that produces keratin. Cysts tend to be hereditary, arise in adulthood, and may occur as multiple lesions.

- **Epidermoid cysts** are the most common type. They are derived from the epithelium of the hair follicle and connect to the surface of the skin with a keratin-filled central pore that looks like a blackhead.
- **Pilar cysts,** the second most common type, have a thicker wall that develops from a stratified epithelium. Pilar cysts lack a central pore.

DESCRIPTION OF LESIONS

- Lesions appear as smooth, discrete, freely moveable, dome-shaped nodules.
- Cysts that have previously been infected, ruptured, drained, or scarred may be more firm and less freely movable.
- Lesions range from 0.5 to 5.0 cm in diameter.
- Often, there is a central pore (seen in epidermoid cysts), from which cheesy-white, malodorous keratin material can be expressed.

DISTRIBUTION OF LESIONS

- Epidermoid cysts occur most often on the face, behind the ears, and on the neck, trunk, scrotum, and labia.
- Pilar cysts are most often located on the scalp.

CLINICAL MANIFESTATIONS

- Cysts are usually asymptomatic, unless they are inflamed or infected.
- Scrotal and pilar cysts may calcify.
- Pilar cysts are generally devoid of overlying scalp hair.

CLINICAL VARIANT

Milia
- Milia (singular, milium) are common epidermal cysts that contain keratin. They can occur in people of any age. They may arise in traumatic scars or in association with certain scarring skin conditions, such as porphyria cutanea tarda.

Description of Lesions
- They are 1.0 to 2.0 mm in diameter and are white to yellow (Figure 21.25).

Distribution of Lesions
- Milia are most often noted on the face, especially around the eyes and on the cheeks and forehead.

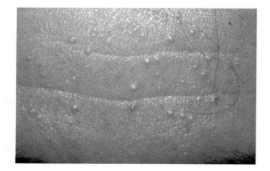

FIGURE 21.25 Milia. These epidermal cysts contain keratin. They are 1.0 to 2.0 mm in diameter and are white to yellow.

DIAGNOSIS OF EPIDERMOID OR PILAR CYSTS

- On palpation, an intact epidermoid or pilar cyst feels smooth; when compressed, it feels like an eyeball or a fully expanded balloon (Figure 21.26). If necessary, a biopsy can be performed to confirm the diagnosis.

 DIFFERENTIAL DIAGNOSIS

- Lipoma should be considered when cystlike lesions are found on the trunk, back of neck, and extremities. However, the consistency of a lipoma is rubbery and somewhat softer than that of a cyst (see Figure 21.29). Lipomas are also irregular in shape.

 MANAGEMENT

Epidermoid and Pilar Cysts
- Complete excision. The entire cyst wall does not have to be completely removed to prevent recurrence.
- Alternatively, a large epidermoid or pilar cyst can be removed through a small hole created by a punch biopsy tool (see Chapter 26, "Basic Dermatologic Procedures," Figure 26.17).
- For incision and drainage, a fluctuant, infected cyst may be incised with a No. 11 blade, drained, and then packed with iodoform gauze.
- The contents of inflamed or so-called "infected" cysts are most often sterile or contain normal skin flora; thus the necessity of pre- or postoperative antibiotics is probably unnecessary.

Milia
- In contrast to closed comedones (which they resemble), milia must first be incised (usually with a No. 11 blade) before their contents can be expressed.
- Alternatively, they can be destroyed with light electrodesiccation.

 HELPFUL HINT

- Ruptured epidermal and pilar cysts are often misdiagnosed as being infected rather than ruptured, and patients are accordingly treated unnecessarily with oral antibiotics.

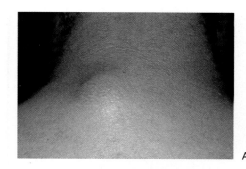
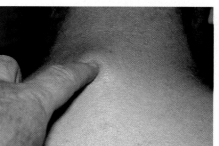

FIGURE 21.26 Epidermoid cyst. These lesions often occur on the back. They appear as smooth, discrete, freely movable, dome-shaped ballotable masses. *A:* Cyst. *B:* Compression of the lesion, which has the same consistency as an eyeball or a fully-inflated balloon.

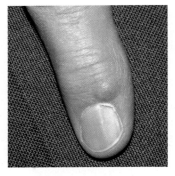

FIGURE 21.27 Digital mucous (myxoid) cyst. Note the longitudinal groove in the nail plate.

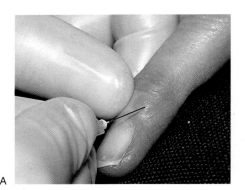

A

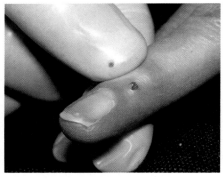

B

FIGURE 21.28 Incision of a digital mucous cyst. *A:* A No. 30 needle can be used to incise and drain the cyst. *B:* Blood-tinged, jellylike mucoid material is revealed.

DIGITAL MUCOUS (MYXOID) CYST

This is not a true cyst, because it lacks an epidermal lining. It is actually a focal collection of clear, gelatinous, viscous mucin (focal mucinosis) that occurs over the distal interphalangeal joint or, more commonly, at the base of the nail.

DESCRIPTION OF LESION

- Pressure from the lesion on the nail matrix (root) results in a characteristic longitudinal groove in the nail plate (Figure 21.27).
- This dome-shaped, rubbery lesion occurs exclusively in adults, particularly in women older than 50 years. Myxoid cysts are believed to be a consequence of osteoarthritis, not of trauma.

MANAGEMENT

This benign lesion may be treated as follows:

- It may be ignored, particularly if it is asymptomatic.
- Lesions have reportedly resolved after several weeks of daily firm compression.
- Incision and drainage (Figure 21.28), cryosurgery with liquid nitrogen, and intralesional triamcinolone injections have been tried with varying results.
- Surgical excision is reserved for the occasional painful, or otherwise troublesome, lesion.

BASICS

A lipoma is a benign, subcutaneous tumor composed of fat cells. **Dercum's disease** is a syndrome of multiple tender lipomas that develop in middle-aged women. **Angiolipomas** may be tender or painful.

DESCRIPTION OF LESIONS

- Lipomas are rubbery, generally asymptomatic masses; they range in size from small nodules (Figure 21.29) to large tumors.
- They are usually irregular in shape and may be greater than 7 cm in length.

DISTRIBUTION OF LESIONS

- Lipomas occur most commonly on the trunk, back of neck, upper arms, and forearms.

DIAGNOSIS

- The diagnosis is made on clinical grounds.
- A biopsy should be performed if the diagnosis is uncertain.

 ## DIFFERENTIAL DIAGNOSIS

- As noted earlier, a lipoma may be confused with an epidermoid cyst. However, the latter feels like an eyeball and has a regular dome shape.

 ## MANAGEMENT

- The lesion may be excised or removed using liposuction.

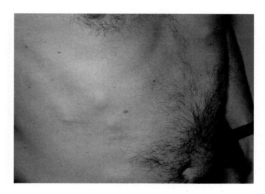

FIGURE 21.29 Lipomas. Multiple rubbery flesh-colored nodules are palpable on this patient.

DERMATOFIBROMA

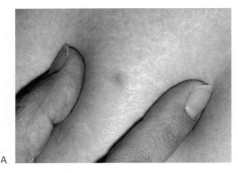

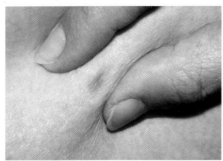

FIGURE 21.30 Dermatofibroma *A:* "dimple" or "collar button" sign is elicited on compression of a lesion *(B).*

BASICS

Also known as *fibrous histiocytoma* and *sclerosing hemangioma,* a dermatofibroma is a common dermal fibrous tumor of unknown cause. Dermatofibromas occur most commonly on the legs, trunk, and arms, especially in women older than 20 years. The lesions are benign growths that are usually brought to medical attention either to rule out skin cancer or because of cosmetic concerns.

DESCRIPTION OF LESIONS

- A lesion may be a papule or a nodule. It may be elevated with a dome shape, flat, or depressed below the plane of the surrounding skin.
- The color can vary, even in a single lesion and can be skin-colored, including chocolate brown, red, or even purple. The surface may be smooth or scaly, depending on whether the lesion has been traumatized (e.g., by shaving).

DIAGNOSIS

- Typically, a dermatofibroma feels like a firm pea or a button that is fixed to the surrounding dermis (accounting for the "dimple" or "collar button" sign) (Figure 21.30).
- It is freely movable over deeper adipose tissue.

 DIFFERENTIAL DIAGNOSIS

- Cysts and lipomas are either compressible or rubbery.
- Melanocytic nevi (moles) are also not as firm as dermatofibromas.
- A malignant melanoma is more variable in shape and size than a dermatofibroma.

 MANAGEMENT

- No treatment is necessary; however, local excision can be performed for biopsy confirmation or cosmetic concerns, or if the lesion is symptomatic.

 POINTS TO REMEMBER

- If there is any doubt about the diagnosis, a biopsy should be performed.
- The patient should be informed that if the lesion is removed, the scar may be more cosmetically objectionable than the original lesion.

COMMON ANGIOMAS

BASICS

- These lesions, which are also known as *Campbell De Morgan spots, ruby spots,* and *senile angiomas,* are extremely common benign vascular neoplasms. The angiomas are found in fair-skinned adults older than 40 years. They are asymptomatic, easily diagnosed, cherry- to plum-colored papules that develop primarily on the trunk (Figure 21.31).
- A venous lake *(venous varix)* is another common benign vascular neoplasm; this lesion usually occurs in patients older than 60 years. Venous lakes are generally macules or papules that are dark blue to purple and may be seen on the lower lip (Figure 21.32), face, ears, and eyelids.
- Angiokeratomas *(Fordyce angiokeratomas)* are most often found on the scrotum (Figure 21.33) or vulva (Figure 21.34), and they are usually first noticed in young adulthood. They consist of multiple red-purple asymptomatic papules ("caviar spots").

 DIFFERENTIAL DIAGNOSIS

- The diagnosis of all these lesions is usually made on clinical grounds. There should be little reason to confuse them with pyogenic granulomas.

 MANAGEMENT

- Reassure the patient that the lesions are benign.
- If the lesions are a cosmetic problem, they may be treated with electrocautery, cryosurgery with liquid nitrogen, or laser therapy.

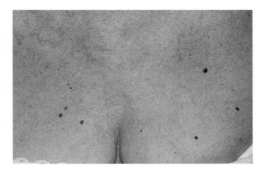

FIGURE 21.31 Multiple cherry angiomas. These cherry- and plum-colored papules are common in fair-skinned persons older than 40 years.

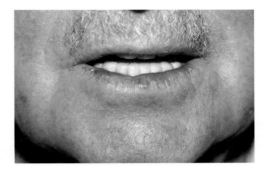

FIGURE 21.32 Venous lake. If the patient is concerned about its appearance, the lesion can be removed with electrocautery or laser destruction.

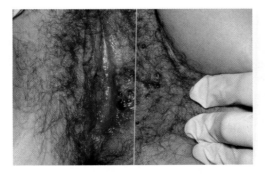

FIGURE 21.34 Angiokeratomas. These lesions are seen here on the vulva.

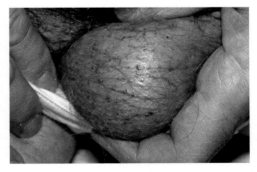

FIGURE 21.33 Angiokeratomas. These red-purple papules are most often found on the scrotum; they are usually first noticed when the patient is a young adult.

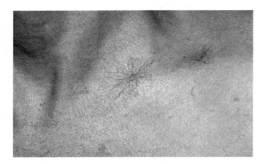

FIGURE 21.35 Spider angioma. This lesion is actually a cluster of telangiectasias, radiating from a central arteriole. Compression of the central arteriole will completely blanch the lesion.

SPIDER ANGIOMA

BASICS

- A spider angioma *(nevus araneus)* is a cluster of telangiectasias, or dilated capillaries, that radiate from a central arteriole (Figure 21.35).
- It is more commonly seen in women and may be associated with pregnancy or oral contraceptive use. Spider angiomas are also seen in patients with hyperestrogenic conditions, such as chronic liver disease. They may also be seen in healthy children.
- Lesions appear as spokelike capillaries radiating from a central arteriole. Compression of the central arteriole completely blanches the lesion. Spider angiomas most often occur on the face and trunk. Lesions are asymptomatic and are generally only a cosmetic problem.

MANAGEMENT

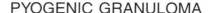

- Light electrocautery or laser destruction of the spider angioma may be performed if the lesion presents a cosmetic problem. Occasionally, lesions regress spontaneously.
- Other types of telangiectasias may serve as a clue to an underlying collagen vascular disease, such as the periungual telangiectasias of systemic lupus erythematosus and dermatomyositis or the telangiectasias seen in scleroderma and the CREST syndrome (calcinosis, Raynaud's phenomenon, esophageal motility disorders, sclerodactyly, and telangiectasia) (see Chapter 25, "Cutaneous Manifestations of Systemic Disease").

PYOGENIC GRANULOMA

BASICS

- A pyogenic granuloma is a benign, rapidly developing, red, purple, or red-brown dome-shaped papule or nodule. Pyogenic granulomas resemble hemangiomas or granulation tissue ("proud flesh").
- They occur more often in young children and adolescents, but pyogenic granulomas may also develop during pregnancy (such a lesion is known as a *granuloma gravidarum*).
- Lesions are generally solitary papules or nodules that range in size from a few millimeters to 3 to 4 cm in diameter (Figure 21.36). The bases of lesions are often surrounded by a collarette of skin.
- Lesions most frequently occur at sites of minor trauma, such as the fingers and toes, but they also may be seen on the trunk.
- During pregnancy, lesions tend to occur on the lips and gums. Pyogenic granulomas present as asymptomatic lesions that tend to bleed after minor trauma. Spontaneous resolution may occur after childbirth.

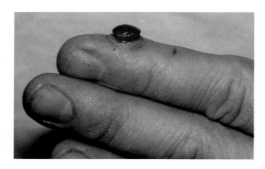

FIGURE 21.36 Pyogenic granuloma. This patient has a typical dusky red nodule with a collarette of skin.

DIAGNOSIS

- The diagnosis is usually based on the typical clinical appearance and biopsy.

 DIFFERENTIAL DIAGNOSIS

- Nodular malignant melanoma
- Kaposi's sarcoma

 MANAGEMENT

- If there is any doubt about the diagnosis, a biopsy should be performed.
- The lesion is generally destroyed by electrocautery, laser therapy, cryosurgery, or excisional surgery. Recurrences are not uncommon if the lesion is not completely removed.

 POINT TO REMEMBER

- The clinical presentation of a rapidly developing, friable, vascular lesion in a child or pregnant woman suggests a pyogenic granuloma.

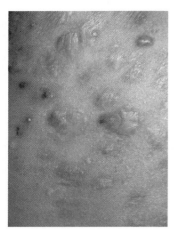

FIGURE 21.37 Hypertrophic scars. These lesions are characteristic of acne scars that occur on the trunk.

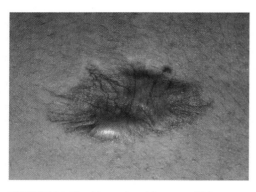

FIGURE 21.38 Hypertrophic scar. This shiny hypertrophic scar shows the effects of intralesional steroid injections: atrophy, telangiectasias, and perilesional hypopigmentation.

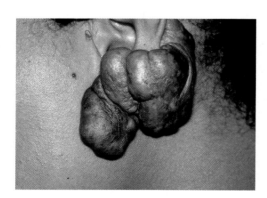

FIGURE 21.39 Keloid. The ear lobes are a common location.

BASICS

- Hypertrophic scars represent an exaggerated formation of scar tissue in response to skin injuries such as lacerations, insect bites, ear piercing, and surgical wounds. They may also result from healed inflammatory lesions of acne (Figure 21.37) or varicella. Hypertrophic scars tend to regress in size over time.
- A keloid is a scar whose size far exceeds that expected from the extent and margins of injury. Keloids do not regress without treatment. They are much more common in blacks than in whites and Asians.

DESCRIPTION OF LESIONS

- Lesions are firm, shiny, hairless papules, nodules, or tumors (Figures 21.38 and 21.39).
- If lesions are inflamed or are of recent onset they may be red or purple.

DISTRIBUTION OF LESIONS

- Hypertrophic scars and keloids are most likely to occur on the ear lobes, chest, shoulders, and upper back (Figure 21.39).

CLINICAL MANIFESTATIONS

- There is cosmetic disfigurement.
- Lesions may itch, or they may be tender or painful.

DIAGNOSIS

- The diagnosis of hypertrophic scars and keloids is made on clinical appearance.

MANAGEMENT

Hypertrophic Scars
- Intralesional steroid injections often help to flatten lesions; they are also useful for diminishing itching.
- Pulsed-dye lasers have been used successfully on some persistent lesions.

Keloids
- As with hypertrophic scars, intralesional steroid injections can help to flatten lesions and can diminish itching and erythema.
- Surgical ablation followed by compression dressings and repeated intralesional steroid injections is sometimes successful.
- Irradiation alone or after surgical treatment has been used in selected cases.
- The use of silicone gel sheeting has not proved effective.

Premalignant and Malignant Skin Neoplasms

Overview

This chapter is intended to help health care providers distinguish skin cancers from precancers and benign growths. The ability to make clinical diagnoses, to identify benign versus malignant lesions, especially in their less classic presentations, is an important skill that comes with focused, repetitive, visual scrutiny.

The therapy of malignant lesions should be undertaken *only* by persons experienced in skin cancer therapy.

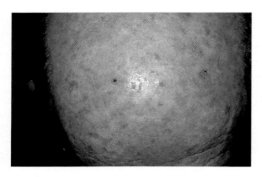

FIGURE 22.1 Solar keratoses. Rough, scaly papules are present on the scalp. This is a typical finding in bald, elderly men with fair complexions who have spent much of their lives working outdoors.

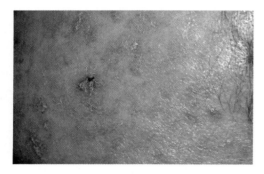

FIGURE 22.2 Solar keratoses. This is a closer view of Figure 22.1.

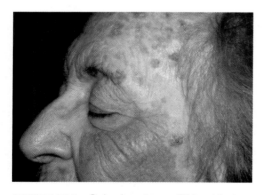

FIGURE 22.3 Solar keratoses. This elderly woman has vitiligo. The solar keratoses occur primarily in areas of unprotected, melanocyte-poor, vitiliginous skin.

BASICS

An aging population that is living longer, in an atmosphere with a declining ozone layer and with more outdoor and leisure time to bask in this ultraviolet environment, has led to a dramatic increase in sun-related skin damage *(dermatoheliosis)* and precursors to skin cancer such as solar keratoses. It is estimated that 60% of predisposed people older than 40 years have at least one solar keratosis, and many of them have new solar keratoses each year.

Solar keratosis, also known as *actinic keratosis,* is the most common sun-related skin growth. Whether this lesion is benign (premalignant) or malignant (squamous cell carcinoma *in situ*) from its onset is controversial. What is accepted, however, is that solar keratoses have the potential to develop into invasive squamous cell carcinomas. It is estimated that one in 20 lesions eventually becomes squamous cell carcinoma. It is also accepted that the invasive carcinomas that develop from these actinic keratoses are of a very slow-growing, indolent, unaggressive type, and the prognosis usually is excellent. Distant metastases are extremely rare. Consequently, among dermatologists, there is an ongoing debate regarding the need to be aggressive or *laissez-faire* in the approach to these lesions.

Solar keratoses are more common in men, particularly those who work, or have worked, in outdoor occupations, such as farmers, sailors, and gardeners, and those who participate in outdoor sports. The incidence is highest in Australia and in the Sun Belt of the United States.

Pathogenesis
- The development of solar keratoses, which is directly proportional to sun exposure, is seen in people who are fair-skinned, burn easily, and tan poorly.
- These lesions are rare in dark-skinned persons.

Histopathology
- Cellular atypia is present, and the keratinocytes vary in size and shape. Mitotic figures are common.

DESCRIPTION OF LESIONS

- They usually appear as multiple discrete, flat or elevated, verrucous, scaly lesions.
- Their texture typically feels rough to the touch (Figures 22.1 through 22.3).
- Lesions typically have an erythematous base covered by a white or yellowish scale (hyperkeratosis).

- Sometimes, they are tan or dark brown *(pigmented solar keratosis)* (Figure 22.4) and are often clinically indistinguishable from a lentigo (see Figure 21.3).
- Lesions are usually 3 to 10 mm in size and can gradually enlarge, thicken, and become more elevated and thus develop into a **hypertrophic solar keratosis** or a **cutaneous horn** (Figures 22.5 and 22.6).
- In time, a solar keratosis may develop into a squamous cell carcinoma.

DISTRIBUTION OF LESIONS

- Solar keratoses are most often seen on a background of sun-damaged skin.
- They are found chiefly on sun-exposed areas: the face, especially on the nose, temples, and forehead.
- They are also commonly noted on the bald areas of the scalp and the tops of the ears in men, the dorsum of the forearms and the dorsum of the hands, the "V" of the neck, and the neck below the occipital hairline and below the ears.
- They may also occur on any area that is chronically or repeatedly exposed to the sun, such as the legs in women.

CLINICAL MANIFESTATIONS

- Solar keratoses are usually asymptomatic, but they may itch and become tender or irritated.
- They are of cosmetic concern to many patients.
- They may regress spontaneously.

CLINICAL VARIANTS

Clinical variants include the following:

- Solar keratosis of the lower lip is known as **actinic cheilitis** (Figure 22.7).
- **Pigmented solar keratosis** (Figure 22.4) is a variant.
- **Hypertrophic (hyperkeratotic) solar keratosis** (Figure 22.5) is another variant.
- Solar keratosis can be associated with an overlying **cutaneous horn** (Figure 22.6). A cutaneous horn is a hornlike projection of keratin. Besides solar keratoses, warts and squamous cell carcinomas *in situ (Bowen's disease)* may also produce a cutaneous horn on their surface.

DIAGNOSIS

- Clinically, small lesions are better felt than seen. Palpation of these scaly growths reveals a gritty, sandpaper-like texture.
- A shave biopsy is performed if the diagnosis is in doubt.

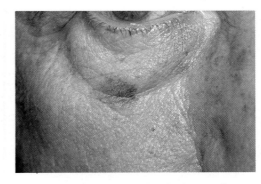

FIGURE 22.4 Pigmented solar keratosis. This lesion is slightly rough to the touch.

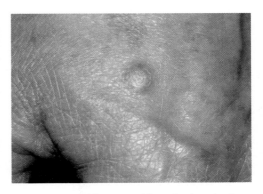

FIGURE 22.5 Hypertrophic solar keratosis. A shave biopsy was necessary to rule out squamous cell carcinoma.

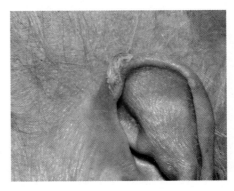

FIGURE 22.6 Cutaneous horn produced by an actinic keratosis. Underlying the cutaneous horn, a biopsy revealed a solar keratosis.

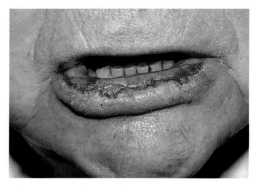

FIGURE 22.7 Actinic cheilitis. This patient is undergoing treatment with topical 5-fluorouracil for multiple solar keratoses of his lower lip.

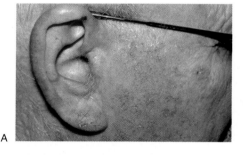

A

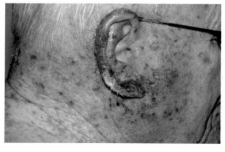

B

FIGURE 22.8 Solar keratoses. *A:* Before treatment, few lesions are clinically visible. *B:* Two weeks after treatment with topical 5-fluorouracil, crusting and erythema are evident in areas that had lesions that were not initially apparent.

 DIFFERENTIAL DIAGNOSIS

Squamous Cell Carcinoma (see later)
- This may be indistinguishable from a solar keratosis.
- Untreated, squamous cell carcinoma becomes indurated, with a tendency to ooze, ulcerate, or bleed.

Seborrheic Keratosis
This lesion is discussed in Chapter 21, "Benign Skin Neoplasms."

- A seborrheic keratosis may, at times, be indistinguishable from a solar keratosis.
- Seborrheic keratosis has a "stuck-on" appearance and a nonerythematous base; it may occur in areas not exposed to the sun.

Basal Cell Carcinoma (see later)
- Classically, this lesion is a pearly, shiny papule with telangiectasias.
- It may be indistinguishable from solar keratosis, particularly when it is small, ulcerated, manipulated, or pigmented.

Verruca Vulgaris (Wart)
- Warts may also be indistinguishable from solar keratoses.

 MANAGEMENT

Prevention begins with educating the patient to limit sun exposure by using sunscreens and wearing protective clothing. *Treatment* is achieved by destruction of solar keratoses (see Chapter 26, "Basic Dermatologic Procedures").

Destructive methods include the following:

- Liquid nitrogen (LN$_2$) is applied to individual lesions for 3 to 5 seconds.
- Biopsy followed by electrocautery of individual lesions or electrocautery alone is performed.
- Topical application of Efudex, a 5-fluorouracil (5-FU) cream, is a method that may be used when lesions are too numerous to treat individually (Figure 22.8). 5-FU interferes with the synthesis of DNA. This medication is applied using enough to cover the entire area with a thin film. This is done twice daily for a period of 2 to 4 weeks for facial lesions. Other body sites require longer treatment; the arms often require from 6 to 8 weeks.
- Alternatively, a 0.5% 5-FU cream (Carac) is applied only once daily. This preparation is reportedly less irritating than the stronger 5% 5-FU agents.
- During this treatment, the lesions become increasingly red and crusted, and subclinical lesions become visible. This situation can result in a very red, disfiguring complexion; however, if the patient completes the treatment, the lesions usually heal within 2 weeks of stopping treatment, the skin becomes smooth, and the majority of the solar keratoses are gone (Figures 22.7 and 22.8).

(continued)

Other Treatments

- Topical tretinoin (Retin-A) has been shown to reverse mild actinic damage to the skin.
- Photodynamic therapy can also be used to treat multiple actinic keratoses. In this treatment, topical 5-aminolevulinic acid accumulates preferentially in the dysplastic cells. On exposure to irradiation with light of appropriate wavelength, oxygen-derived free radicals are generated, and cell death results.
- Chemical peels and dermabrasion are also used in patients with numerous facial solar keratoses.
- Imiquimod (Aldara) cream is currently being evaluated as a topical treatment for solar keratoses. This agent is a local inducer of interferon; it may be applied at home by the patient.
- Diclofenac sodium 3% (Solarase) gel is a nonsteroidal antiinflammatory preparation that has been introduced as a topical treatment for solar keratoses. This agent appears to be less irritating than the standard 5-FU products; however, its efficacy does not match theirs.

 POINT TO REMEMBER

- If a lesion persists or recurs, despite treatment, it should be examined by biopsy.

 HELPFUL HINTS

- The number of solar keratoses is directly related to cumulative sun exposure. Childhood exposure of sun damage is "accumulated like interest on money in the bank"; some of this damage seems to be reversed and prevented by sun avoidance and sun protective measures.
- Sunscreens should also be applied to the lower lip to prevent actinic cheilitis.
- Topical 5-FU treatment can be likened to using a "smart bomb" in which the "bomb," in this case 5-FU, targets only the "enemy," the rapidly growing dysplastic cells.

 SEE PATIENT HANDOUTS, PAGES 485 AND 491

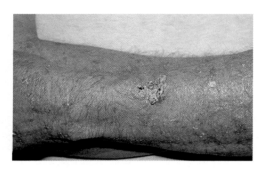

FIGURE 22.9 Nodular squamous cell carcinoma. The surrounding, smaller lesions are solar keratoses.

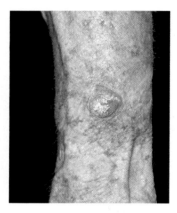

FIGURE 22.10 Squamous cell carcinoma. This reddish nodule is indistinguishable from basal cell carcinoma.

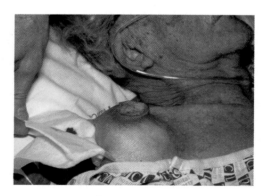

FIGURE 22.11 Squamous cell carcinoma. This neglected tumor has ulcerated.

BASICS

- Squamous cell carcinoma is a malignant tumor of keratinocytes. It is the second most common type of skin cancer. Squamous cell carcinoma is diagnosed much less frequently than basal cell carcinoma and it occurs in an older age group. Most squamous cell carcinomas arise in a solar keratosis.
- As with solar keratosis and basal cell carcinomas, squamous cell carcinoma is related to sun exposure and is noted more frequently in those with a greater degree of outdoor activity.
- Although very rare in dark-skinned persons, squamous cell carcinoma may occur for causes other than sun exposure. For example, it may arise in an old burn scar, at the site of radiation therapy, human papilloma virus infection (see Figure 19.18) or in a lesion of cutaneous lupus erythematosus.

Histopathology

- In the *in situ* type of squamous cell carcinoma *(Bowen's disease)*, only the full thickness of the epidermis is involved. Atypical keratinocytes (squamous cells) show a loss of polarity and an increased mitotic rate. The basement membrane remains intact.
- An invasive squamous cell carcinoma penetrates into the dermis. It has various levels of anaplasia and may manifest relatively few to multiple mitoses and may display varying degrees of differentiation such as keratinization.

Squamous cell carcinoma occurs in several clinical variants that vary in their aggressiveness:

- *In situ* squamous cell carcinoma (Bowen's disease)
- Squamous cell carcinoma arising in a solar keratosis
- Squamous cell carcinoma occurring on mucous membranes

The risk for metastasis of squamous cell carcinoma depends on its degree of differentiation, depth of penetration, and location:

- Lesions on mucous membranes have the highest risk for metastasis.
- Tumors that are induced by ionizing radiation or those that arise in old burn scars or in inflammatory lesions also are more likely to metastasize.

DESCRIPTION OF LESIONS

- Papules, plaques, or nodules (Figure 22.9) grow slowly.
- Lesions are scaly or ulcerated.
- A squamous cell carcinoma may appear as a reddish brown nodule (Figure 22.10). It may, at times, be indistinguishable from a basal cell carcinoma or a hypertrophic solar keratosis.
- Tumors may ulcerate when they are neglected (Figure 22.11).

DISTRIBUTION OF LESIONS

- Lesions occur in the same locations as do solar keratoses—sun-exposed areas such as the face, dorsa of the forearms and hands, and the "V" of the neck.
- In women, lesions tend to occur on the legs as well as other relatively sun-exposed locations.

CLINICAL MANIFESTATIONS

- Slow-growing, firm papules with the ability to produce scale (keratinization) tend to be more clearly differentiated and less likely to metastasize.
- Softer, nonkeratinizing lesions are less well differentiated and are more likely to spread.

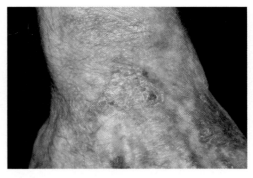

FIGURE 22.12 Bowen's disease *(in situ squamous cell carcinoma)*. This resembles a scaly psoriatic or eczematous plaque.

CLINICAL VARIANTS

Clinical variants include Bowen's disease *(squamous cell carcinoma in situ)* (Figure 22.12), a solitary lesion that resembles a scaly psoriatic or eczematous plaque.

- This lesion often arises in sites that are not exposed to the sun such as the trunk or extremities. When the lesion occurs on the penis, it is known as **erythroplasia of Queyrat.**
- **Bowen's disease** and frank squamous cell carcinoma are two of the few skin cancers that should be considered as a diagnosis in African-American, Afro-Caribbean, and African blacks. This non–sun-related skin cancer tends to arise on the extremities *de novo* (Figure 22.13), in an old scar (Figure 22.14), or in a lesion of discoid lupus erythematosus.

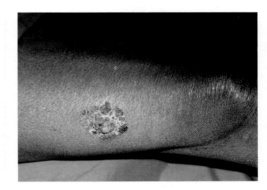

FIGURE 22.13 Bowen's disease in an African-American woman. This lesion arose *de novo.*

DIAGNOSIS

- An early lesion of squamous cell carcinoma is difficult to distinguish from a precursor solar keratosis.
- The diagnosis is generally made by shave or excisional biopsy.

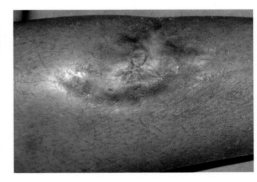

FIGURE 22.14 Squamous cell carcinoma arising in a burn scar. This lesion has a significant chance to metastasize.

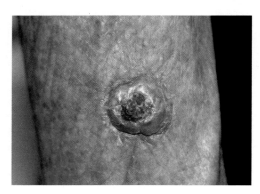

FIGURE 22.15 Keratoacanthoma. This nodule arose over a period of 2 weeks. Note the typical crusting in the center.

 DIFFERENTIAL DIAGNOSIS

Solar Keratosis (Actinic Keratosis)
- This lesion is often indistinguishable from squamous cell carcinoma (see earlier).

Basal Cell Carcinoma
This lesion is discussed later in this chapter.

- Basal cell carcinomas are generally pearly and telangiectatic.
- They are more common in a younger age group.
- Basal cell carcinoma may be indistinguishable from squamous cell carcinoma, particularly if the lesion is ulcerated.

Keratoacanthoma
- This lesion also may be indistinguishable from squamous cell carcinoma (Figure 22.15).
- It is fast growing.
- Usually, it has a typical central crater.

 MANAGEMENT

- Electrocautery and curettage for small lesions of squamous cell carcinoma and squamous cell carcinoma *in situ* (Bowen's disease) are done in a fashion similar to that performed for basal cell carcinoma treatment (see later).
- Like superficial basal cell carcinomas, selected squamous cell carcinomas may be treated rapidly using cryosurgery with LN_2.
- Total excision, the preferred method of therapy for squamous cell carcinoma, permits histologic diagnosis of the tumor margins.
- Micrographic (Mohs') surgery is useful for excessively large or invasive carcinomas, for recurrent lesions, for lesions with poorly delineated clinical borders, for squamous cell carcinomas within an orifice (e.g., ear canals or nostrils), and for carcinomas in locations where preservation of normal tissue is extremely important (e.g., tip of the nose, eyelids, ala nasi, ears, lips, and glans penis) (see later).
- Radiation therapy is used for those patients who are physically debilitated or who are unable to, or refuse to undergo, excisional surgery.

 POINT TO REMEMBER

- Squamous cell carcinoma arising on a mucous membrane such as the glans penis (erythroplasia of Queyrat) or lip, arising from a chronic ulcer, or one arising in an immunocompromised patient should be regarded as potentially metastatic.

 SEE PATIENT HANDOUTS, PAGES 489 AND 491

BASICS

A keratoacanthoma is a unique lesion with a characteristic clinical appearance. If ignored, lesions often regress spontaneously. There is controversy about the benign versus malignant nature of this lesion. A keratoacanthoma resembles a squamous cell carcinoma histologically and is considered by some dermatologists and dermatopathologists to be a low-grade variant of a squamous cell carcinoma and believe that it should be treated as such. These lesions occur in persons older than 65 years.

DESCRIPTION OF LESIONS

- Keratoacanthoma usually occurs as a single, dome-shaped erythematous or skin-colored nodule with a central keratin core with an overlying crust (Figures 22.15 and 22.16).
- It attains a diameter of 1.0 to 2.5 cm.

DISTRIBUTION OF LESIONS

- Lesions appear on the face, ears, neck, dorsa of hands, and forearms.

CLINICAL MANIFESTATIONS

- Lesions arise quickly, usually taking 3 to 4 weeks.
- Spontaneous regression may result in scarring.

DIAGNOSIS

- An excisional or incisional biopsy is often recommended so that the complete architecture of the lesion can be evaluated histologically. (An insufficient biopsy, such as a shave biopsy, may result in a histology that is indistinguishable from a squamous cell carcinoma.) These lesions often appear in difficult areas to perform an excisional biopsy such as the nose and external ears; thus a deep shave biopsy is often adequate to obtain sufficient tissue.

 DIFFERENTIAL DIAGNOSIS

- Squamous cell carcinoma
- Verruca vulgaris

MANAGEMENT

- Excisional removal
- Deep shave biopsy in selected cases
- Intralesional 5-fluorouracil

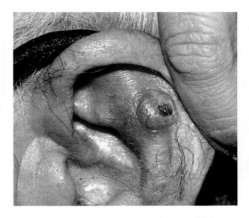

FIGURE 22.16 Keratoacanthoma. This nodule arose over a period of 4 weeks. Note typical crusting in the center.

BASAL CELL CARCINOMA

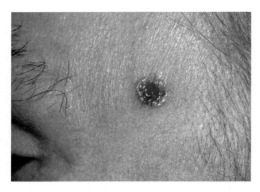

FIGURE 22.17 Nodular basal cell carcinoma. A pearly papule with ulceration ("rodent ulcer") is noted.

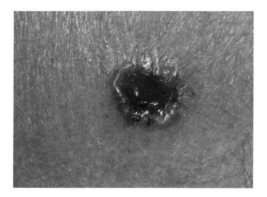

FIGURE 22.18 Nodular basal cell carcinoma. This is a close-up view of Figure 22.15, showing rolled borders with telangiectasia.

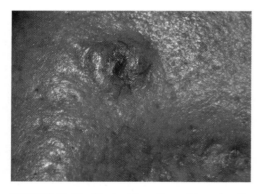

FIGURE 22.19 Typical location of basal cell carcinoma. Note the central crust.

BASICS

The same risk factors that predispose to solar keratoses and squamous cell carcinomas are responsible for the development of basal cell carcinomas. Although this lesion qualifies as a cancer, its morbidity, if recognized and treated early, is usually inconsequential. Basal cell carcinoma is usually slow growing and very rarely metastasizes, but it can cause significant local invasion and destruction if it is neglected or treated inadequately.

Histopathology
Cells of nodular basal cell carcinoma typically have large, hyperchromatic oval nuclei and little cytoplasm. Cells appear rather uniform, and, if present, mitotic figures are usually scant. Nodular tumor aggregates may be of varying sizes, but tumor cells tend to align more densely in a palisade pattern at the periphery of these nests. Cleft formation, known as retraction artifact, commonly occurs between basal cell carcinoma nests and stroma because of shrinkage of mucin during tissue fixation and staining.

Risk Factors
Risk factors for basal cell carcinoma include the following:

- Age older than 40 years
- Male sex
- Positive family history of basal cell carcinoma
- Light complexion (like squamous cell carcinomas and solar keratoses, basal cell carcinomas are rare in blacks and Asians) with poor tanning ability
- Long-term sun exposure

DESCRIPTION OF LESIONS

- The classic lesion, the nodular basal cell carcinoma, is also the most common type (Figures 22.17 and 22.19). Nodular basal cell carcinomas occur most commonly on the head, neck, and upper back and have some of the following features:
- A pearly, shiny, papule or nodule
- A semitranslucent appearance
- A rolled (raised) border
- Telangiectases over the surface, thus accounting for a history of bleeding with minor trauma
- Erosion or ulceration ("rodent ulcer")

- Brownish to blue-black pigmentation *(pigmented basal cell carcinoma)* is seen in more darkly pigmented persons (Figures 22.20 and 22.21)

DISTRIBUTION OF LESIONS

- Lesions occur on the head and neck in 85% of all affected persons.
- Lesions occur on sun-exposed areas (e.g., the face, especially on the nose, cheeks, forehead, periorbital area, lower face, and the back of the neck).

CLINICAL MANIFESTATIONS

- Lesions are often ignored, asymptomatic, and slow growing.
- Very mild trauma, such as face washing or drying with a towel, may cause bleeding.
- In time, lesions may ulcerate (e.g., "the sore that will not heal").

CLINICAL VARIANTS

Clinical variants include the following:

Superficial Basal Cell Carcinoma
- A superficial basal cell carcinoma occurs as a scaly pink to red-brown patch with a threadlike border (Figure 22.22).
- The lesions tend to be indolent, asymptomatic, and the least aggressive of basal cell carcinomas.
- Lesions are often multiple, occurring primarily on the trunk and proximal extremities.
- When solitary, a lesion of superficial basal cell carcinoma may resemble psoriasis, eczema, a seborrheic keratosis, or Bowen's disease (squamous cell carcinoma *in situ*).
- There is no clear association between superficial BCC and sun exposure.

Morpheaform Basal Cell Carcinoma
This is the least common and most aggressive form of basal cell carcinoma.

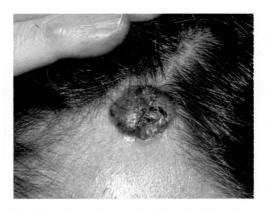

FIGURE 22.20 Pigmented basal cell carcinoma. This lesion could easily be mistaken for a melanoma. Note the pearly surface.

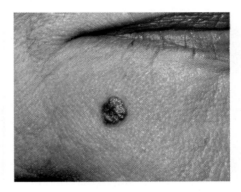

FIGURE 22.21 Pigmented basal cell carcinoma. Note the pearly, waxy surface.

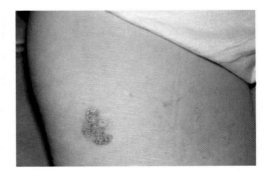

FIGURE 22.22 Superficial basal cell carcinoma. This lesion resembles a psoriatic plaque as well as Bowen's disease.

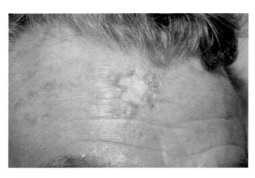

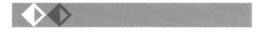

FIGURE 22.23 Morpheaform basal cell carcinoma. A whitish atrophic plaque is present, with surrounding telangiectasias and pearly papules surrounding the atrophic plaque.

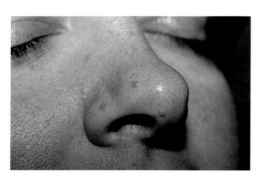

FIGURE 22.24 Angiofibromas *(fibrous papules of the nose)*. These lesions are often confused with basal cell carcinomas.

- Lesions appear as whitish, scarred atrophic plaques with surrounding telangiectasia (Figure 22.23).
- The margins of these lesions are often difficult to evaluate clinically; similar to icebergs, what is seen on the surface is not always what lies under the surface.
- Consequently, morpheaform basal cell carcinomas are generally more difficult to treat than other basal cell carcinomas.
- A morpheaform basal cell carcinoma may be mistaken for scar tissue.

DIAGNOSIS

- The diagnosis is generally made by shave or excisional biopsy.
- A shave biopsy suffices for the diagnosis of most basal cell carcinomas (see Chapter 26, "Basic Dermatologic Procedures").

 DIFFERENTIAL DIAGNOSIS

- Squamous cell carcinoma
- Solar keratosis
- Sebaceous hyperplasia (see Chapter 21, "Benign Skin Neoplasms")
- Angiofibroma *(fibrous papule of the nose)* (Figure 22.24), which may be clinically indistinguishable from basal cell carcinoma
- Seborrheic keratosis, which may be indistinguishable from a pigmented basal cell carcinoma

MANAGEMENT

Prevention is achieved by sun avoidance, use of sunscreens with a sun protection factor (SPF) of at least 15, and wearing of protective clothing. People should learn skin self-examination and should have annual skin examinations by a physician. *Treatment* (see Chapter 26, "Basic Dermatologic Procedures") is achieved by the following means:

- Electrodesiccation and curettage. The overall cure rate exceeds 90% for low-risk basal cell carcinomas. This method is quick and simple and is less expensive than most other procedures.
- Cryosurgery with LN$_2$. Superficial basal cell carcinomas may be treated rapidly using this method. However, nodular lesions, particularly selected eyelid lesions and those on the ear are ideally treated with a temperature probe before cryosurgery is performed. Successful treatment is highly dependent on the experience of the operator.
- Excision, permitting histologic diagnosis of margins. Cosmetic results compare favorably with those of curettage; however, surgical excision is more time-consuming and costly than curettage.

(continued)

- Micrographic (Mohs') surgery for morpheaform, recurrent, or large lesions, as well as for lesions in "danger zones" (e.g., the nasolabial area, around the eyes, behind the ears, in the ear canal, and on the scalp). Mohs' micrographic surgery is a microscopically controlled method of removing skin cancers that allows for controlled excision and maximum preservation of normal tissue. Excisions are repeated in the areas proven to be cancerous until a complete cancer-free plane is reached. Mohs' surgery is time-consuming and expensive, and it may require extensive reconstruction of surgical wounds; however, it provides the most reliable method of determining adequate margins, it has a very high cure rate of 98% to 99% for basal cell carcinomas, and it preserves the maximum amount of normal tissue around the cancer.
- Radiation therapy for elderly debilitated patients or for those who are physically unable to undergo excisional surgery. The disadvantages include the potential for late radiation changes in the skin, as well as the inability to examine skin margins because tissue is not obtained.

 POINTS TO REMEMBER

- Basal cell carcinoma is, by far, the most common type of skin cancer.
- As with squamous cell carcinoma and solar keratoses, basal cell carcinomas are induced by ultraviolet radiation in susceptible persons.
- Almost 50% of patients with basal cell carcinoma will have another one within 5 years.
- Recurrent basal cell carcinomas are generally more aggressive than primary lesions.
- Patients with basal cell carcinoma have an increased risk for melanoma.

 HELPFUL HINTS

- Patients should always be undressed for adequate examination of the skin.
- A topical immunomodulator, a 5% imiquimod cream (Aldara), is being used for the treatment of multiple superficial basal cell carcinomas.
- Avoidance of exposure to ultraviolet radiation is encouraged. Preventive measures include carefully planning outdoor activities before 10 a.m. and after 4 p.m., wearing a broad-brimmed hat during outdoor activities, and using SPF 15 or greater sunscreens.

 SEE PATIENT HANDOUTS, PAGES 487 AND 491

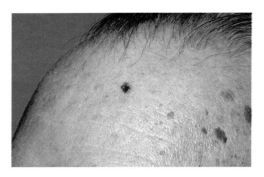

FIGURE 22.25 *In situ* melanoma. Note jet-black coloration of the lesion. Compare with surrounding seborrheic keratoses.

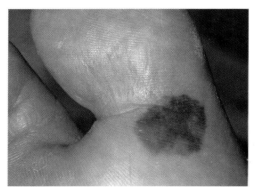

FIGURE 22.26 Acral lentiginous melanoma. Note the pronounced variegation pigmentation of this lesion. (Courtesy of Charles Miller, M.D., San Diego Naval Hospital.)

BASICS

Malignant melanoma (Figures 22.25 and 22.26) is a cancer of melanocytes, the cells that produce pigment. The lesion generally occurs in the skin and, much less commonly, in the eyes, ears, gastrointestinal tract, leptomeninges of the central nervous system, and oral and genital mucous membranes. Malignant melanoma is one of the only skin diseases that can be fatal if neglected, consequently, early recognition and prompt removal of a melanoma can save a life.

The incidence of malignant melanoma has markedly increased over the past several decades; it currently represents 1% to 2% of all cancer-related deaths. It is the most common cancer in women aged 25 to 29 years and is second only to breast cancer in women aged 30 to 34 years.

Pathogenesis

- Primary cutaneous melanoma may develop in precursor melanocytic nevi (common acquired, congenital, and atypical or dysplastic types), although more than 50% of cases are believed to arise *de novo* without a preexisting pigmented lesion.
- Malignant melanoma tends to occur at sites of intermittent intense sun exposure (i.e., on the trunk in male patients and on the arms, lower legs, and back in female patients). The disease shows an increased worldwide incidence in locations nearer the equator—the highest incidence in Australia and New Zealand—and this suggests a causative role for ultraviolet radiation.
- Two genodermatoses, *xeroderma pigmentosum* and *familial atypical mole melanoma syndrome,* confer a 500-fold or greater relative risk for developing melanoma.

Risk Factors

Persons at greatest risk for melanoma include the following:

- They are generally older than 20 years, particularly older than 60 years.
- They have a light complexion, an inability to tan, and a history of sunburns.
- They have moles that are numerous, changing, or atypical *(dysplastic nevi)*.
- They have a personal or family history of melanoma (first-degree relatives).
- They have a personal or family history of basal or squamous cell carcinomas.

Malignant melanoma is very rare in dark-skinned persons and Asians. However, when it does occur, it tends to be present on acral areas (e.g., the hands and feet).

Histopathology

Superficial spreading melanoma, lentigo maligna melanoma, and acral lentiginous melanoma have an *in situ* (radial growth) phase characterized by increased numbers of intraepithelial melanocytes, which are large and atypical, are arranged haphazardly at the dermal-epidermal junction, show upward (pagetoid) migration, and lack the biologic potential to metastasize. Invasion into the dermis may confer metastatic potential and is characterized by a distinct population of melanoma cells with mitoses and nuclear pleomorphism within the dermis (papillary, reticular) and, possibly, the subcutaneous fat.

DISTRIBUTION OF LESIONS

- In white women, the most common lesion sites for **superficial spreading melanoma** are the upper back, the lower leg between the knees and ankle, and the arms. Lesions are relatively fewer on covered areas such as under bras and swimsuits.
- In white men, the most common lesion sites for superficial spreading melanoma are the upper back, anterior torso, and the upper extremity.
- In both white women and white men, other types of melanoma (e.g., **lentigo maligna melanoma**) may occur on the head, neck, and sun-exposed arms. **Nodular melanomas** are seen on the legs and trunk.
- In African-American and Asian men and women, the **acral lentiginous melanoma** is found on the plantar foot, followed by subungual and palmar sites.

CLINICAL MANIFESTATIONS

Warning Signs

- New, changing, or unusual moles. A changing mole is the most common sign of melanoma.
- Symptomatic moles (e.g., moles that itch, burn, or are painful). The lesions are generally asymptomatic, unless inflammation or invasion occurs.
- An initial slow horizontal growth phase, if left untreated, is followed in months or years by a vertical growth phase, which indicates invasive disease and potential metastasis.

Prognosis

Five-year survival is based on the thickness of the tumor. The scale shown in Table 22.1 is known as **Breslow's measurement.**

Other important prognostic factors include the sex of the patient (women have a better prognosis than men), age (the prognosis worsens with increasing age), and the presence of ulceration or regional or distant spread. Prognosis may also be determined by the grade of the melanoma, as determined by its location in the dermis using **Clark's levels** (Table 22.2).

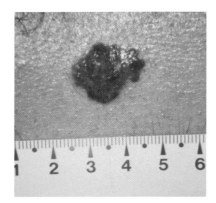

FIGURE 22.27 Superficial spreading melanoma. Note the "ABCD" features: asymmetry, notched border, varied colors, and diameter of more than 6 mm.

Superficial Spreading Melanoma

This is by far the most common type of malignant melanoma (Figures 22.27 and 22.28). It may arise *de novo* or in a preexisting nevus.

The lesions of superficial spreading melanoma may conform to some (or all) of the "ABCD" criteria for melanoma, in which the primary lesion is a macular lesion or an elevated plaque that displays the following:

A: Asymmetry
B: Border that is irregular or notched
C: Color that is varied (may have brown, black, pink, blue gray, white, or admixtures of these colors)
D: Diameter greater than 6 mm (the size of a pencil eraser)

DIAGNOSIS

- Clinical diagnosis is based on ABCD criteria.
- Elliptic excisional biopsy should include all of the visible lesion.

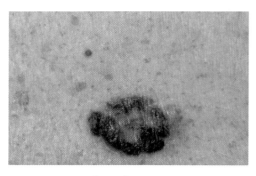

FIGURE 22.28 Superficial spreading melanoma. Note the central area (whitish gray) of regression.

 DIFFERENTIAL DIAGNOSIS

See Chapter 21, "Benign Skin Neoplasms."

Seborrheic Keratosis
- Seborrheic keratosis, particularly if it is variegated in color or jet black (Figure 22.29), should be considered.

Basal Cell Carcinoma
- Pigmented basal cell carcinoma may be clinically indistinguishable from superficial spreading melanoma or other types of malignant melanoma (Figures 22.20 and 22.21).

Dysplastic or Atypical Nevus
- A dysplastic nevus or a melanocytic nevus with an atypical appearance may also be clinically indistinguishable from malignant melanoma (Figure 22.30).

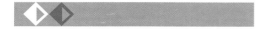

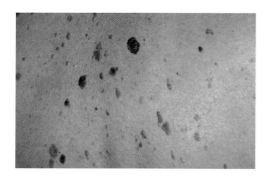

FIGURE 22.29 Seborrheic keratoses. These "stuck-on" appearing lesions are most often confused with malignant melanoma by clinicians who are not dermatologists. The darkest lesion is also a seborrheic keratosis.

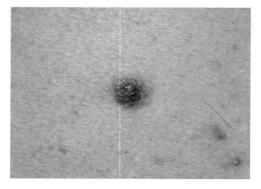

FIGURE 22.30 Dysplastic nevus. Note the raised center and indistinct border; such a nevus is sometimes called a *sunny-side-up egg lesion.*

In general, to determine the diagnosis, a biopsy is necessary. If any form of malignant melanoma is suspected, an excisional biopsy should be performed.

OTHER VARIANTS

Nodular Melanoma

The lesion of a nodular melanoma arises *de novo* as a nodule or plaque. It occurs in 15% to 20% of patients (Figure 22.31). Because of their rapid vertical growth phase, lesions invade early.

Nodular melanoma lesions have the following characteristics:

- They are blue, blue black, or nonpigmented (as in *amelanotic melanoma*); their color is more uniform than that of superficial spreading melanoma (Figure 22.32).
- They may ulcerate and bleed with minor trauma.
- They occur most commonly on the legs and trunk.
- They may be indistinguishable from a pyogenic granuloma (see Figure 21.36).

Lentigo Maligna and Lentigo Maligna Melanoma

Lentigo maligna is a type of lentigo that is considered a malignant melanoma *in situ* (Figure 22.33). Lesions are characterized by the following:

- They occur most often on the faces of fair-skinned older individuals (average age 65 years)
- They grow slowly over 5 to 20 years.
- They have an irregular color and border.
- When a lentigo maligna invades the dermis, it is then referred to as a **lentigo maligna melanoma** (Figure 22.34).

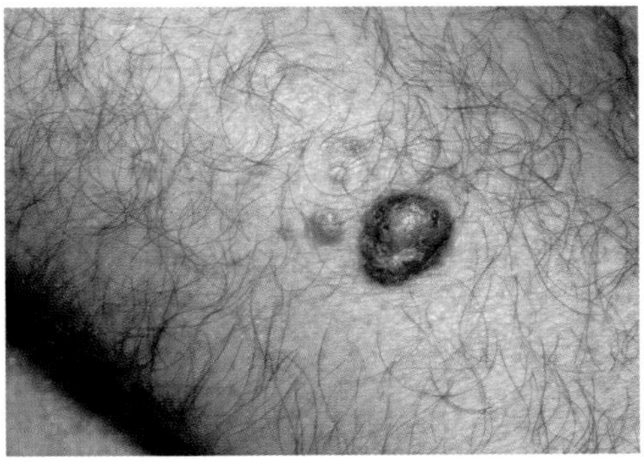

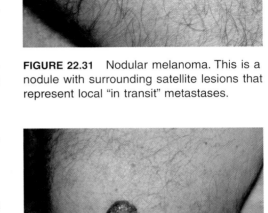

FIGURE 22.31 Nodular melanoma. This is a nodule with surrounding satellite lesions that represent local "in transit" metastases.

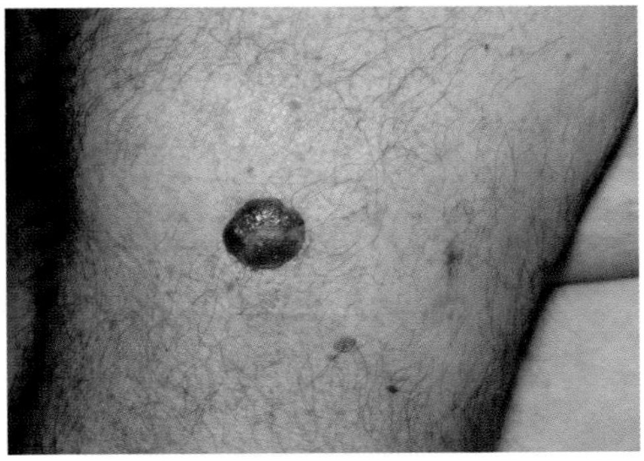

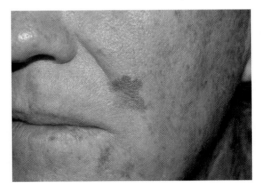

FIGURE 22.32 Nodular amelanotic melanoma. This lesion arose *de novo*; it has a great probability of metastasizing.

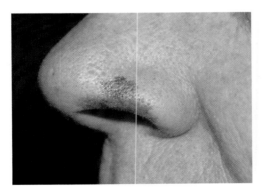

FIGURE 22.34 Lentigo maligna melanoma. Biopsy of this lesion demonstrated invasion into the dermis.

FIGURE 22.33 Lentigo maligna. Note the irregular color and irregular border of this malignant melanoma *in situ*.

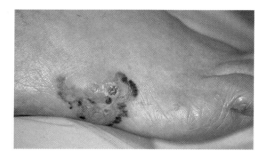

FIGURE 22.35 Melanoma. This patient was referred by a podiatrist who was treating the lesion as a wart; the lesion did not resolve with destructive therapy. It was, in fact, a level V melanoma (melanoma cells were located in the subcutaneous tissue). (Courtesy of Art Huntley, M.D., University of California at Davis.)

Acral Lentiginous Melanoma

Acral lentiginous melanoma is the least common subtype of melanoma. These lesions have the following features:

- They occur most often in blacks and Asians.
- They appear on areas that do not bear hair, such as the palms, soles, and periungual skin.

CLINICAL MANIFESTATIONS

- Acral lentiginous melanoma has a tendency toward early metastasis (Figure 22.35).
- A subungual acral lentiginous melanoma presenting as diffuse nail discoloration or a longitudinal pigmented band within the nail plate is potentially confused with subungual hematoma or **junctional nevus** (Figures 22.36 and 22.37). Pigment spread to the proximal or lateral nail folds (*Hutchinson's sign,* a hallmark of acral lentiginous melanoma) (Figure 22.38).

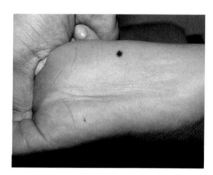

FIGURE 22.36 Junctional nevus. This fairly common lesion may present a worrisome quandary (to biopsy or not to biopsy). It is extremely rare for a lesion such as this to be a melanoma (especially in a child).

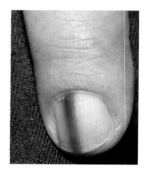

FIGURE 22.37 Junctional nevus. Note the even linear bands of pigmentation in this patient's nail bed.

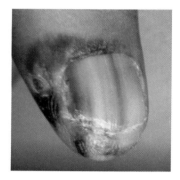

FIGURE 22.38 Acral lentiginous melanoma. Hutchinson's sign shows uneven pigmentation spreading beyond the nail into surrounding skin.

MANAGEMENT

- Elliptic excision should include the entire visible lesion down to the subcutaneous fat.
- Surgical margins of 5 mm currently are recommended for melanoma *in situ*.
- For lesions with a thickness of less than 1 mm, a 1-cm margin of normal skin is usually adequate.
- For thicker lesions, the margin should be more than 1 cm. The margin size is based on the histologic type and the anatomic location of the lesion.
- Elective lymph node dissection is not recommended for lesions that are less than 1 mm thick, unless lymph nodes are palpable. The decision whether to perform elective lymph node dissection on thicker lesions (1 to 4 mm) is controversial. A negative sentinel node biopsy (dissecting the lymph node closest to the site of the primary melanoma) may allow for a less invasive procedure.
- Amputation, regional lymph node dissection, and regional chemotherapy perfusion are often necessary for acral lentiginous melanomas.
- In more advanced stages of malignant melanoma, chemotherapy and radiation therapy have not been very effective for achieving remission of metastatic disease (Figures 22.39 and 22.40).
- Vaccines, interleukin-2, arterial limb perfusion, and immunotherapy are more promising adjuncts to surgery. In fact, an injectable recombinant interferon alfa 2B (Intron A) has been shown to improve the 5-year survival rate significantly in patients with thick lesions, lymph node involvement, or both.

Long-Term Management

- Patients who have had malignant melanoma should be followed every 3 months for the first 2 years and annually thereafter.
- At each visit, the patient's entire cutaneous surface and lymph nodes should be examined.
- Patients with invasive disease require an annual chest x-ray film, complete blood count, and liver function studies.

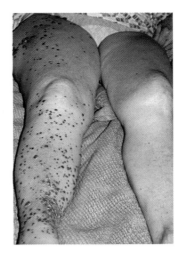

FIGURE 22.39 Metastatic malignant melanoma. Note the lymphedema and multiple metastatic nodules on this patient's leg.

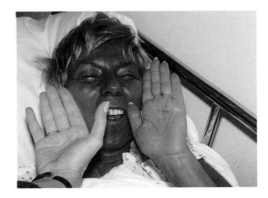

FIGURE 22.40 Metastatic malignant melanoma. The unusual brown-blue coloration is the result of widespread melanin pigmentation in the tissues.

POINTS TO REMEMBER

- Anyone who has a history of melanoma needs lifelong skin surveillance, because 3% of these patients will develop a second malignant melanoma within 3 years.
- Sun protection should be stressed in those with a personal or family history of melanoma. The need to protect children (beginning at an early age) from excessive sun exposure should also be emphasized.
- Patients should be taught self-examination.
- All family members should be examined.
- Any lesion that looks suspicious must be examined by biopsy.
- An amelanotic melanoma is easily overlooked because of its lack of pigmentation.
- Removal of thin lesions (less than 0.76 mm) is curative in almost all patients.
- Early detection and removal are paramount because the treatments for metastatic melanoma are limited and the prognosis is guarded.

HELPFUL HINTS

- Early detection of thin cutaneous melanoma is the best means of reducing mortality.
- Trauma from rubbing or irritation does not cause malignant degeneration of moles.
- Total skin examination that includes the legs should be performed when evaluating a female patient for possible skin cancer.

SEE PATIENT HANDOUT, PAGE 491

TABLE 22.1. BRESLOW'S MEASUREMENT

TUMOR THICKNESS (mm)	5-YEAR SURVIVAL (%)
<0.75	98–99
0.76–1.50	94
1.51–2.25	83
2.26–3.00	72–77
>3.00	<50

TABLE 22.2. CLARK'S LEVELS

GRADE	LOCATION IN DERMIS
I	*In situ* disease confined to the epidermis
II	Melanoma cells in papillary dermis
III	Melanoma cells filling papillary dermis
IV	Melanoma cells in reticular dermis
V	Melanoma cells in subcutaneous fat

PART TWO
Systemic Conditions and the Skin

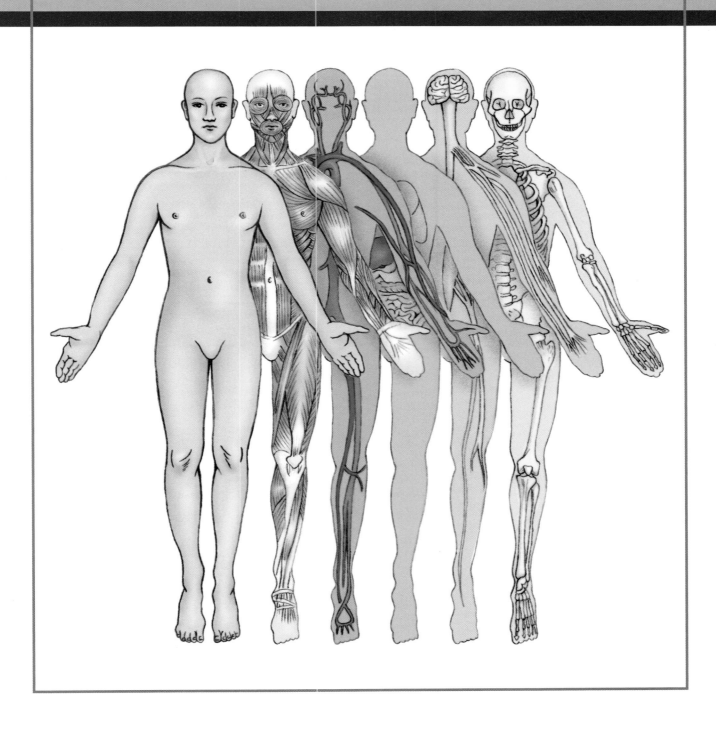

Skin and Hair During Pregnancy

Overview

During pregnancy, various skin changes occur. Many of these changes are so frequently seen that they are considered normal. Pregnancy can also alter the course of certain preexisting skin conditions or systemic diseases that have cutaneous involvement, for example:

- Systemic lupus erythematosus and scleroderma may flare.
- Acne may improve, or it may worsen.
- Dyshidrotic eczema may appear *de novo,* or a flare-up of preexisting lesions may occur.
- Condylomata acuminatum may enlarge considerably and may proliferate.

It should always be kept in mind, however, that many common skin diseases unrelated to pregnancy should be considered when evaluating a pregnant patient with a skin disorder.

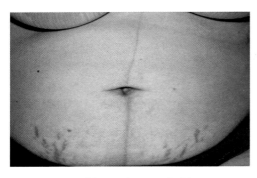

FIGURE 23.1 Linea nigra and striae gravidarum. The linea alba darkens during pregnancy, but the normal color usually returns after delivery. In contrast, although the purplish color of striae gravidarum will fade over time, the striae themselves are permanent.

HYPERPIGMENTATION

Hyperpigmentation is presumed to be secondary to increased levels of estrogens and melanocyte-stimulating hormone. It frequently manifests as follows:

- Darkening of the linea alba (which becomes the *linea nigra*). There may also be darkening of the nipples and surrounding areolae, as well as darkening of the axillae, thighs, umbilicus, perineum, and external genitalia (Figure 23.1).
- Melasma (For a more complete discussion, see Chapter 14, "Pigmentary Disorders"). The "mask of pregnancy" (formerly known as *chloasma*) occurs in more than 50% of women. It is worsened by exposure to the sun. Melasma is also seen in women taking oral contraceptives and, on occasion, *de novo* in women in whom no explanation is obvious.
- Darkening of preexisting freckles and nevi.

MANAGEMENT

- For patients with melasma caused by pregnancy, it is usually best to keep sun exposure to a minimum and to wait for fading, which often takes place spontaneously. Treatment of persistent nongestational melasma consists of diligent sun avoidance and, frequently, the use of skin bleaching creams (see Chapter 14, "Pigmentary Disorders").
- Darkened freckles, nevi, and linea nigra usually regress after termination of the pregnancy.
- Pregnancy does not appear to affect the survival rate adversely in women who have preexisting malignant melanoma.

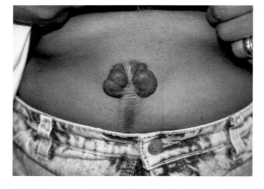

FIGURE 23.2 Keloid. This lesion is growing well beyond the border of cesarian section scar.

CONNECTIVE TISSUE CHANGES

- Striae gravidarum (*striae cutis distensae* related to pregnancy) or "stretch marks" are thought to be caused by the combination of increased adrenocortical activity and rapid tissue growth and distention, which result in tearing of the collagen matrix of the dermis and a weakness of elastic fibers. Typically, striae are reddish pink to violaceous linear atrophic bands that are located on the abdomen, hips, buttocks, and breasts. The striae are permanent, but the purplish color most often fades with time.
- Proliferation and enlargement of skin tags, with some persisting after pregnancy.
- Occasional growth of preexisting keloids. For example, this may occur in the scars of an abdominal hysterectomy or a cesarian section (Figure 23.2). Growth of preexisting keloids is not an uncommon problem in black women.

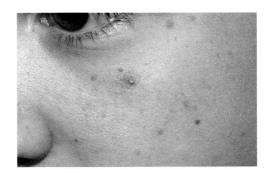

FIGURE 23.3 Spider telangiectasias. These can result from the high levels of estrogens in pregnancy.

MANAGEMENT

- There is no proven effective treatment for striae.
- If desired, skin tags may be easily removed (see Chapter 21, "Benign Skin Neoplasms").
- Keloids may diminish in size postpartum; if they do not, treatment with intralesional steroids may be helpful (see Chapter 21, "Benign Skin Neoplasms").

VASCULAR PHENOMENA

- Spider telangiectasias. These can result from the high levels of estrogens in pregnancy (Figure 23.3).
- Scattered petechiae in the lower extremities. These are the result of increased capillary fragility and increased hydrostatic pressure in this region.
- Palmar erythema, flushing, and increased sweating (Figure 23.4).
- Venous varicosities of the legs and feet
- Hemorrhoids
- Edema of the leg, face, or eyelids

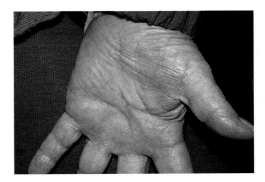

FIGURE 23.4 Palmar erythema. Flushing and increased sweating may also occur.

MANAGEMENT

- Most vascular phenomena resolve post partum. However, varicosities may persist and may worsen with further pregnancies.

HAIR CHANGES

- Telogen effluvium. Hair loss may occur from 1 to 5 months post partum and is generally followed by total regrowth. Rarely, the regrowth may not be as thick as prepregnancy hair growth.
- Hirsutism. Mild degrees of hirsutism are common. The face is frequently affected, although hair growth may be pronounced on the extremities as well. Hirsutism normally regresses after delivery, but it may recur in subsequent pregnancies.

MANAGEMENT

- Because both telogen effluvium and hirsutism usually resolve spontaneously, no specific management is needed. However, excessive hirsutism warrants investigation for an androgen-secreting tumor (see Chapter 11, "Hirsutism").

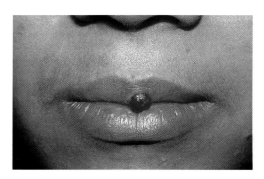

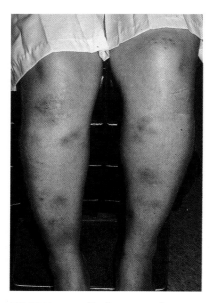

FIGURE 23.5 Pyogenic granuloma. During pregnancy, lesions tend to occur on the lips and gums.

FIGURE 23.6 Erythema nodosum. These tender nodules occurred during pregnancy and resolved postpartum.

OTHER FINDINGS

Skin conditions during pregnancy can also include the following:

- Increased nail fragility, brittleness, and distal separation of the nail plate (onycholysis) may occur.
- Edema and hyperemia of the gums ("pregnancy gingivitis") have been noted.
- Pyogenic granulomas often develop on the lips and gums and usually regress shortly post partum (Figure 23.5).
- Erythema nodosum, an apparently autoimmune skin condition, is usually associated with infections, sarcoidosis, malignant diseases, and drugs, but it can also be precipitated by pregnancy alone (Figure 23.6).
- Erythema multiforme has a variety of causes, including pregnancy.

MANAGEMENT

Pregnancy Gingivitis
- Good dental hygiene (adequate brushing and flossing) is essential, because the problem is exacerbated by plaque and calculus.

Pyogenic Granulomas
- Treatment may be deferred until after delivery or performed during pregnancy, if necessary. Options include cryodestruction, electrodesiccation, and excisional surgery (see Chapter 21, "Benign Skin Neoplasms").

Erythema Nodosum
- Erythema nodosum tends to clear post partum and to recur in subsequent pregnancies. Treatment is with bed rest and mild analgesics.

Erythema Multiforme
- Like erythema nodosum, erythema multiforme resulting from pregnancy tends to clear spontaneously and is managed symptomatically. Underlying causes other than pregnancy (e.g., infection) should be sought and treated.

For further discussion of these conditions, see Chapter 25, "Cutaneous Manifestations of Systemic Disease."

SPECIFIC DERMATOSES OF PREGNANCY

BASICS

The specific dermatoses of pregnancy are a group of cutaneous eruptions that are unique to pregnancy. Historically, these eruptions have been variously classified, resulting in overlapping and confusing terminology. The following discussion should help to simplify the approach to these entities.

PRURITIC URTICARIAL PAPULES AND PLAQUES OF PREGNANCY

A common dermatosis of late pregnancy, pruritic urticarial papules and plaques of pregnancy (PUPPP) is, as its name suggests, a pruritic eruption consisting of urticarial papules that coalesce into plaques (Figure 23.7). Initially, the papules are found in the striae cutis distensae (i.e., stretch marks) of the abdomen, and they generally spare the area surrounding the umbilicus. Later, they can be found on the thighs and buttocks, where they coalesce to form plaques.

The itching, which can become quite intense, generally begins in the last few weeks of the third trimester of pregnancy. It can be sufficiently discomforting to require potent topical—and sometimes oral—corticosteroids.

The natural history of PUPPP is, in most cases, spontaneous resolution within a few days of delivery. It does not appear to increase infant morbidity. Recurrences in subsequent pregnancies are unlikely, and if they do appear, they tend to be less severe.

Some dermatologists broaden the clinical description of PUPPP to include the following:

- A rash resembling that of a drug eruption
- A targetlike rash that resembles erythema multiforme
- A vesicular eruption

These dermatologists thus suggest that PUPPP be renamed *polymorphic eruption of pregnancy.*

PRURITUS GRAVIDARUM

A common, benign, generalized itching, pruritus gravidarum begins in the later stages of pregnancy. The patient's complaints often seem to be out of proportion to the visible changes on the skin. There are no primary skin lesions, and the condition clears after delivery. Pruritus gravidarum is considered by some investigators to be possibly a variation of PUPPP without lesions.

Management of pruritus gravidarum is aimed at symptomatic control of pruritus with the use of bland emollients and topical antipruritic agents. Oral antihistamines are sometimes effective.

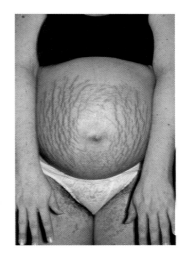

FIGURE 23.7 Pruritic urticarial papules and plaques of pregnancy. Lesions are located in the stretch marks. Note the periumbilical sparing.

RECURRENT CHOLESTASIS OF PREGNANCY

Also known as *intrahepatic cholestasis of pregnancy*, recurrent cholestasis of pregnancy is characterized by generalized itching and jaundice. It is caused by hyperbilirubinemia and bile acid accumulation in the skin. This condition generally occurs during the second or third trimester of pregnancy, although onset in the first trimester has also been reported. It initially manifests as severe, generalized pruritus that is followed by the clinical appearance of jaundice. The degree of itching correlates with levels of serum and skin bile acid. There are no primary skin lesions; however, excoriations may result from the patient's scratching.

Treatments for recurrent cholestasis of pregnancy are the same as for pruritus gravidarum: bland emollients, topical antipruritic agents and, sometimes, oral antihistamines. The condition clears after delivery, but it may recur in future pregnancies. The incidence of premature birth and low birth weight appears to be increased in the children of women with recurrent cholestasis of pregnancy.

HERPES GESTATIONIS

Herpes gestationis is a rare, intensely pruritic vesicobullous autoimmune dermatitis that may be clinically confused with PUPPP (Figure 23.8). The diagnosis can be confirmed by using direct immunofluorescent testing of the skin, which is positive in herpes gestationis.

The skin lesions of herpes gestationis are polymorphic, ranging from urticarial papules or plaques to bullae that are small and vesicular or large and tense. The term *herpes* derives from the grouped herpetiform clustering of blisters that sometimes occurs; there is no relation to herpesvirus infection.

Treatment generally requires systemic corticosteroids in gradually tapered doses. In mild cases, topical corticosteroids and oral antihistamines may be sufficient.

Some reports have suggested that women with herpes gestationis may have an increased risk for fetal morbidity and mortality, as well as an increased chance of giving birth prematurely and of having a baby with a lower birth weight; however, the extent, if any, of this increased risk remains controversial. Rarely, a neonate may develop transient blisters.

Postpartum flares are common. Symptoms may recur with menses or with administration of oral contraceptives, findings suggesting that hormonal factors play a strong role. Herpes gestationis often recurs in subsequent pregnancies, with earlier and more florid consequences; however, it has been known to skip an ensuing pregnancy.

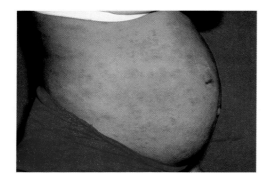

FIGURE 23.8 Herpes gestationis. The multiple urticarial plaques on the abdomen of this patient closely resemble the pruritic urticarial papules and plaques of pregnancy.

OTHER CONDITIONS

- *Pruritic folliculitis of pregnancy* manifests as a papular, acnelike eruption. Some dermatologists consider this condition a variant of acne.
- *Impetigo herpetiformis*, an extremely rare dermatosis, is considered a form of generalized pustular psoriasis.

CHAPTER 24

Cutaneous Manifestations of HIV Infection

Mary Ruth Buchness

Overview

- The first organ that may be affected in human immunodeficiency virus (HIV) infection is the skin. Before the advent of highly active antiretroviral therapy (HAART), the inevitable decrease in CD4 cells with disease progression was accompanied by a variety of HIV-associated skin diseases. HIV infection was often suspected initially based on the occurrence of cutaneous diseases, such as Kaposi's sarcoma (KS) or severe molluscum contagiosum, or in a patient with particularly severe or recalcitrant manifestations of a common skin disease, such as psoriasis.
- With the use of HAART, the number and frequency of cutaneous manifestations have plummeted in the United States and other countries. Furthermore, in patients with advanced HIV infection, the cutaneous manifestations often remit spontaneously when HAART is started. Nonetheless, some patients have viral resistance to these drugs or personal or economic reasons for not taking HIV medications, and in this group, the severe cutaneous manifestations of advanced HIV infection may still be seen.
- Acute HIV infection is characterized by a rash resembling measles (Figure 24.1), fever, lymphadenopathy, sore throat, and malaise.
- As the number of CD4 cells decreases to fewer than 200 during the course of infection, signaling the onset of acquired immunodeficiency syndrome (AIDS), skin manifestations become more severe and increase in number.

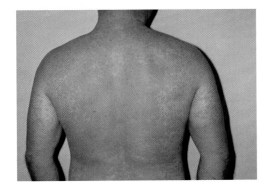

FIGURE 24.1 Acute human immunodeficiency virus infection. This fleeting eruption is characterized by a rash resembling measles.

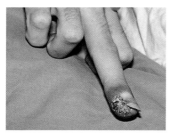

FIGURE 24.2 Herpes simplex. Shown here is human immunodeficiency virus–associated chronic ulcerated herpes simplex that is resistant to acyclovir. This patient is receiving intravenous foscarnet.

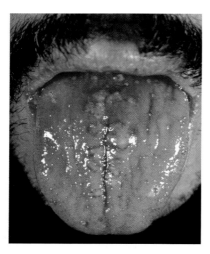

FIGURE 24.3 Herpes simplex. Mucosal papules are present in this patient with acquired immunodeficiency syndrome.

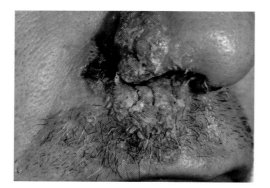

FIGURE 24.4 Herpes simplex. Crusted wartlike papules are noted.

BASICS

- In the immunocompromised host, the clinical manifestations and course of herpes simplex virus (HSV) infection differ in patients with defective cell-mediated immunity, as seen in HIV infection (see Chapter 6, "Superficial Viral infections," and Chapter 19, "Sexually Transmitted Diseases," for a full discussion of HSV infections in immunocompetent hosts).
- Recurrent lesions may affect mucous membranes and possibly become chronic, centrifugally expanding ulcerations. These ulcerations last 1 month or more in an HIV-positive patient and are an AIDS-defining diagnosis.
- Lesions may become resistant to acyclovir, or they may develop into chronic keratotic papules. Because acyclovir resistance is associated with prior treatment of suboptimal doses, it is important not to undertreat HIV-positive patients who also have HSV infections.

DESCRIPTION OF LESIONS

- Initially, there are the typical grouped vesicles on an erythematous base, which evolve into pustules, erosions, and crusts.

Ultimately, the following lesions may occur:

- Chronic digital ulcerations (Figure 24.2) may be seen.
- Mucosal erosions or papules (Figure 24.3) may be present.
- Patients may have centrifugally expanding ulcerations with scalloped borders.
- Keratotic or wartlike papules or plaques (Figure 24.4) may occur.

DISTRIBUTION OF LESIONS

- Intraoral areas, including the tongue, buccal mucosa, palate, and gingivae may be involved.
- Chronic ulcerative lesions in perianal areas may occur, especially in male homosexual patients. These lesions can extend into the intergluteal cleft (Figure 24.5).
- Keratotic lesions may occur in any location.

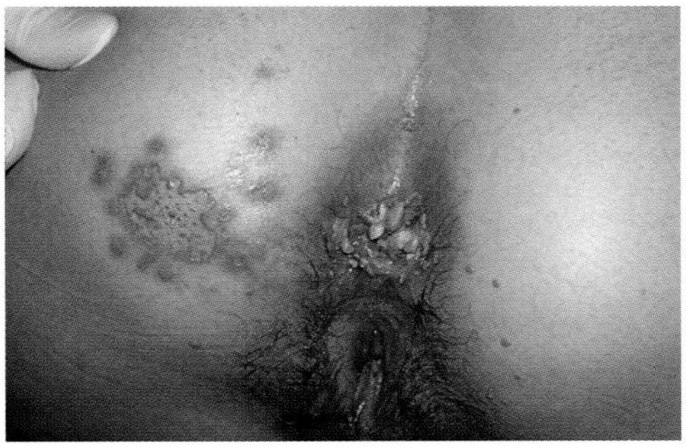

CLINICAL MANIFESTATIONS

- Lesions may be more severe and more extensive than in immunocompetent hosts.
- Severe or chronic erosions, ulcerations, or keratotic lesions should alert the clinician to the presence of advanced immunosuppression.

DIAGNOSIS

See Chapter 6, "Superficial Viral infections," and Chapter 19, "Sexually Transmitted Diseases," for more detailed discussions.

 DIFFERENTIAL DIAGNOSIS

Herpes Zoster
- Lesions of herpes zoster may involve only part of a dermatome and may be clinically indistinguishable from HSV lesions.
- When in doubt, sufficient doses of antiviral medications are recommended for herpes zoster infection. Avoid underdosing.

Decubitus Ulcer
- These lesions affect bony prominences in debilitated patients and do not extend to the intergluteal cleft.

Cutaneous Cytomegalovirus Infection
- In cytomegalovirus infection, perianal ulcers develop as an extension of gastrointestinal involvement. Skin biopsy shows characteristic viral inclusion bodies.
- In the keratotic type of cytomegalovirus infection, disseminated infection is associated with retinal findings, so an ophthalmologic examination is essential.

FIGURE 24.5 Herpes simplex. Chronic ulcerated lesions and scattered intact vesicles are present in a patient with acquired immunodeficiency syndrome.

Disseminated *Mycobacterium avium-intracellulare* Complex

• Patients may have oral ulcerations.
• This infection is associated with severe systemic disease and fever in HIV-infected patients.

Disseminated Histoplasmosis

• Patients may have oral and cutaneous ulcerations.
• Disseminated histoplasmosis is associated with systemic disease.

MANAGEMENT

Recalcitrant Herpes Simplex

• If the patient has malabsorption or if lesions do not respond to other treatment, acyclovir (5 to 10 mg/kg every 8 hours) is infused over 1 hour. The dosage interval should be increased in patients with renal failure.

Acyclovir Resistance

• Failure to respond to intravenous acyclovir indicates acyclovir resistance.
• Acyclovir resistance can be prevented by avoiding undertreatment and intermittent treatment.
• Foscarnet (40 mg/kg intravenously every 8 hours, is used in acyclovir-resistant patients.
• Strains that recur after treatment with foscarnet are usually acyclovir sensitive.

POINTS TO REMEMBER

• Long-term suppressive therapy with acyclovir has been associated with acyclovir resistance.
• Treatment should continue until clinical lesions resolve completely.
• Clinicians should be careful not to underdose with antiviral agents.

BASICS

- Herpes zoster is most common in elderly patients and in immuno-compromised persons, although it may occur in anyone who has a history of chickenpox.
- See Chapter 6, "Superficial Viral Infections," for a more detailed discussion.

DESCRIPTION OF LESIONS

- Grouped vesicles or bullae on an erythematous base affect all or part of a dermatome.
- Lesions evolve into pustules and crusts and may erode. Chronic ulcerations and crusted or verrucous lesions may occur.
- Severe scarring may result (Figure 24.6).

DISTRIBUTION OF LESIONS

- Any dermatome can be affected.
- Disseminated herpes zoster virus may occur. Occasional dissemination may lead to 25 or more lesions outside of the primary and two contiguous dermatomes (Figure 24.7). The disease usually begins with typical dermatomal herpes zoster virus that becomes widespread and chronic. The eruption may be indistinguishable from varicella.

CLINICAL MANIFESTATIONS

- Prodromal symptoms of pain and itching may be severe enough to lead to a suspicion of serious illness. For example, the prodromal pain of thoracic zoster has led to critical care unit admission to rule out myocardial infarction.
- Regional adenopathy may occur.
- Varicella pneumonia may develop.
- Cutaneous lesions may become chronic in patients with AIDS.

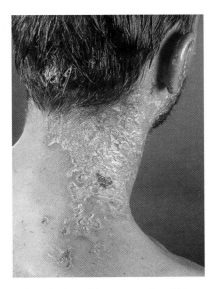

FIGURE 24.6 Herpes zoster. This patient developed severe scarring from his infection.

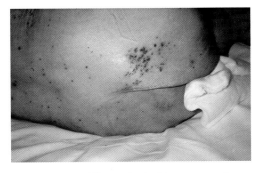

FIGURE 24.7 Disseminated herpes zoster. Note the initial dermatomal involvement on the buttock. (Courtesy of Herbert A. Hochman, M.D.)

MANAGEMENT

Recalcitrant Herpes Zoster
- Intravenous acyclovir (10 mg/kg every 8 hours) is given for 10 to 14 days.
- Dosage intervals are increased in patients with renal failure.
- If lesions improve but persist beyond 10 to 14 days, treatment is continued until all lesions resolve.

Acyclovir Resistance
- If lesions fail to resolve, the virus may be resistant to acyclovir.
- Acyclovir-resistant varicella-zoster virus infection responds to foscarnet (40 mg/kg every 8 hours until lesions resolve).

POINTS TO REMEMBER

- Undertreatment may lead to viral resistance.
- Patients with herpes zoster can transmit the virus as chickenpox to nonimmune persons.

HIV-ASSOCIATED MOLLUSCUM CONTAGIOSUM

BASICS

- Molluscum contagiosum is caused by a poxvirus; the condition is most commonly seen in immunocompetent children and less commonly in healthy adults.
- Multiple and extensive facial lesions, as well as lesions with atypical morphology, should alert the practitioner to the possibility of HIV infection.
- See Chapter 6, "Superficial Viral Infections," for further discussion.

DESCRIPTION OF LESIONS

- Papules may be dome-shaped or, more commonly, are atypical in appearance.
- Size may be up to, or greater than, 1 cm *(giant molluscum contagiosum)*.
- Lesions may lack central umbilication or may have several umbilications.
- Lesions on hairy areas tend to penetrate hair follicles.
- Lesions may be extensive (hundreds to thousands in number) in patients with advanced AIDS.
- Patients receiving HAART tend to have rare molluscum, with the more typical morphology seen in immunocompetent hosts.
- The appearance of new lesions may follow a downward fluctuation in immunity caused by a concurrent infection, such as influenza.

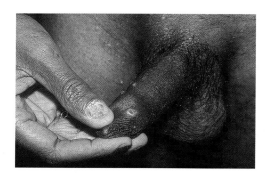

FIGURE 24.8 Molluscum contagiosum. This patient has "giant" molluscum lesions on the shaft of his penis as well as other scattered smaller lesions. Also note onychomycosis of his thumbnail.

DISTRIBUTION OF LESIONS

- All areas of the body may be affected, but lesions are most common on the face and genitals (Figure 24.8).
- In men, possible extensive involvement of the beard area may result from shaving (see Figure 6.17).

CLINICAL MANIFESTATIONS

- There is occasional tenderness or inflammation.
- Lesions are often a great cosmetic concern to patients.

DIFFERENTIAL DIAGNOSIS

Disseminated Cryptococcosis

- Cutaneous lesions may be clinically identical to those of molluscum contagiosum (Figure 24.9).
- Affected patients are usually systemically ill, although cutaneous involvement may be the first sign of illness.
- Crush preparation with India ink shows encapsulated yeast.
- When in doubt, lesions can be identified by biopsy.
- Patients with cutaneous dissemination have neurologic involvement, and a faster diagnosis can be made by cerebrospinal fluid examination.

Disseminated Histoplasmosis

- This is a less common cause of molluscum contagiosum–like lesions than cryptococcosis.
- Cutaneous histoplasmosis is always indicative of systemic infection.

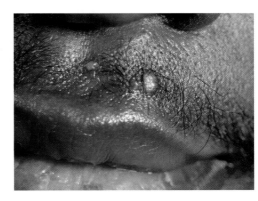

FIGURE 24.9 Disseminated cryptococcosis. Note the resemblance of these papules to those of molluscum contagiosum.

 MANAGEMENT

- Treatment is individualized for each patient. No specific treatment is universally more effective than any other.
- Topical tretinoin is a useful adjunctive treatment in cases of molluscum contagiosum of the beard.
- Surgical treatment is with curettage or liquid nitrogen cryosurgery.
- Trichloroacetic acid 25% to 75% may be applied to individual lesions.
- Podofilox (Condylox) 5% may be applied to lesions twice per day, 3 days per week.
- Imiquimod 5% (Aldara) cream may be effective and should be used daily if possible.
- Treatment is long term and is unlikely to eradicate all lesions unless the patient's immunity improves. Lesions may remit spontaneously after the patient is started on HAART, and knowing this will sometimes influence a reluctant patient to start and adhere to treatment for HIV infection.

 POINT TO REMEMBER

- Cutaneous lesions of disseminated cryptococcosis and histoplasmosis may look identical to lesions of molluscum contagiosum.

HIV-ASSOCIATED (EPIDEMIC) KAPOSI'S SARCOMA

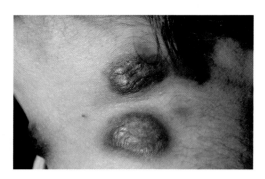

FIGURE 24.10 Epidemic Kaposi's sarcoma. Note the resemblance to the lesions of bacillary angiomatosis in Figure 24.18.

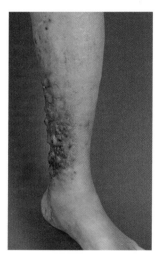

FIGURE 24.11 Epidemic Kaposi's sarcoma. Multiple papules and nodules are present on this patient's leg.

BASICS

- Epidemic KS is an AIDS-defining diagnosis.
- Because it is found almost exclusively in men who have had homosexual contact, KS is thought to be sexually transmitted.
- KS is exceedingly rare in women, and women with KS are presumed to have had sexual contact with bisexual men.
- KS is associated with infection of human herpesvirus 8 (HHV-8), which has been detected in saliva and in semen of affected patients.
- Lesions may resolve spontaneously as immunity improves. A similar phenomenon has been observed in immunocompromised renal transplant recipients.

DESCRIPTION OF LESIONS

- Violaceous macules, papules, or nodules occur (Figures 24.10 and 24.11).
- Limb edema with subtle violaceous discoloration of the skin may be present.

DISTRIBUTION OF LESIONS

- Lesions are most common acrally, on the nose, penis, and extremities.
- Mucous membranes may be affected.
- Lesions may be disseminated in advanced HIV infection.

CLINICAL MANIFESTATIONS

- Lesions are most commonly asymptomatic.
- Edema occurs with lymphatic involvement, usually in the extremities, but sometimes it affects the face.
- Oral lesions can cause pain, difficulty with eating, and loss of teeth.

 DIFFERENTIAL DIAGNOSIS

- Pyogenic granuloma
- Bacillary angiomatosis
- Disseminated *M. avium-intracellulare* complex (see earlier)

MANAGEMENT

- All forms of KS regress spontaneously with successful treatment of immunodeficiency with HAART.

Disseminated Cutaneous Kaposi's Sarcoma
- Disseminated involvement that does not regress with HAART requires systemic chemotherapy.

Lymphangitic Kaposi's Sarcoma
- Lymphatic involvement that does not respond to HAART requires systemic chemotherapy.
- Intermittent sequential compression boots can be used to decrease edema and to increase the comfort level of the patient.

Localized Cutaneous or Mucosal Kaposi's Sarcoma
- Radiation therapy is used, particularly for facial lesions.
- Intralesional vinblastine is given at doses of 0.1 to 0.6 mg/mL.
- Liquid nitrogen cryosurgery is used for macular lesions.
- A retinoid gel, alitretinoin (Panretin), applied three to four times daily as tolerated, is useful for macular lesions.

POINTS TO REMEMBER

- KS in an HIV-infected patient is an AIDS-defining diagnosis.
- Treatment of individual lesions does not prevent the occurrence of new lesions.
- Lesions may resolve spontaneously in patients receiving effective antiretroviral therapy, so it is beneficial to delay surgical treatment until the patient has been receiving HAART for several months.

BASICS

- HIV-associated eosinophilic folliculitis, also known as eosinophilic pustular folliculitis, is an extremely pruritic rash that is seen in the later stages of HIV infection.
- Eosinophilic folliculitis appears to be a hypersensitivity reaction because of the large numbers of eosinophils that are seen in the skin, but no consistent association with specific allergens has been reported.
- Very few patients with eosinophilic folliculitis respond to antihistamines.
- HIV-infected patients have high circulating levels of interleukin 4 and 5, the cytokines that are chemotactic for eosinophils, so a seemingly allergic manifestation such as eosinophilic folliculitis may be a result of the general immunologic derangement in these patients.
- Eosinophilic folliculitis has become rare since the use of HAART has decreased the number of cases of advanced HIV infection.

DESCRIPTION OF LESIONS

- Primary lesions are urticarial papules measuring 3 to 5 mm that look like insect bites.
- Pustules may be present, but they are not the predominant lesions.
- In many cases, only excoriations are present because of the intense pruritus (Figure 24.12).
- Patients with long-standing eosinophilic folliculitis may develop lichenification secondary to repeated scratching.

DISTRIBUTION OF LESIONS

- Lesions may occur anywhere, but they are prominent on the "seborrheic areas" of the skin (e.g., scalp, face, chest, and upper back).

CLINICAL MANIFESTATIONS

- Severe pruritus may interfere with the patient's ability to function.

DIAGNOSIS

- Skin biopsy shows perifollicular and follicular infiltration by eosinophils.
- Occasional peripheral eosinophilia may be present.

FIGURE 24.12 HIV-associated eosinophilic folliculitis. Intensely pruritic excoriated and nonexcoriated papules are present on this patient's upper back.

DIFFERENTIAL DIAGNOSIS

Bacterial Folliculitis
See also Chapter 5, "Superficial Bacterial Infections," for a more complete discussion.
- Bacterial folliculitis may be clinically indistinguishable from eosinophilic folliculitis.
- Gram's stain and bacterial culture should be performed.

Pityrosporum Folliculitis
- Pityrosporum folliculitis may be clinically indistinguishable from eosinophilic folliculitis.
- Potassium hydroxide preparation of pus shows yeast and hyphae.
- Periodic acid–Schiff stain of skin biopsy specimen shows yeast and hyphae.

Arthropod Bite Reaction
- Arthropod bite reaction may be clinically and histologically indistinguishable from eosinophilic folliculitis.
- Lesions are less likely to be folliculocentric.
- The patient's history should include possible exposure to arthropods (e.g., fleas, lice, scabies, bed bugs, and mosquitoes).

MANAGEMENT
- Topical steroids, antihistamines, and antibiotics are usually ineffective.
- Ultraviolet B phototherapy is effective. Patients should be referred to a qualified phototherapy center. In the summer, sunlight is effective.
- Isotretinoin (40 mg per day) is usually effective. Treatment must be continued for at least 3 months and may need to be continued on a long-term basis. Once the lesions have resolved, an attempt to taper the dosage to the lowest effective dose should be made. Cholesterol and triglyceride levels require monitoring on a monthly basis because of the side effect of hyperlipidemia. Because the protease inhibitors also cause hyperlipidemia, patients may need to be started on a cholesterol-lowering medication concomitantly.
- Itraconazole (200 mg twice daily) may be effective.

POINT TO REMEMBER
- Eosinophilic folliculitis, as described herein, is almost always associated with HIV infection.

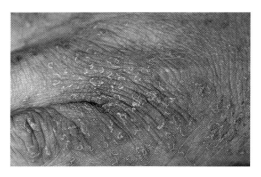

FIGURE 24.13 Norwegian scabies in a patient with acquired immunodeficiency syndrome. Note the crusted papules and the white linear burrows.

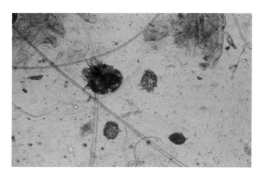

FIGURE 24.14 Scabies. Mites, ova, and fecal pellets are shown.

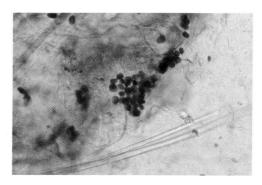

FIGURE 24.15 Scabies. Fecal pellets are shown here.

BASICS

- Norwegian scabies is an infestation with *Sarcoptes scabiei* var. *hominis* in an immunocompromised host.
- Immunocompetent hosts are able to limit the number of mites (10 to 12) that remain in the epidermis.
- The rash and itching are the result of a delayed hypersensitivity response to the mite, its eggs, and its fecal products.
- Immunocompromised hosts are not able to contain the population of mites and may be infested with millions of mites. These patients may not itch because of their defective cell-mediated immunity.
- HIV-infected patients with Norwegian scabies infestation pose a significant risk for transmission of scabies to household contacts and medical personnel.
- See Chapter 20, "Bites, Stings, and Infestations," for a more complete description of this condition.

DESCRIPTION OF LESIONS

- Fine white linear lesions from female mites may be visualized burrowing into the skin (Figure 24.13).
- Crusted, keratotic plaques are characteristic in Norwegian scabies.
- Atypical acral lesions may be seen in HIV-infected patients.

DIAGNOSIS

- Mineral oil preparation is done by scraping the epidermal surface of a burrow with a scalpel that has been dipped in mineral oil. The scraping is examined with a low-power microscope. Mites, ova, or fecal pellets are seen (Figures 24.14 and 24.15).

DIFFERENTIAL DIAGNOSIS

Psoriasis

- Psoriatic lesions tend to be located on extensor aspects of the extremities.
- Predominance of scale in the finger webs should lead to suspicion of Norwegian scabies.

Solar Keratoses

- Norwegian scabies on sun-exposed areas in elderly patients can mimic solar keratoses (Figure 24.16).

MANAGEMENT

Scabicides

- Permethrin 5% (Elimite) cream is applied, after a warm bath, to all skin surfaces from head to toe, including the palms and soles and scalp in small children; it is left on for 8 to 12 hours, usually overnight, and is washed off the next morning. *or*
- Lindane 1% (Kwell) lotion is applied from head to toe after bathing. Treatment should be continued once weekly until there is no evidence of residual lesions. Lindane is not as effective as permethrin and may cause neurologic toxicity, particularly in children and in elderly patients.

Keratolytic Agents

- Keratolytic agents, such as 10% to 40% salicylic acid, remove crusts and allow penetration of the scabicides.
- Ivermectin, 0.2 mg/kg by mouth, has been shown to be effective in eradicating infection. It is not approved by the United States Food and Drug Administration for this use.

POINTS TO REMEMBER

- Norwegian scabies is an infestation with millions of scabies mites and is highly contagious. Failure to treat patients promptly has led to epidemics affecting dozens of people.
- Because of the immunodeficiency in patients with Norwegian scabies, prolonged treatment may be necessary.
- Household contacts and medical staff who come into contact with the patient or the patient's bedclothes should undergo treatment as for scabies in an immunocompetent host, regardless of symptoms.

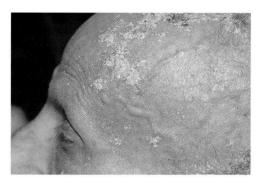

FIGURE 24.16 Norwegian scabies in a patient with acquired immunodeficiency syndrome. The lesions resemble solar keratoses.

HIV-ASSOCIATED CONDYLOMA ACUMINATUM

BASICS

- HIV-infected patients appear to have an increased susceptibility to malignant degeneration when they are infected with oncogenic subtypes of human papillomavirus, with the development of anal cancers in homosexual men and cervical cancer in women.
- Condylomata are difficult to eradicate in immunocompromised hosts. A cause of recurrent perianal warts is the presence of internal condylomata, and affected patients should be referred to a rectal surgeon. For a detailed discussion of the diagnosis and management of condyloma acuminatum, see Chapter 19, "Sexually Transmitted Diseases."

SYPHILIS

BASICS

- An intact cell-mediated immune system is necessary to "cure" the infection.
- Unusual manifestations of syphilis have been reported in patients with coinfection with HIV. These include negative serologic examination for syphilis in the presence of active secondary syphilis, relapse after treatment that should have been adequate, fulminant cutaneous lesions with induration and necrosis (Figure 24.17), and fulminant neurosyphilis resulting in permanent neurologic deficits.
- See Chapter 19, "Sexually Transmitted Diseases," for a more detailed discussion.

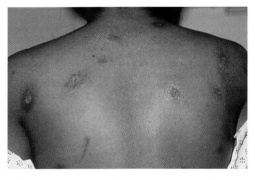

FIGURE 24.17 Syphilis in a patient with acquired immunodeficiency syndrome. Note the necrotic lesions.

 POINTS TO REMEMBER

- If syphilis is suspected in an HIV-infected patient and the serologic test is negative, then a skin biopsy should be performed.
- The only medication for the treatment of syphilis that adequately penetrates the blood–brain barrier is intravenous aqueous penicillin, which should be given at a dosage of 2 to 4 million units every 4 hours for 10 to 14 days in cases of suspected or proven neurosyphilis. Patients allergic to penicillin should undergo desensitization.

HIV-ASSOCIATED BACILLARY ANGIOMATOSIS

BASICS

- Bacillary angiomatosis, which was first reported in 1983, is seen almost exclusively in HIV-positive patients with advanced disease. Cases have been extremely rare in recent years.
- Bacillary angiomatosis is caused by the bacilli *Bartonella henselae* and *B. quintana*.
- Bacillary angiomatosis is a systemic infection, and lesions have been described in nearly every organ of the body.
- Untreated bacillary angiomatosis can be fatal.

DESCRIPTION OF LESIONS

- Lesions may occur as erythematous dome-shaped papules and nodules (Figure 24.18); they can also be flatter, violaceous lesions, subcutaneous nodules, or rarely, necrotic tumors.

DISTRIBUTION OF LESIONS

- Bacillary angiomatosis can occur on any location of the skin or internally.

CLINICAL MANIFESTATIONS

- There may be associated fever.
- Untreated lesions can lead to respiratory obstruction, gastrointestinal bleeding, and local or systemic infection.
- Deaths have been reported from laryngeal obstruction and disseminated intravascular coagulopathy.

DIAGNOSIS

- Skin biopsy shows a lesion resembling pyogenic granuloma, with characteristic clusters of bacilli.
- Culture is available only in research centers.

◇◆ DIFFERENTIAL DIAGNOSIS

- Pyogenic granuloma (see Figure 21.36) may be clinically identical to lesions of bacillary angiomatosis.
- Epidemic KS (HIV-associated) should be considered.

MANAGEMENT

- Doxycycline (100 mg twice per day) *or*
- Erythromycin (250 to 500 mg four times per day)
- Treatment until lesions have resolved (usually 3 to 4 weeks)

HIV-ASSOCIATED ORAL HAIRY LEUKOPLAKIA

BASICS

- Oral hairy leukoplakia is a marker of HIV infection that is thought to be caused by Epstein–Barr virus infection of the oral mucosa. It is rarely seen in patients receiving HAART.
- See Chapter 12, "Disorders of the Mouth, Lips, and Tongue," for a detailed discussion.

DESCRIPTION OF LESIONS

- White plaques resembling "corrugated cardboard" (Figure 24.19) are fixed to the mucosa; they are not friable, as in candidiasis (see Figure 12.10).

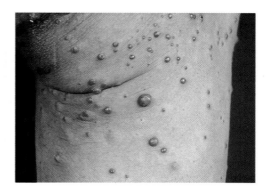

FIGURE 24.18 Bacillary angiomatosis. Dome-shaped papules and nodules are present.

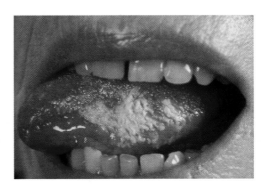

FIGURE 24.19 Oral hairy leukoplakia. White plaques resembling "corrugated cardboard" are fixed to the mucosa.

DISTRIBUTION OF LESIONS

- Lesions most often appear on the lateral aspects of the tongue.

CLINICAL MANIFESTATIONS

- Lesions are usually asymptomatic.
- Patients occasionally complain of a burning sensation of the tongue.

  DIFFERENTIAL DIAGNOSIS

Oral Candidiasis (Figure 24.20)

- Candidiasis ("thrush") is also seen in immunocompromised patients and in neonates.
- Curdlike or erosive lesions can easily be removed with gauze or a tongue blade.
- Lesions are more common on the dorsal aspect of the tongue, oropharynx, angles of mouth, and buccal mucosa.
- The potassium hydroxide preparation shows yeast.

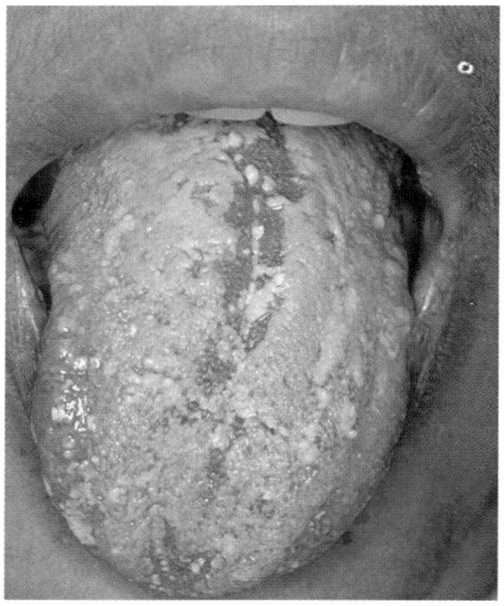

MANAGEMENT

- Treatment is necessary only in symptomatic cases.
- Surgical excision can be performed, but lesions recur at the margins.
- Acyclovir (3.2 g per day) is given with recurrence of lesions on cessation of treatment. The use of acyclovir for oral hairy leukoplakia may result in the development of acyclovir-resistance of concurrent HSV infection.
- Topical tretinoin 0.05% solution may be applied for 15 minutes once daily using a gauze sponge.
- Podophyllin 25% solution is applied sparingly to one side of the tongue at a time and is allowed to air dry. This is repeated once weekly.

HIV-ASSOCIATED APHTHOUS ULCERS

BASICS

- Aphthous ulcers may be severe in HIV-infected patients (Figure 24.21).
- The pain may interfere with the patient's ability to eat.
- Mucosal pain leads to difficulties with eating and drinking, with resultant weight loss and dehydration.
- See the discussion of mucous membranes in Chapter 12, "Disorders of the Mouth, Lips, and Tongue" (see Figures 12.1 and 12.2).

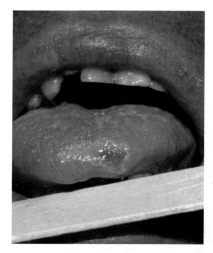

FIGURE 24.20 Oral candidiasis. These curdlike lesions can easily be removed with gauze.

FIGURE 24.21 Aphthous ulcer in a patient with acquired immunodeficiency syndrome. This lesion is quite painful.

MANAGEMENT

- Topical steroids may be applied directly to the ulcerations.
- Stomatitis elixir, consisting of equal parts of magnesium carbonate or magnesium hydroxide suspension, viscous lidocaine, diphenhydramine elixir 12.5 mg/5 mL, and 1 g tetracycline powder, to be swished and spat out of the mouth as needed, is useful for pain.
- Thalidomide (100 mg by mouth twice per day) is effective, with notable toxic effects of sedation, neutropenia, peripheral neuropathy, and teratogenicity.

HIV-ASSOCIATED DRUG ERUPTIONS

BASICS

- Drug eruptions are common in the HIV-infected population because of the large number of medications taken by these patients. The most commonly implicated medications are sulfamethoxazole-trimethoprim, to which at least 60% of patients with AIDS develop an allergy, followed by the aminopenicillins.
- When the drug allergy causes a typical morbilliform eruption, it is possible to continue the offending medication and treat the patient's symptoms with antihistamines and topical steroids. More serious drug eruptions are characterized by urticaria, mucosal involvement, target lesions, erythroderma, and tenderness of the skin. Any of these signs or symptoms requires prompt discontinuation of the offending medication.
- Mucosal involvement and target lesions are indicative of erythema multiforme or Stevens–Johnson syndrome, whereas erythroderma and skin tenderness are seen in toxic epidermal necrolysis (Figure 24.22). The nonnucleoside reverse transcriptase inhibitor nevirapine has been associated with severe cases of Stevens–Johnson syndrome. For a complete discussion of drug eruptions, see Chapter 17, "Drug Eruptions."

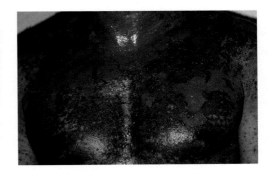

FIGURE 24.22 Drug eruption. Toxic epidermal necrolysis has resulted from treatment with nevirapine.

HIV-ASSOCIATED PRURITUS

BASICS

- Pruritus is a common and troubling symptom in HIV-infected patients. It often has a multifactorial origin.
- Many patients use antibacterial or deodorant soaps with the mistaken belief that they will decrease the risk for infection. In fact, these soaps dry the skin and make the patients itchy and them more susceptible to cutaneous infection because of the excoriations that result.
- Patients may become itchy because of subclinical drug eruptions or as a medication-related side effect.
- Patients may be colonized with S. aureus, which is known to be a cause of pruritus in HIV-infected patients.

MANAGEMENT

- Careful history taking and a physical examination rule out dermatologic disease as the cause.
- Patients should discontinue use of deodorant and antibacterial soaps; superfatted soaps are the least drying.
- Patients should be instructed to limit bathing to once per day.
- Emollients should be applied after the patient has bathed and pats dry; ointments are more emollient than creams, which are more emollient than lotions.
- Patients need to try different preparations to find which is most cosmetically acceptable and effective.
- Patients who do not obtain relief with over-the-counter moisturizers often do well with ammonium lactate 12% lotion.
- Antiitch preparations containing calamine, pramoxine, menthol, camphor, and oatmeal may be soothing.
- Sedating antihistamines are useful, especially before bedtime.
- Topical steroids should be prescribed for dermatitis, which may result from dry skin.
- Ultraviolet B phototherapy is palliative.

For further discussion of pruritus, see Chapter 15, "Pruritus: The Itchy Patient."

HIV-ASSOCIATED SEBORRHEIC DERMATITIS

BASICS

- Seborrheic dermatitis is a scaly skin condition that affects up to 5% of the human population.
- In immunocompetent patients, it may be associated with an overgrowth of saprophytic *Pityrosporum* yeast on the scalp and face; it is not known whether the same is true in HIV-infected patients.
- The frequency and severity of seborrheic dermatitis are increased in HIV-infected patients, for unknown reasons.
- Seborrheic dermatitis appears commonly in hospitalized patients, probably because of the changes in hygiene (e.g., inability to shampoo the hair) experienced during illness.

For description and distribution of lesions, as well as management, see Chapter 4, "Inflammatory Eruptions of Unknown Cause."

POINT TO REMEMBER

- Seborrheic dermatitis is common in HIV-infected patients, and the sudden onset of severe, recalcitrant, seborrheic dermatitis should lead to an inquiry regarding risk factors and HIV testing.

HIV-ASSOCIATED PSORIASIS

BASICS

- Psoriasis is a scaly skin disease that affects 1% to 2% of the general population.
- Psoriasis is not more common in HIV-infected patients, but it may present in a more severe or unusual form and may be recalcitrant to the usual treatments.
- The most severe manifestation is Reiter's disease (see Chapter 25, "Cutaneous Manifestation of Systemic Disease"), with psoriatic lesions, arthritis, urethritis, and conjunctivitis. A new onset of severe psoriasis in a patient at risk for HIV should lead to HIV testing.
- The combination of treatment with methotrexate and sulfonamides can lead to fatal bone marrow suppression.
- The use of systemic steroids for treatment of psoriasis may result in life-threatening pustular psoriasis.
- See Chapter 3, "Psoriasis," for a more complete discussion.

CHAPTER 25

Cutaneous Manifestations of Systemic Disease

Peter G. Burk and Herbert P. Goodheart

Overview

- Many different skin lesions are seen in conjunction with endocrine diseases. Some of these cutaneous lesions are directly related to the degree of endocrine dysfunction and may be caused by an excess or lack of a hormone acting on a specific tissue, such as warm and moist skin associated with hyperthyroidism and dry and cool skin associated with hypothyroidism.
- In a disease such as diabetes, it may be difficult to link these skin findings to a specific degree of endocrine dysfunction (e.g., necrobiosis lipoidica diabeticorum with hyperglycemia).

DIABETES MELLITUS

BASICS

- Diabetes mellitus is a disease characterized by a disturbance in the production of insulin or resistance to insulin activity, which results in abnormal glucose metabolism.
- The clinical results of diabetes include cellular changes, such as microangiopathy of small blood vessels. This causes organ damage including retinal disease, renal dysfunction, and possibly cutaneous lesions.
- Diabetes mellitus can also affect immune function and can result in increased bacterial, fungal, and yeast infections.

DESCRIPTION OF LESIONS

- **Necrobiosis lipoidica diabeticorum** (NLD) is characterized by yellow-red to brown, translucent plaques with epidermal atrophy and telangiectasia (Figure 25.1). As the lesion progresses, the center becomes depressed and yellow (Figure 25.2). Ulceration is not uncommon.
- **Perforating folliculitis** (Kyrle's disease) consists of firm, rough hyperkeratotic papules, which are often hyperpigmented in dark-skinned people (Figure 25.3).

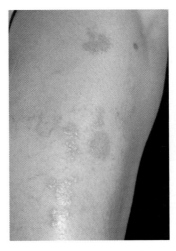

FIGURE 25.1 Necrobiosis lipoidica diabeticorum. This diabetic patient has early lesions that consist of yellow–red plaques. Epidermal atrophy and telangiectasias tend to occur later.

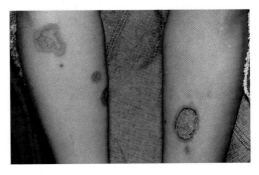

FIGURE 25.2 Necrobiosis lipoidica diabeticorum. This diabetic patient has more advanced lesions than those seen in Figure 25.1. Epidermal atrophy and telangiectasias are seen here.

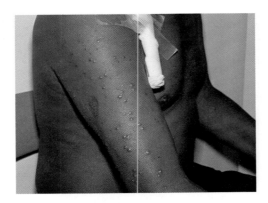

FIGURE 25.3 Perforating folliculitis (Kyrle's disease). Hyperkeratotic papules are present on extensor areas of the upper extremity. This patient has diabetes with Kimmelstiel–Wilson disease and is undergoing renal dialysis.

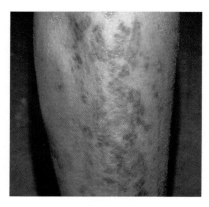

FIGURE 25.4 Diabetic dermopathy. Small, brownish, atrophic, scarred, hyperpigmented plaques are seen.

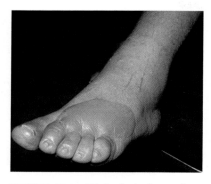

FIGURE 25.5 Diabetic bullous disease. A large, tense blister is noted in a characteristic location.

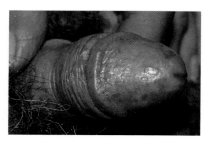

FIGURE 25.6 Candidal balanitis. This diabetic patient has erythematous erosions. The KOH examination revealed pseudohyphae (see Figures 26.8 and 26.9).

- **Diabetic dermopathy** is characterized by small (less than 0.5 cm), brownish, atrophic, scarred, hyperpigmented plaques (Figure 25.4).
- **Diabetic bullous disease** manifests as large, tense subepidermal blisters (Figure 25.5).
- **Acanthosis nigricans** sometimes occurs in insulin-resistant diabetes (see Chapter 14, "Pigmentary Disorders").
- **Cutaneous candidiasis** may also occur (Figure 25.6) (see Chapter 7, "Superficial Fungal Infections").
- **Eruptive xanthomas** are seen as skin markers for various primary genetic disorders such as certain types of hyperlipidemias or secondary to diabetes (see later).
- **Disseminated granuloma annulare** consists of annular dermal papules (see Chapter 4, "Inflammatory Eruptions of Unknown Cause"), and occurs both in patients with clinical diabetes and sometimes in individuals with only abnormal glucose levels.
- **Diabetic neuropathic ulcers** *(mal perforans)* (Figure 25.7) may occur.
- **Scleredema of Buschke-Löwenstein** (rare) is a sclerotic, thickened plaque seen on the upper back.

DISTRIBUTION OF LESIONS

- NLD is seen most commonly on the pretibial areas, but it may appear on other sites.
- Perforating folliculitis is found most commonly on the extensor surfaces of the lower extremities.
- Diabetic dermopathy occurs primarily on the anterior lower legs.
- Bullous diabetic lesions most often occur on the lower extremities, especially the ankles and feet.
- Diabetic neuropathic ulcers are noted at sites of pressure (e.g., the heel) in areas of poor sensory function and poor circulation.

CLINICAL MANIFESTATIONS

- NLD is seen more frequently in type-1 than in type-2 diabetes and may occur before the onset of clinical diabetes. Lesions may ulcerate. A minority of patients have no clinical evidence or family history of diabetes; in these patients, the term *necrobiosis lipoidica* is used.
- Perforating folliculitis, which can itch intensely, is seen primarily in patients with long-standing severe diabetes who have microangiopathy and neuropathy. There is a high incidence of perforating folliculitis in patients with diabetes who are undergoing long-term hemodialysis.

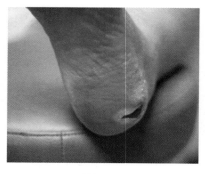

FIGURE 25.7 Diabetic ulcer of the heel (mal perforans). These lesions are noted at sites of pressure, such as the heel in this patient.

- Diabetic dermopathy occurs in patients with type-1 and type-2 diabetes. It is typically a late manifestation of diabetes and is usually asymptomatic.
- Bullous diabetic lesions occur most frequently in patients with severe neuropathy.
- Diabetic neuropathic ulcers are usually painless as a result of peripheral neuropathy.

DIAGNOSIS

- The diagnosis of most of these entities can generally be made on clinical grounds.
- Skin biopsy of the various clinical manifestations may be necessary to confirm the diagnosis.

Laboratory Evaluations
- Serum glucose levels and glycosylated hemoglobin A_1 are determined to confirm the diagnosis of diabetes mellitus.
- Skin biopsies of lesions of necrobiosis lipoidica and granuloma annulare demonstrate palisading granulomas with degeneration of collagen.
- Skin biopsy of perforating folliculitis demonstrates basophilic material in the dermis with transepidermal elimination.
- Skin biopsies of diabetic dermopathy show thickening of blood vessels and mild perivascular infiltrate.
- Diabetic bullous lesions have subepidermal blistering on hematoxylin and eosin staining of skin biopsy tissue; direct immunofluorescence of skin biopsies in these lesions is negative for immunoglobulins.
- Diabetic neuropathic ulcers are rarely examined by biopsy.

 DIFFERENTIAL DIAGNOSIS

- NLD lesions can be similar to morphea and other localized sclerosing lesions.
- Perforating folliculitis can be differentiated from other keratotic papules by the size and distribution of lesions.
- Diabetic dermopathy must be differentiated from lesions caused by trauma.
- Bullous diabetic lesions can be differentiated from bullous pemphigoid by the characteristic location of lesions and negative direct immunofluorescence of skin biopsies.

 MANAGEMENT

- Long-term clinical control of glucose levels in diabetes mellitus reduces microangiopathy and subsequent organ damage that leads to retinopathy, nephropathy, neuropathy, and other tissue damage.
- High-potency topical steroids or intralesional steroid injections are used in the management of NLD and granuloma annulare.
- Topical antibiotic therapy is recommended for bullous diabetic lesions until the blisters heal.
- Becaplermin (Regranex), a recombinant human platelet-derived growth factor, is available in gel form for topical therapy (in conjunction with good ulcer care) and is reported to promote healing of diabetic neuropathic foot ulcers.

THYROID DISEASE

BASICS

• Thyroid hormones profoundly influence the growth and differentiation of epidermal and dermal tissues.
• Abnormal levels of thyroid hormone produce striking changes in the texture of the skin, hair, and nails.
• Some of the associated skin alterations in thyroid disease are the result of a deficiency or a high toxic level of tissue thyroid hormone; other skin disorders seen with thyroid disease such as vitiligo and alopecia areata are associated clinical findings that are not directly related to thyroid hormone function, but are seen frequently in patients with thyroid disease.
• Findings such as pretibial myxedema are caused by a circulating autoimmune γ-globulin, which acts as a thyroid-stimulating hormone.
• Hyperthyroidism may be caused by Graves' disease, subacute thyroiditis, toxic goiter, and thyroid carcinoma (rare). Hypothyroidism may be caused by iodine deficiency (cretinism), Hashimoto's thyroiditis, pituitary dysfunction with thyroid-stimulating hormone deficiency, and surgical or radiation ablation of the thyroid.
• Patients with thyroid disease may be hyperthyroid at one point in their clinical course and hypothyroid at another time.

DESCRIPTION OF LESIONS

Hyperthyroid skin lesions may include the following:

• Warm, moist, and velvety skin
• Alopecia with diffuse hair loss
• Nail changes with onycholysis *(Plummer's nails)*
• Hyperpigmentation
• Pretibial myxedema lesions—flesh-colored, waxy infiltrated translucent plaques (Figure 25.8)

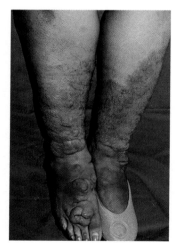

FIGURE 25.8 Pretibial myxedema lesion. This patient is hyperthyroid. Note the red–brown plaques on her shins and the dorsum of her right foot.

Hyperthyroid findings may include the following:

- Nervousness and tremor
- Weight loss
- Tachycardia with atrial fibrillation
- Proximal muscle weakness
- Graves' disease
- Exophthalmos with protruding eyes (Figure 25.9)

Hypothyroid skin lesions may include the following:

- Myxedema of the skin with generalized thickening and a dry, coarse feel; yellow skin secondary to carotenemia
- Hair changes—coarse, sparse hair; lateral third of eyebrows lost

The following conditions may be associated with thyroid disease:

- Alopecia areata
- Vitiligo
- Connective tissue diseases
- Multiple endocrinopathy syndrome
- Urticaria

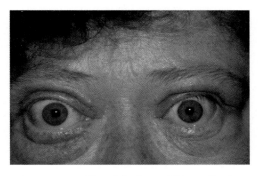

FIGURE 25.9 Exophthalmos. This patient has Graves' disease. Note the lid retraction and proptosis.

DISTRIBUTION OF LESIONS

- Pretibial myxedema (Graves' disease) lesions are found most frequently on the lower legs.

CLINICAL MANIFESTATIONS

- Hyperthyroid skin changes that result from the hypermetabolic state (e.g., warm, moist, flushed skin) occur during the active thyrotoxic stage of thyroiditis, during active Graves' disease, and in patients with toxic goiters. These skin changes may gradually resolve when the patient returns to a euthyroid state.
- Graves' disease lesions (pretibial myxedema) occur in up to 4% of patients with this disease. The skin lesions and eye lesions usually do not resolve even after treatment of the thyroid disease brings a return to a euthyroid state.
- Hypothyroid skin changes (e.g., cool, dry skin) are related to the length and severity of the clinical hypothyroid state. These skin lesions gradually improve some months after returning to euthyroid state.

DIAGNOSIS

- Diagnosis of both hyperthyroid and hypothyroid disease is made by specific thyroid function tests.
- Graves' disease is diagnosed clinically and with confirmatory thyroid function tests.

Laboratory Evaluations

- Elevated thyroid-stimulating hormone levels are the most sensitive screening test for hypothyroidism.
- Thyroid serum hormone levels can be most accurately measured by obtaining free thyroxine and free triiodothyronine levels.
- Antithyroglobulin antibodies and antithyroid microsomal antibodies are often positive in Graves' disease and Hashimoto's thyroiditis.
- Long acting thyroid stimulater is elevated in 50% of patients with Graves' disease.
- Skin biopsies in Graves' disease show increased staining of hyaluronic acid with mucin stains in the reticular and papillary dermis.

 DIFFERENTIAL DIAGNOSIS

- Pretibial myxedema must be differentiated from other skin diseases with increased mucin production, such as papillary mucinosis and scleredema.

 MANAGEMENT

- Functional symptoms (e.g., increase or decrease of sweating, dry skin, hair and nail changes) of hyperthyroidism and hypothyroidism may improve after appropriate treatment of thyroid disease and return to a euthyroid state.
- Treatment of pretibial myxedema lesions can be attempted with high-potency topical steroids and intralesional steroids, although the response generally is poor.

XANTHOMAS

BASICS

- Abnormalities of lipid metabolism, with high circulating levels of various lipoproteins, can result in deposition of cholesterol and other lipids in the skin, tendons, and other organs.
- Xanthomas result from the deposition of cholesterol and other lipids found in tissue macrophages in the skin and tendons. There is also a high correlation between abnormal lipoproteinemia and the development of atherosclerosis.
- Lipoprotein abnormalities have been classified into primary (genetic) lipoproteinemia and secondary lipoproteinemia resulting from underlying diseases.
- **Primary lipoproteinemias** are phenotypic expressions of various genetic disorders of lipid metabolism with the following characteristics:
  – Type I, familial lipoprotein lipase deficiency: elevated chylomicrons
  – Type IIA, familial hypercholesterolemia: elevated low-density lipoproteins
  – Type IIB, familial hyperlipidemia: elevated low-density lipoproteins and very low-density lipoproteins
  – Type III, familial dysbetalipoproteinemia: elevated intermediate-density lipoproteins
  – Type IV, endogenous familial hypertriglyceridemia: elevated triglycerides
  – Type V, familial combined hyperlipidemia: elevated chylomicrons and elevated very low-density lipoproteins
- **Secondary hyperlipoproteinemias** result from disturbances in cholesterol and triglyceride metabolism caused by cholestatic liver disease, diabetes mellitus, pancreatitis, multiple myeloma, and nephrotic syndrome. These disorders may mimic any of the genetic lipoprotein abnormalities and may produce similar xanthomatous deposits in tissues.

DESCRIPTION OF LESIONS

- **Eruptive xanthomas** are smooth, yellow, papular lesions (2 to 5 mm). There is sometimes a red halo around the lesions (Figure 25.10).
- **Planar xanthomas** are flat to slightly palpable yellow lesions.
- **Xanthelasma** *(xanthoma palpebrarum)* is a form of planar xanthoma (Figure 25.11).
- **Tuberous xanthomas** are small (0.5 cm) to large (3 to 5 cm), firm yellow papules and nodules (Figure 25.12).
- **Tendinous xanthomas** are subcutaneous thickenings around tendons and ligaments.

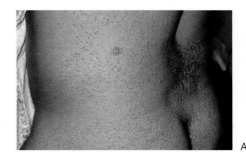

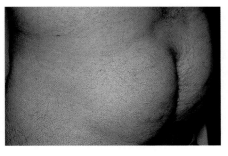

FIGURE 25.10 Eruptive xanthomas. *A:* This 28-year-old male patient has a triglyceride level of 31,000 and a cholesterol level of 580 mg/dL. *B:* This is the same patient after 2 months of a low-fat diet and a cholesterol-lowering drug.

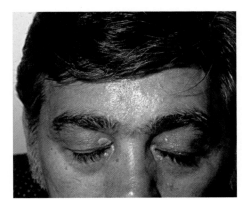

FIGURE 25.11 Xanthelasma. Periorbital yellow–orange plaques are present on the upper inner eyelids. This patient was normolipemic when this photograph was taken.

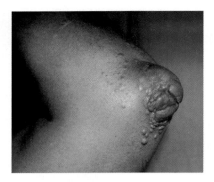

FIGURE 25.12 Tuberous xanthomas. These are firm papulonodules in a patient with hyperlipidemia type II.

Laboratory Evaluations
- Fasting blood levels of triglycerides and cholesterol should be determined.
- Lipoprotein electrophoresis demonstrates specific lipoprotein abnormalities.
- Skin biopsy of xanthomas demonstrates collections of lipids in foamy macrophages in the dermis.
- Serum glucose levels and glycosylated hemoglobin A_1 are determined to rule out diabetes mellitus.
- Serum amylase levels to rule out pancreatitis.
- Serum protein electrophoresis to rule out multiple myeloma.

DISTRIBUTION OF LESIONS

- Eruptive xanthomas appear most frequently over the knees, elbows, and buttocks.
- Planar xanthomas are found in the palmar creases but may also be generalized.
- Xanthelasma lesions are usually found on the eyelids and medial canthus.
- Tuberous xanthomas are found on the elbows, knees, and buttocks.
- Tendinous xanthomas affect the Achilles tendon, extensor tendons of the wrists, elbows, and knees.

CLINICAL MANIFESTATIONS

- Eruptive xanthomas appear suddenly over the extensor surfaces and pressure points. These lesions are usually seen in association with high levels of triglycerides (2,000 to 4,000 mg/dL). Uncontrolled diabetes mellitus and acute pancreatitis are both common underlying causes of eruptive xanthomas.
- Planar xanthomas are usually asymptomatic. Palmar xanthomas are seen with type III lipoproteinemia. Diffuse planar xanthomas are found in patients with multiple myeloma.
- Xanthelasma lesions grow slowly over years. More than 50% of patients with xanthelasma have normal lipoprotein levels.
- Tuberous xanthomas also are slow growing. They are associated with familial hypercholesterolemia but can also occur in patients with high triglyceride levels.
- Tendinous xanthomas occur in patients with hypercholesterolemias.

DIAGNOSIS

- The diagnosis is made by clinical evaluation of skin and subcutaneous lesions.
- Skin biopsy is confirmatory for xanthomas.

 DIFFERENTIAL DIAGNOSIS

- Eruptive xanthomas must be differentiated from cutaneous sarcoid papules and cutaneous histiocytosis.
- Tuberous xanthomas can be confused with rheumatoid nodules and subcutaneous granuloma annulare.

 MANAGEMENT

- Patients with lipid disorders and xanthomas must be appropriately evaluated for primary and secondary lipoprotein abnormalities. Treatment of the underlying cause may reverse both eruptive and tuberous xanthomas over time.
- Dietary restrictions and cholesterol-lowering drugs may reverse some changes associated with hypercholesterolemia.
- Xanthelasmas of the eyelids can be removed by application of 25% to 50% trichloroacetic acid or by local electrodesiccation.

Inflammatory Skin Disorders That May Be Associated with an Underlying Systemic Disease

EXFOLIATIVE DERMATITIS

BASICS

Exfoliative dermatitis (ED), known as *erythroderma* in the United Kingdom, refers to a total, or almost total, redness or scaling of the skin. It is an uncommon disorder seen more often in male patients; 50 years is the average age of occurrence. When seen in children, ED most often is secondary to severe atopic dermatitis. In adults, psoriasis is the most frequently associated skin disease (see Chapter 3, "Psoriasis").

ED may appear suddenly or gradually, occasionally accompanied by fever, chills, and lymphadenopathy. It may be seen in the following situations:

- It may be a stage in the natural history of severe eczematous dermatitis or psoriasis.
- Less commonly, it is a finding in the following skin disorders:
  - Allergic contact dermatitis
  - Stasis dermatitis with secondary autoeczematization
  - Pityriasis rubra pilaris (a rare disorder of keratinization)
  - Graft-versus-host disease
  - Seborrheic dermatitis (Leiner's disease) in infants
  - Pemphigus foliaceus
  - Lichen planus
  - Papulosquamous dermatitis of acquired immunodeficiency syndrome
- ED may occur as a reaction to the following drugs: sulfonamides, penicillins, antimalarials, lithium, phenothiazines, barbiturates, gold, allopurinol, nonsteroidal antiinflammatory drugs (NSAIDs) including aspirin, captopril, codeine, and phenytoin.
- It may be a complication or presenting symptom of the following malignant diseases:
  - Mycosis fungoides (cutaneous T-cell lymphoma)
  - Sézary syndrome (leukemic variant of mycosis fungoides)
  - Hodgkin's disease
  - Non-Hodgkin's lymphoma and leukemia
- It is an idiopathic phenomenon in 20% to 30% of cases without any preceding dermatosis or systemic disease.

DESCRIPTION OF LESIONS

- Marked generalized erythema is followed by scaling (Figure 25.13).
- Pruritus may be severe.
- There is edema and increased warmth of the skin.
- Lymphadenopathy, usually a reactive type *(dermatopathic lymphadenopathy),* is often present.

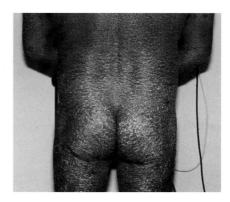

FIGURE 25.13 Generalized exfoliative dermatitis. This patient has a severe widespread type of psoriasis.

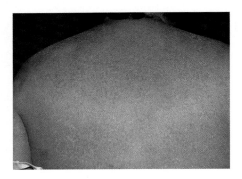

FIGURE 25.14 Exfoliative erythroderma. This patient has widespread erythema and scaling.

DISTRIBUTION OF LESIONS

- ED usually begins in a limited area; however, it may rapidly become generalized.

CLINICAL MANIFESTATIONS

- The course of ED depends on its underlying origin. ED resulting from a drug eruption may clear in days to weeks, whereas, in some cases, the disease may persist for many years, with exacerbations and remissions and with no diagnosis ever being made.
- The prognosis of acute, severe episodes, particularly in elderly persons or in persons with preexisting heart disease, is more guarded.
- Unlike toxic epidermal necrolysis, ED spares mucous membranes. Unless patients have a known preexisting skin condition or concurrent physical evidence of a skin disease such as psoriasis, the clinical appearance and symptoms of most cases of ED tend to be similar, consisting of the following:
  - Erythema is followed by scaling (Figure 25.14).
  - Pruritus may develop.
  - Edema and increased warmth of skin are usually present.
  - Lymphadenopathy, usually a reactive type *(dermatopathic lymphadenopathy)*, secondary to the marked inflammatory changes in the skin, may be seen; however, lymphoma should be considered, particularly if the lymph nodes are large or unilateral.
  - Thermoregulatory disturbances are manifested by fever or, more frequently, by hypothermia. If widespread inflammation occurs, the barrier efficiency of the skin may be impaired secondary to extensive vasodilatation.
  - Protein loss secondary to a massive shedding of scale may occur, with resultant hypoalbuminemia.
  - Rarely, high-output cardiac failure may develop, particularly in patients with a history of cardiac disease.

The following chronic changes may also be seen:

- Scaling of palms and soles *(keratoderma)* may occur.
- Thickening and lichenification of the skin may be noted.
- Patients may have scalp involvement, occasionally producing non-scarring alopecia.
- Nail dystrophy, onycholysis (separation of the nail plate from the nail bed), or nail shedding may occur.
- Pigmentary changes (postinflammatory hypopigmentation or hyperpigmentation) may be noted.
- Persistent generalized erythema may occur.
- Patients may have conjunctivitis, keratitis, or ectropion.

DIAGNOSIS

- The diagnosis of ED is made on a clinical basis. The diagnosis of the underlying cause is often elusive. Clinical findings, such as the characteristic lichenification and crusting of atopic dermatitis or nail pitting that suggests psoriasis, may be found.
- Eliciting a history of drug ingestion or a preexisting dermatosis may be valuable.
- Laboratory testing can provide serologic evidence of Sézary's syndrome or leukemia.
- Patch testing during a period of remission may uncover a contact allergen.

Histopathology

- Histologic findings of the various causes are similar and are generally nondiagnostic; however, a diligent search for lymphoma, particularly mycosis fungoides, must be pursued with repeated skin biopsies.

 DIFFERENTIAL DIAGNOSIS

- Toxic epidermal necrolysis is a potentially fatal condition that involves the skin and mucous membranes. Marked erythema is quickly followed by sloughing of the skin. This condition is often the result of a severe drug reaction (see Figure 24.22).

 MANAGEMENT

- Treatment is directed toward the underlying cause, if it is known. For example, suspected etiologic drugs or contactants should be eliminated.
- Bed rest, cool compresses, lubrication with emollients, antipruritic therapy with oral antihistamines, and low- to intermediate-strength topical steroids are used.
- In severe cases, patients frequently require hospitalization, where measures such as fluid replacement, temperature control, expert topical skin care, and systemic corticosteroids may be used.

Exfoliative Dermatitis Secondary to Psoriasis

For a further discussion of psoriasis, see Chapter 3, "Psoriasis."

- Possible precipitating factors (e.g., ultraviolet exposure) or drugs that are suspected to provoke ED (e.g., antimalarials) should be avoided.
- Systemic and topical steroids are helpful, except they may worsen psoriasis and have been known to precipitate ED or an acute fulminant form of pustular psoriasis, known as pustular psoriasis of Von Zumbusch. This worsening of psoriasis tends to occur after steroid withdrawal.
- If conservative therapy fails, methotrexate, cyclosporine, and retinoids (e.g., acitretin) are additional therapeutic options.

 POINTS TO REMEMBER

- In its more severe manifestations, ED is a medical and dermatologic emergency. Consultation and ongoing management, using the expertise of both disciplines, are often necessary.
- In many cases, the underlying cause is never established.

Laboratory Evaluations

The following are possible positive laboratory findings:

- Anemia (usually the anemia of chronic disease)
- Decreased serum levels of protein and albumin
- Leukocytosis
- Eosinophilia
- Elevated sedimentation rate
- Elevated immunoglobulin E level (possibly supporting the diagnosis of atopic dermatitis)
- Leukemia (found by peripheral blood smear)
- Imaging studies with computed tomography or magnetic resonance imaging are needed if lymphoma or Hodgkin's disease is suspected

REITER'S SYNDROME

BASICS

- Reiter's syndrome (RS) is an idiopathic inflammatory process affecting the skin, joints, and mucous membranes. The classic triad of **urethritis, conjunctivitis,** and **arthritis** is found in only 40% of cases at the time of the initial clinical presentation.

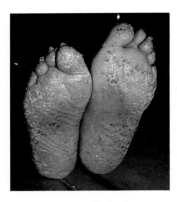

FIGURE 25.15 Reiter's syndrome. Keratoderma blennorrhagicum. Scaly, red–brown, inflammatory, pustular psoriasislike lesions are present on the soles.

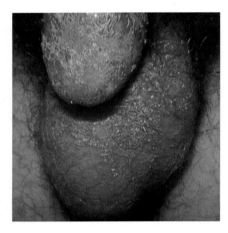

FIGURE 25.16 Reiter's syndrome. In circinate balanitis, psoriasiform lesions occur on the glans penis and the scrotum.

Laboratory Evaluations
- HLA-B27 is positive in 75% of patients.
- Antinuclear antibody (ANA) and rheumatoid factor are usually negative.
- The histopathologic features of skin lesions in RS are indistinguishable from those of psoriasis.
- HIV testing should be done.

- RS is seen most commonly in young white males of European origin.
- Initial symptoms often occur after nongonococcal urethritis (e.g., chlamydial infection) or infection with an enteric pathogen (e.g., *Shigella* and *Yersinia*).
- Human leukocyte antigen (HLA)-B27 is frequently positive in patients with RS and portends a poorer prognosis.

DESCRIPTION OF LESIONS

Skin lesions are often indistinguishable from psoriasis; however, RS often manifests certain characteristic findings such as the following:

- Keratoderma blennorrhagicum (Figure 25.15) consists of scaly, red, inflammatory psoriasislike lesions on the palms and soles. The lesions may have a thick scale and may be pustular.
- Scaling red plaques or erosions may be found on the glans penis *(circinate balanitis)* (Figure 25.16).
- Nail changes may include findings such as those seen in psoriasis— onycholysis and subungual hyperkeratosis; furthermore, subungual pustules with resultant shedding of nails may occur.
- Oral lesions are usually painless, irregularly shaped, white plaques on the tongue that resemble geographic tongue.

DISTRIBUTION OF LESIONS

- Keratoderma blennorrhagicum is most often noted on the palms and soles.
- Psoriasislike plaques may be seen on the scalp, elbows, knees, buttocks, shaft of the penis, and scrotum.

CLINICAL MANIFESTATIONS

- RS is a multisystemic disease that may present with fever, malaise, dysuria, arthralgias, and red irritated eyes with accompanying cutaneous lesions.
- Frequently, RS has a self-limited course, but it may become a chronic, relapsing condition.
- RS is common in patients with human immunodeficiency virus (HIV) disease.
- The arthritis of RS is asymmetric oligoarthritis that commonly involves large joints (elbows, knees); it may also involve smaller joints. Sacroiliitis and ankylosing spondylitis may occur.
- Ocular disease may include conjunctivitis with intense red conjunctival injection and, less commonly, iritis and keratitis.
- Urethritis is a nonspecific urethral inflammation with a purulent exudate and dysuria.

DIAGNOSIS

- The diagnosis is generally made on clinical grounds.

DIFFERENTIAL DIAGNOSIS

Psoriasis with Arthritis
- Psoriasiform skin lesions
- Arthritis similar to that seen in RS
- No ocular symptoms
- No urethritis

Behçet's Syndrome
- Painful oral ulcers
- Arthritis
- Iritis
- Vasculitic skin lesions

Candidal Balanitis
- Positive potassium hydroxide examination or fungal culture

 MANAGEMENT

Mild Cases
- RS may be treated with topical steroids for the skin lesions.
- NSAIDs are prescribed for pain.

Severe Cases
- Oral methotrexate is sometimes used on a weekly basis for severe cases.
- Oral steroids may be necessary; however, tapering of steroids can produce an extreme flare of the pustular lesions.
- Oral retinoids such as Accutane 13-*cis*-retinoic acid (Accutane) and acitretin (Soriatane) have also been used to treat skin lesions.

POINT TO REMEMBER

- During initial or recurrent episodes, most patients with RS do not manifest the complete triad of urethritis, conjunctivitis, and arthritis.

ERYTHEMA NODOSUM

BASICS

- Erythema nodosum (EN) is an acute inflammatory reaction of the subcutaneous fat. It is considered a delayed hypersensitivity reaction to various antigenic stimuli.
- EN is three times more common in female than male patients and has a peak incidence between 20 and 30 years of age.
- Sarcoidosis, streptococcal infections, pregnancy, and the use of oral contraceptives are the most common causes of EN in the United States.
- In children, streptococcal pharyngitis is the most likely underlying cause.
- Approximately 40% of cases are idiopathic.

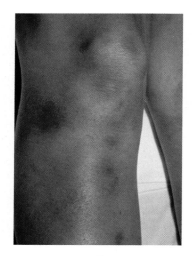

FIGURE 25.17 Erythema nodosum. These are acute red, tender nodules.

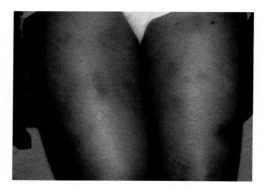

FIGURE 25.18 Erythema nodosum. These are healing "contusiform" lesions.

Laboratory Evaluations
- Usually, a complete blood count, erythrocyte sedimentation rate, throat culture, antistreptolysin titer, purified protein derivative skin test, and chest film are all that are necessary.
- A excisional skin biopsy will show panniculitis with infiltration of lymphocytes in the septa of the fat.
- Further tests, such as gastrointestinal tract evaluation and serum angiotensin-converting enzyme determination, can be performed if suggested by the review of systems and physical examination.

Besides sarcoidosis and pregnancy, EN is associated with a variety of conditions: deep fungal infections (in endemic areas), including coccidioidomycosis, histoplasmosis, and blastomycosis; tuberculosis; *Yersinia enterocolitica* infection; inflammatory bowel disease, including ulcerative colitis and Crohn's disease; malignant disease, including lymphoma and leukemia; postradiation therapy; and Behçet's syndrome. Drugs such as sulfonamides, penicillin, gold, amiodarone, and opiates also have been implicated as causes of EN.

DESCRIPTION OF LESIONS

- Lesions begin as bright red, deep, extremely tender nodules (Figure 25.17).
- During resolution, lesions become dark brown, violaceous, or bruise-like macules ("contusiform") (Figure 25.18).

DISTRIBUTION OF LESIONS

- EN tends to occur in a bilateral distribution on the anterior shins, thighs, knees, and arms.

CLINICAL MANIFESTATIONS

- Malaise, fever, arthralgias, and periarticular swelling of the knees and ankles may accompany the panniculitis.
- Other symptoms may also be present, depending on the cause of EN.
- Spontaneous resolution of lesions occurs in 3 to 6 weeks, regardless of the underlying cause.
- Generally, EN indicates a better prognosis in patients who have sarcoidosis.

DIAGNOSIS

- The diagnosis of EN is usually made on clinical grounds, but a biopsy may be helpful for confirmation.

MANAGEMENT

- Treatment is symptomatic, consisting of bed rest, leg elevation, NSAIDs, or iodides.
- Systemic corticosteroids, which often bring dramatic improvement, can be used if an infectious cause is excluded.
- Treatment or avoidance of the underlying cause, if discovered, should be attempted.

PYODERMA GANGRENOSUM

BASICS

Pyoderma gangrenosum (PG) is an uncommon condition of uncertain origin. It is a unique, painful, inflammatory, ulcerative process of the skin. It is often seen in association with certain systemic diseases including ulcerative colitis, regional enteritis, rheumatoid arthritis, and leukemia; however, some investigators believe it to be a distinct disease.

DESCRIPTION OF LESIONS

- PG skin ulcers are 2 to 10 cm in diameter.
- They are deep ulcerations with an erythematous to violaceous border. The border is often undermined (a probe can be placed under the overhanging edge of the lesion).
- Lesions may be multiple.
- Lesions heal with scarring (Figure 25.19).

DISTRIBUTION OF LESIONS

- PG skin ulcers are most commonly found on the lower extremities (shins and ankles).

CLINICAL MANIFESTATIONS

- PG lesions can appear as a rapidly expanding, painful, skin ulcer.
- Patients often have associated oligoarticular arthritis.
- Ulcerations of PG occur after trauma or injury to the skin in 30% of patients; this process is termed *pathergy*.

Diseases associated with PG include the following:

- Ulcerative colitis
- Regional enteritis (Crohn's disease)
- Rheumatoid arthritis
- Myelogenous leukemia

In 50% of patients, no underlying systemic disease is present.

DIAGNOSIS

- The diagnosis of PG is made by excluding other causes of similar-appearing cutaneous ulcerations including infection, stasis ulcers, malignant disease, vasculitis, collagen vascular diseases, diabetes, and trauma, as described later in the section on differential diagnosis.

 DIFFERENTIAL DIAGNOSIS

Cutaneous Malignant Diseases
- Basal cell carcinoma
- Squamous cell carcinoma

Infectious Processes
- Bacterial infections
- Deep fungal infections
- Herpes simplex virus infections

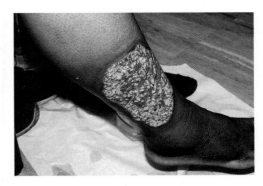

FIGURE 25.19 Pyoderma gangrenosum. This large ulceration is beginning to heal with a craterlike (cribriform) scar.

Laboratory Evaluations
- Skin biopsy of the edge of the ulcer may be performed to rule out other causes of skin ulcers, such as infections or malignant disease; however, the pathologic findings for PG are nonspecific.
- Bacterial, fungal, and viral cultures of the ulcer are done if clinically indicated.
- Workup for systemic disease should include complete blood count with differential, sedimentation rate, sequential multichannel autoanalyzer 20, ANA, Venereal Disease Research Laboratory test, rheumatoid factor, and a chest radiograph.
- Serum or urine protein electrophoresis, peripheral smear, and bone marrow aspirate are performed if indicated, to evaluate for hematologic malignant diseases.
- A gastrointestinal series for inflammatory bowel disease should be done if clinically indicated.

Inflammatory Processes
- Collagen vascular diseases
- Polyarteritis nodosa
- Behçet's disease
- Wegener's granulomatosus
- Antiphospholipid antibody syndrome

MANAGEMENT

- The diagnosis and treatment of underlying associated diseases do not necessarily promote the healing of PG.

Topical and Intralesional Therapy
- Local compresses, antiseptic washes, and topical antibiotics may be useful.
- Superpotent topical corticosteroids, cromolyn sodium 2% solution, nitrogen mustard, and 5-aminosalicyclic acid may be tried.
- Intralesional steroid injections (triamcinolone acetonide, 10 mg/mL) are administered into the edge of the ulcer.

Systemic Therapy
- Oral steroids for several weeks to months (starting at 60 to 80 mg prednisone daily and tapering the steroid slowly). Systemic steroids may be given alone or in combination with dapsone, azathioprine, or chlorambucil. In patients with steroid-resistant PG, oral cyclosporine has been shown to be effective.
- The following drugs have also met with some success: mycophenolate mofetil, tacrolimus, cyclophosphamide, thalidomide, and nicotine.
- Intravenous therapy can be administered using pulsed methylprednisolone, pulsed cyclophosphamide, and immunoglobulin.

Other Therapy
- Hyperbaric oxygen has been used.

POINT TO REMEMBER

- Surgical débridement of PG lesions should be avoided, if possible, because of the pathergic phenomenon that may occur with surgical manipulation or grafting. This can result in further wound enlargement.

BASICS

- Sarcoidosis is an example of a systemic disease in which cellular granulomatous infiltrates produce dermal skin lesions.
- Sarcoidosis is a chronic multisystemic disease of unknown origin. Most often, it presents with bilateral hilar adenopathy, pulmonary infiltration, eye lesions, and arthralgias; less commonly, there is involvement of the spleen and salivary and lacrimal glands, as well as gastrointestinal and cardiac manifestations.
- Sarcoidosis is seen most commonly in young adults, particularly in blacks in the United States and South Africa. It is also more common in Scandinavians.
- Of patients with sarcoidosis, 20% to 35% have cutaneous involvement.

DESCRIPTION OF LESIONS

Specific lesions of cutaneous sarcoid include the following:

- Dermal papules, nodules, or plaques that are brown or violaceous (Figures 25.20 and 25.21).
- Lesions may be annular, serpiginous, or atrophic.
- Lesions can also appear on dorsa of hands, fingers, toes, and forehead.
- *Lupus pernio*, a distinct variant, consists of reddish purple plaques around the nose, ears, lips, and face.
- Subcutaneous nodules *(Darier–Roussy nodules)*. These lesions that are usually nontender, firm, oval, flesh-colored or violaceous 0.5- to 2-cm nodules found on the extremities or trunk.

Nonspecific cutaneous lesions associated with sarcoid include the following:

- Erythema nodosum (EN) may occur in acute sarcoidosis (see the earlier discussion of EN).
- Ichthyosis may be noted.

DISTRIBUTION OF LESIONS

- Lesions tend to be located periorifically (e.g., around the eyelids, nasal ala, tip of nose, earlobes, and lips).
- Lesions may occur in old scars anywhere on the body. Scars from previous trauma, surgery, venipuncture, or tattoo may become infiltrated and may be red or purple.
- Scalp lesions may produce scarring alopecia.
- Ichthyosiform and EN lesions tend to occur on the pretibial area.

CLINICAL MANIFESTATIONS

- Skin lesions are generally asymptomatic; however, they are often of great cosmetic concern because they occur commonly on the face.
- EN associated with sarcoidosis generally resolves spontaneously and suggests a better prognosis.
- *Löfgren's syndrome* (EN and arthritis) is a clinical variant of sarcoidosis.

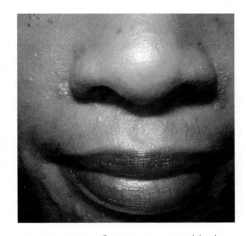

FIGURE 25.20 Cutaneous sarcoidosis. The subtle dermal papules seen around this patient's nose and mouth could easily be mistaken for acne.

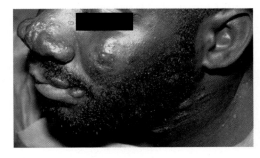

FIGURE 25.21 Cutaneous sarcoidosis. Dermal nodules are seen in a periorificial distribution (i.e., around the mouth, eyes, and nares). Note the sarcoidal lesions arising in the scars of this patient's neck.

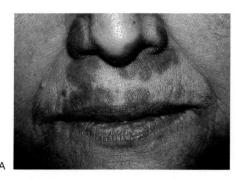
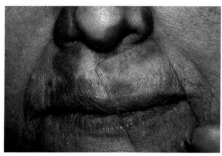

A

B

FIGURE 25.22 *A* and *B:* Cutaneous sarcoidosis. Reddish-violaceous plaques display an "apple jelly" coloration on diascopy performed with a glass slide.

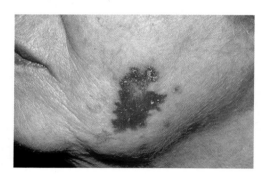

FIGURE 25.23 Lupus vulgaris. This reddish dermal plaque has been slowly growing for 20 years. On diascopy, yellow–brown "apple jelly" nodules were demonstrated.

DIAGNOSIS

- "Apple jelly" nodules are seen on blanching lesions with a glass slide (diascopy) (Figure 25.22). These nodules represent the gross appearance of granulomas.
- Skin biopsy demonstrates noncaseating granulomas (sarcoidal granulomas).
- A chest radiograph may demonstrate bilateral hilar adenopathy and other characteristic changes.

Abnormal laboratory evaluations may include the following:

- Elevated angiotensin-converting enzyme levels
- Hypergammaglobulinemia
- Hypercalcemia

 DIFFERENTIAL DIAGNOSIS

Granuloma Annulare
- This condition is discussed in Chapter 4, "Inflammatory Eruptions of Unknown Cause."

Cutaneous Tuberculosis (Figure 25.23)
- This is also known as *lupus vulgaris*.

 MANAGEMENT

- Potent topical steroids are applied under occlusion, if necessary.
- Intralesional steroid injections can help to flatten lesions.
- Oral antimalarial agents such as hydroxychloroquine and chloroquine are administered for therapeutically unresponsive or widespread disease.
- Oral corticosteroids should be used only on a short-term basis.
- If corticosteroids are not effective, immunosuppressants such as methotrexate and azathioprine may be effective. Other agents that have been used to treat cutaneous sarcoidosis include cyclosporine, oral isotretinoin, allopurinol, and thalidomide. Chlorambucil also has been reported to be effective, but the risk for malignant disease is great with this medication.

HELPFUL HINTS

- Systemic steroids should not be routinely used to treat cutaneous lesions; rather, potent topical steroids, intralesional steroids, or oral antimalarials should be tried first. If possible, systemic steroids are best reserved for more serious systemic involvement.
- Oral antimalarials can lead to irreversible retinopathy and blindness. Eye examination is necessary before and during antimalarial therapy.
- Granulomatous acne rosacea may mimic sarcoidosis clinically and histopathologically. It is referred to as *lupus miliaris disseminatus faciei.*

SYSTEMIC LUPUS ERYTHEMATOSUS

BASICS

- **Systemic lupus erythematosus** (SLE) is a chronic, idiopathic, multisystemic, autoimmune disease associated with polyclonal B-cell activation. Fibrinoid degeneration of connective tissue and the walls of blood vessels associated with an inflammatory infiltrate involving various organs may result in arthralgia or arthritis, kidney disease, liver disease, central nervous system disease, gastrointestinal disease, pericarditis, pneumonitis, myopathy, and splenomegaly, as well as skin disease.
- The cutaneous manifestations of SLE result from the production of multiple autoantibodies that deposit immune complexes at the dermal–epidermal junction.
- Current investigators have reclassified lupus skin lesions into three distinct groups:
  - **Acute cutaneous lupus erythematosus** (ACLE) lesions are strongly associated with active SLE; however, ACLE lesions may occasionally be seen in **subacute cutaneous lupus erythematosus** (SCLE).
  - **SCLE** comprises the second category.
  - **Chronic cutaneous lupus erythematosus** (CCLE) traditionally had been referred to as discoid lupus erythematosus (DLE).
- SLE is seen in a 9:1 female-to-male ratio; it is more common in blacks and Hispanics.
- Approximately 10% of patients with SLE have a first-degree relative with the disease. An association of lupus and HLA-DR2 and DR4 has been seen.

The following 4 of the 11 American Rheumatologic Association criteria for lupus are related to the skin and are considered lupus-specific lesions:

- The classic malar or "butterfly" rash (Figure 25.24) is a persistent erythema over the cheeks that tends to spare the nasolabial creases. Sometimes, this is the initial symptom of lupus, and it often occurs after sun exposure.
- Photosensitivity (Figure 25.25) occurs as an exaggerated or unusual reaction to sunlight. The reaction may resemble a drug eruption.
- Discoid lesions (CCLE) (Figure 25.26) are erythematous lesions that evolve into scaly, atrophic scarring plaques. Such discoid lesions affect 10% to 15% of patients with SLE.
- Oral ulcerations (see Figure 12.7) develop, often on the hard palate or nasopharynx.

Lupus nonspecific lesions that may be seen in SLE and other connective tissue diseases include the following:

- The "spider" type of telangiectasia is usually seen in SLE, scleroderma, and dermatomyositis. Macular (matlike) telangiectasias usually occur in scleroderma.
- Periungual telangiectasias are seen in SLE, as well as in dermatomyositis and scleroderma.
- Palmar telangiectasias are usually seen in SLE.
- Vasculitis, palpable purpura, and vasculitic ulcers usually occur in SLE and scleroderma.
- Raynaud's phenomenon is associated with SLE and scleroderma.

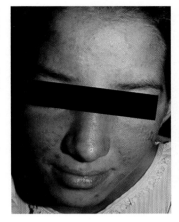

FIGURE 25.24 Systemic lupus erythematosus. A "butterfly rash" is evident. Note the sparing of the nasolabial creases.

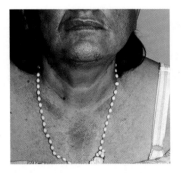

FIGURE 25.25 Systemic lupus erythematosus. Photodistribution at the "V" of the neck is noted. Note the violaceous color suggestive of connective tissue disease.

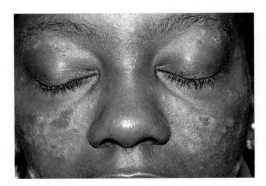

FIGURE 25.26 Chronic cutaneous lupus erythematosus. Lesions of discoid lupus erythematosus consist of erythematous, scaly, disc-shaped scarring plaques.

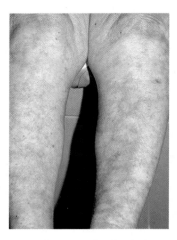

FIGURE 25.27 Systemic lupus erythematosus. Livedo reticularis is present.

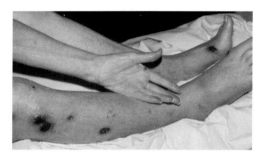

FIGURE 25.28 Systemic lupus erythematosus. Vasculitic ulcers are seen on the legs.

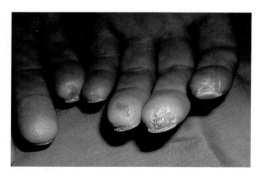

FIGURE 25.29 Systemic lupus erythematosus. Necrotic, painful, vasculitic ulcers are present on the fingertips.

- Livedo reticulitis, panniculitis, thrombophlebitis, urticaria, urticarial vasculitis, frontal alopecia ("lupus hair"), and diffuse nonscarring, alopecia, palmar erythema, and bullae are associated primarily with SLE.

DISTRIBUTION OF LESIONS

- ACLE lesions tend to occur in sun-exposed areas such as the face, dorsa of the forearms, the hands, and the "V" of the neck.
- CCLE (discoid LE) lesions may occur on the head, neck, or oral mucosa, or they may be widespread (see later).
- On the lower extremity, livedo reticularis (Figure 25.27) and vasculitic ulcers (Figure 25.28) may be seen.
- On the dorsal hands, violaceous plaques that spare the skin overlying the joints are characteristic of SLE. Conversely, in dermatomyositis, the joints are affected (*Gottron's papules*). Ulcerated vasculitic lesions on the fingertips may also develop (Figure 25.29).

CLINICAL MANIFESTATIONS

- Fatigue, fever, and malaise may be the presenting nonspecific symptoms.
- Signs or symptoms are related to the specific organ or area involved (e.g., arthralgia).
- Flare of lupus is common during pregnancy.
- The following hematologic abnormalities may be associated with SLE: idiopathic thrombocytopenic purpura, hemolytic anemia, leukopenia, and clotting abnormalities, which may be related to the anticardiolipin syndrome. Other associated conditions and symptoms include rheumatoid arthritis, Sjögren's syndrome, seizures, and the occurrence of multiple spontaneous abortions.

CLINICAL VARIANT

Drug-Induced Lupus Erythematosus
- The clinical and serologic picture of drug-induced lupus erythematosus is often indistinguishable from that of SLE.
- A syndrome resembling SLE can be induced by certain drugs: hydralazine, procainamide, phenytoin, isoniazid, quinidine, β-blockers, sulfasalazine, and lithium; however, patients with drug-induced lupus syndromes have cutaneous lesions much less commonly than is seen in SLE.
- Arthralgia or arthritis, generally affecting the small joints, is often the only clinical symptom. Myalgia, pleuritis, pericarditis, fever, and hepatosplenomegaly may occur; however, the classic SLE-type lesions of butterfly rash and mucosal ulcerations, for example, are usually absent in drug-induced lupus erythematosus. CNS manifestations and renal involvement are rare.
- In 90% of patients, ANAs are present in a homogenous or speckled pattern.
- Withdrawal of the offending drug, followed by a regression of symptoms, helps to confirm the diagnosis.

DIAGNOSIS

According to the American Rheumatologic Association, a person has SLE if four or more of the following criteria are present:

1. "Butterfly" rash
2. CCLE (discoid LE) lesions
3. Photosensitivity
4. Oral ulcers
5. Arthritis in two or more joints
6. Serositis
7. Renal disorder
8. Neurologic disorder
9. Hematologic disorder
10. Immunologic disorder: anti-DNA, anti-Smith antibody, or a false-biologic-positive syphilis serologic result
11. ANAs

 DIFFERENTIAL DIAGNOSIS

Facial Lesions
Rosacea
- Presence of acnelike papules and pustules in addition to malar erythema
- Absence of systemic complaints
- Negative ANA titers

Seborrheic Dermatitis
- Ready response to topical steroids
- Lack of systemic complaints
- Negative ANA titers

Other Conditions
- Other connective tissue diseases, such as scleroderma and dermatomyositis
- Other photosensitivity conditions, such as polymorphous light eruption
- Other causes of renal, hematologic, and CNS disease

 MANAGEMENT

Sun-Related Symptoms
- Excessive sun exposure should be avoided; the patient should be counseled in the use of broad-spectrum sunscreens.

Cutaneous DLE
- See the later discussion of the management of CCLE.

Severely Ill Patients
- Systemic steroids are given.
- Administration of oral antimalarials, dapsone, gold, retinoids, thalidomide, and immunosuppressive drugs such as azathioprine and cyclophosphamide may be helpful.
- Thalidomide and intravenous γ-globulin are used in selected cases.

Laboratory Evaluations
- ANA titers are positive in 95% of patients with SLE.
- Anti-dsDNA (antibody to native double-stranded DNA) is present in 60% to 80% of patients and is more specific for SLE.
- Anti-Sm antibody has a strong specificity for SLE.
- Antiphospholipid antibodies are present in 25% of patients.
- The erythrocyte sedimentation rate is elevated.
- Hypocomplementemia occurs in 70% of patients and is noted especially when there is renal involvement in active SLE.
- The lupus band test involves the direct immunofluorescence of uninvolved, non–sun-exposed skin. When positive, it is suggestive of the presence of renal disease. This test has been largely supplanted by the aforementioned serologic tests.

SUBACUTE CUTANEOUS LUPUS ERYTHEMATOSUS

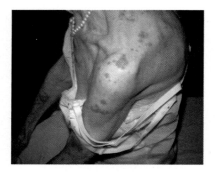

FIGURE 25.30 Subacute and cutaneous lupus erythematosus. This patient has scaly, annular lesions. (Courtesy of Herbert A. Hochman, M.D.)

BASICS

- Subacute cutaneous lupus erythematosus (SCLE) tends to be less severe than SLE and rarely progresses to renal or CNS involvement.
- SCLE is characterized by photodistributed erythematous lesions that are nonscarring.
- SCLE occurs most commonly in young and middle-aged white women.
- Patients may have some of the American Rheumatologic Association criteria for SLE, but serious disease with renal involvement is uncommon.

DESCRIPTION OF LESIONS

- Lesions are papulosquamous and closely resemble psoriasis or pityriasis rosea.
- Lesions are often annular and heal without scarring (Figure 25.30).

DISTRIBUTION OF LESIONS

- There is a distribution of lesions on the upper trunk, the "V" of the neck, and the extensor surfaces of the arms and hands.
- The face is often spared in SCLE.

DIAGNOSIS

- Anti-SS-A (anti-Ro) and anti-SS-B (anti-La) antibodies are often found, although the absence of these antibodies does not exclude the diagnosis.
- Low titers of ANA may be present.

CLINICAL MANIFESTATIONS

- Fatigue, malaise, and arthralgias may be noted.
- Sjögren's syndrome, idiopathic thrombocytopenic purpura, urticarial vasculitis, and morphea also have been reported in association with SCLE.

 DIFFERENTIAL DIAGNOSIS

- Psoriasis
- Pityriasis rosea

 MANAGEMENT

- Treatment of SCLE is much like that of CCLE, and it focuses mainly on the avoidance of excessive sun exposure and the use of broad-spectrum sunscreens and topical steroids, oral antimalarials, dapsone, gold, retinoids, thalidomide, and immunosuppressive drugs.
- Because patients with SCLE have a better prognosis than patients with SLE, the clinician must weigh the potential toxicities of these agents against their benefits before initiating therapy.

CHRONIC CUTANEOUS LUPUS ERYTHEMATOSUS

BASICS

- CCLE consists of scarring plaques.
- DLE is, by far, the most common form of CCLE.
- Other CCLE variants include *hypertrophic lupus erythematosus, lupus erythematosus panniculitis*, and *lupus profundus*.

DISCOID LUPUS ERYTHEMATOSUS

BASICS

- DLE is a chronic, scarring, photosensitive dermatosis. DLE may occur in patients (approximately 25%) with SLE.
- If the initial workup of patients who present solely with localized lesions of DLE shows no evidence of SLE, then those patients are considered to be at low risk (less than 5%) for SLE to develop.

DESCRIPTION OF LESIONS

- Lesions begin as well-defined erythematous plaques that evolve into atrophic disc-shaped plaques, characterized by scale, accentuated hair follicles, follicular plugging, and a combination of hypopigmentation and hyperpigmentation.
- DLE often involves the scalp and produces scarring alopecia (Figure 25.31).

DISTRIBUTION OF LESIONS

- Patients with DLE often are divided into two groups: those with localized disease and those with widespread disease. Localized DLE occurs when the head and neck only are affected, whereas widespread DLE occurs when other areas are affected (Figure 25.32). SLE is more likely to develop in patients with widespread involvement of DLE.

CLINICAL MANIFESTATIONS

- Lesions of DLE are relatively asymptomatic, but they may itch or be tender.
- Rarely, squamous cell carcinoma develops in hypertrophic chronic lesions.

DIAGNOSIS

- The clinical appearance is confirmed by a punch biopsy of the skin.

 DIFFERENTIAL DIAGNOSIS

- **Sarcoidosis** should be considered.
- **Lichen planus** is another possible diagnosis.

CCLE variants include the following:

- Hypertrophic lupus erythematosus is a warty-appearing form of CCLE.

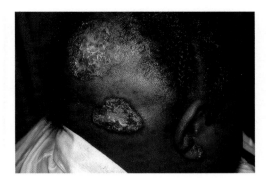

FIGURE 25.31 Chronic cutaneous lupus erythematosus. Lesions of discoid lupus erythematosus have caused scarring alopecia in this patient who has no evidence of systemic lupus erythematosus.

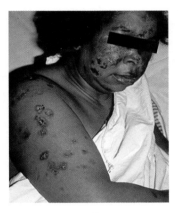

FIGURE 25.32 Chronic cutaneous lupus erythematosus. Widespread lesions of discoid lupus erythematosus are noted.

- Lupus erythematosus panniculitis is an inflammation of subcutaneous tissue.
- When lupus panniculitis occurs with a lesion of CCLE overlying it, it is referred to as **lupus profundus.**

MANAGEMENT

- Excessive sun exposure should be avoided.
- Broad-spectrum sunscreens that block both ultraviolet A and ultraviolet B are used.
- Potent topical steroids are generally effective for treating isolated lesions. Facial lesions should be treated with low- to medium-potency agents. If necessary, high-potency or superpotent agents may be used for short periods.
- Intralesional steroid injections are helpful in CCLE lesions that are refractory to topical therapy.
- Systemic agents may be indicated when lesions are widespread or unresponsive to topical or intralesional therapy. Agents such as the antimalarials hydroxychloroquine (Plaquenil) and chloroquine comprise the first line of systemic therapy. Systemic steroids, dapsone, oral retinoids, gold, clofazimine, methotrexate, thalidomide, tetracycline or erythromycin combined with niacinamide, and mycophenolate mofetil have proved to be helpful in selective cases.

POINTS TO REMEMBER

- Patients with widespread involvement are more likely to develop SLE.
- Most patients with CCLE do not have and will not develop SLE. Even so, many patients who are given the diagnosis of CCLE describe themselves as having "lupus" and are convinced that they have the more serious disease.

NEONATAL LUPUS ERYTHEMATOSUS

BASICS

- Neonatal lupus erythematosus (NLE) is a rare autoimmune syndrome that affects 1% to 2% of infants born of mothers who are anti-Ro (SS-A) antibody positive.
- Mothers may or may not show any of the signs or symptoms of connective tissue disease at the time of birth of the affected infant; however, some features of Sjögren's syndrome or lupus erythematosus (e.g., dry mouth, dry eyes, or arthralgias) do ultimately develop in most of these women. This situation may occur many years after the birth of the child; however, in most of these women, SLE does not develop.

DESCRIPTION OF LESIONS

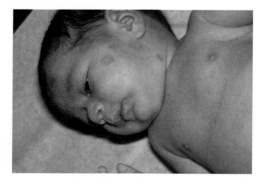

FIGURE 25.33 Neonatal lupus erythematosus. These annular erythematous plaques that look like "ringworm" began shortly after birth in this 3-month-old infant of an Ro-positive mother.

- The rash of NLE is a benign, self-limited eruption that appears at birth and tends to disappear by approximately 6 months of age.
- The rash is characterized by annular (ringlike) erythematous plaques or smaller erythematous patches that generally occur at birth or several days thereafter (Figure 25.33).

CLINICAL MANIFESTATIONS

- NLE is characterized by either benign skin disease or congenital heart block, or both, in about 10% of the cases.
- Involvement of joints, kidneys, and CNS is rare, and the criteria of the American Rheumatologic Association for SLE are not fulfilled.
- Congenital heart block presents a 20% mortality risk and often requires the insertion of a pacemaker. The onset of heart block generally occurs a few weeks before term and is seen at birth.
- Unlike the skin lesions, the cardiac problems associated with NLE are permanent.

MANAGEMENT

Cutaneous Manifestations
- Low-potency, nonfluorinated topical steroids are given.
- Sun exposure should be avoided.

Heart Block
- Experimental therapy using dexamethasone, which crosses the placental barrier, has been used to treat heart block *in utero* with minimal success.
- Pacemaker implantation is frequently required.

DERMATOMYOSITIS

BASICS

- Dermatomyositis is an inflammatory skin and muscle disease that is related to polymyositis; in fact, both conditions are considered to be the same disease except for the presence or absence of the rash. Cutaneous manifestations without detectable muscle disease are known as *amyopathic dermatomyositis*.
- The female-to-male ratio is 2:1.
- An autoimmune origin, which may be initiated by a virus in genetically susceptible people, has been proposed as a possible cause of dermatomyositis. As a result, antibodies that attack the skin and muscle are produced.
- An overlap syndrome with scleroderma or lupus *(mixed connective tissue disease)* is characterized by the presence of antiribonucleoprotein (anti-RNP) antibodies.
- Adults with dermatomyositis appear to have an increased risk for malignant diseases. The skin disease often follows the clinical course of exacerbations and remissions of the cancer. Most malignant diseases are the common cancers (e.g., colon and breast cancer) that occur in a general aging population.

DESCRIPTION AND DISTRIBUTION OF LESIONS

- The **heliotrope rash** consists of red or violaceous coloration around the eyes and is associated with periorbital edema (Figure 25.34). (The change in color may be a subtle clinical finding, particularly in dark-skinned patients.)

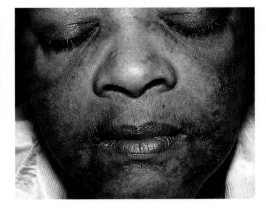

FIGURE 25.34 Dermatomyositis. The heliotrope rash around the eyes is associated with periorbital edema.

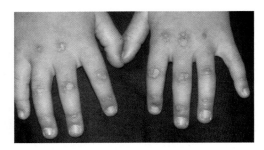

FIGURE 25.35 Dermatomyositis. Gottron's papules are violaceous, flat-topped papules located on the joints of the fingers.

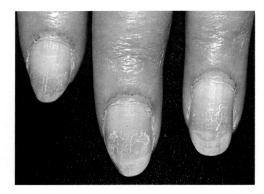

FIGURE 25.36 Dermatomyositis. Periungual telangiectasias are present.

- **Gottron's papules** consist of erythematous or violaceous, flat-topped papules on the dorsa of the hands (Figure 25.35). Lesions are located on the joints of the fingers; they begin as papules and later become atrophic and hypopigmented.
- **Poikiloderma** is a characteristic rash of dermatomyositis, consisting of telangiectasia, atrophy, hyperpigmentation, and hypopigmentation. Poikiloderma occurs on the extensor aspects of the body, upper back, forearms, and "V" of the neck. Atrophic lesions occur particularly on the knees and elbows.
- **Periungual telangiectasias** are shown in Figure 25.36.

CLINICAL MANIFESTATIONS

- Progressive, bilateral, symmetric, proximal muscle weakness develops, as suggested by difficulty with brushing or combing hair and standing from a seated position.
- Muscle tenderness or pain is usually not a complaint.
- Photosensitivity is evidenced in areas of poikiloderma.
- Arthralgias occur in one-third of patients.
- There may be features of an overlap syndrome.
- Pulmonary fibrosis affects 10% of patients, particularly in the presence of anti-Jo 1 or anti-PL 12 antibodies.
- Evidence of vasculitis (e.g., palpable purpura or ulcers) may be present.
- Calcinosis cutis is seen in the juvenile form of dermatomyositis.
- Myocardial disease may be an associated finding.
- Dysphagia may occur.

DIAGNOSIS

- The findings on skin biopsy are often nonspecific, but generally are suggestive of a connective tissue disease.
- Elevation of creatine phosphokinase levels is often a reliable indicator of muscle involvement.
- Aldolase levels may be increased.
- Electromyography may aid in the diagnosis.
- Muscle biopsy may aid in the diagnosis as well.
- The presence of autoantibodies, such as anti-DNA, anti-RNP, and anti-Ro, may be found. Anti-M-1 antibody is highly specific for dermatomyositis, but it is present in only 25% of patients.

 DIFFERENTIAL DIAGNOSIS

- SLE should be considered.
- Mixed connective tissue disease or overlap syndrome is another possibility.
- When only the muscle is involved, other myopathies should be considered.

 MANAGEMENT

Skin
- Avoidance of excessive sun exposure
- Use of broad-spectrum sunscreens
- Antimalarial drugs: hydroxychloroquine, 5 mg/kg per day for 4 to 6 weeks; then titrate according to clinical response
- Low-dose oral methotrexate

(continued)

Systemic Symptoms
- Physical therapy
- Systemic steroids (when used for systemic symptoms, may also improve skin conditions)
- Immunosuppressive therapy, including low-dose oral methotrexate
- Cyclosporine
- Cyclophosphamide
- Azathioprine
- Plasmapheresis
- Interferons
- Intravenous high-dose γ-globulin

 POINT TO REMEMBER

- The adult form of dermatomyositis may be associated with internal malignant diseases; patients older than age 50 years should be evaluated with this possibility in mind.

SCLERODERMA AND MORPHEA

BASICS

- Scleroderma is an autoimmune connective tissue disease in which excess collagen results from an increase in number and activity of fibroblasts. Induration and thickening of the skin and subcutaneous tissues result. This process is triggered by vascular inflammation and infiltration of activated T4 cells.
- The origin of scleroderma is unknown. As in lupus, scleroderma may be seen either in a systemic or localized cutaneous form.

Classification
- Morphea, or *localized scleroderma*, is limited to the skin and has rarely been reported to progress to systemic scleroderma. The female-to-male ratio is 3:1.
- Systemic scleroderma may be divided as follows:
  - **CREST syndrome** (defined later), which accounts for 90% of the cases of systemic sclerosis, is a relatively benign variant with a delayed appearance of visceral involvement.
  - **Progressive systemic sclerosis** is a chronic multisystem disease that affects the skin and internal organs and has a very poor prognosis.
  - In systemic sclerosis, the female-to-male ratio is 4:1.

DESCRIPTION OF LESIONS

Morphea
- A localized, indurated, hairless plaque has a characteristic "lilac" border (Figure 25.37).
- Patients may have a single plaque or multiple plaques.
- White, ivory, or hyperpigmented permanent scars result when lesions heal.

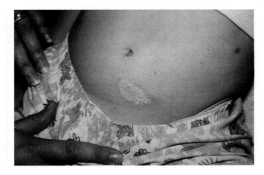

FIGURE 25.37 Morphea. The ivory-colored plaque has a "lilac" border.

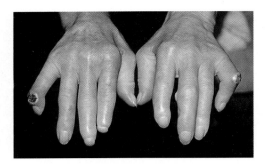

FIGURE 25.38 Scleroderma with acrosclerosis and sclerodactyly. The patient has tapered shiny, stiff, waxy fingers. Note the painful vasculitic lesions on the fingertips.

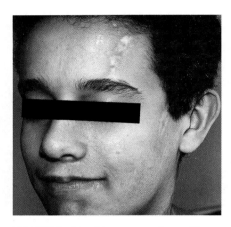

FIGURE 25.39 Linear morphea. *Coup de sabre* lesions are present.

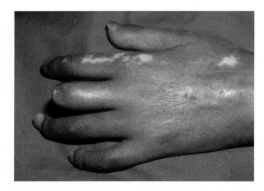

FIGURE 25.40 Scleroderma. Note the shortened finger resulting from distal bone resorption.

CREST Syndrome and Progressive Systemic Sclerosis

- Acrosclerosis refers to ill-defined, indurated fibrotic skin, which occurs peripherally and gradually involves the forearms.
- Sclerodactyly consists of thickened, sausage-shaped digits in which the skin becomes tight and bound down. Gradually, the skin becomes shiny, stiff, waxy, and atrophic (Figure 25.38).

DISTRIBUTION OF LESIONS

- In morphea, lesions are commonly found on the trunk; they may become widespread *(generalized morphea)* or linear *(linear morphea)*, which may have the characteristic frontoparietal distribution *(coup de sabre)* (Figure 25.39).
- In CREST syndrome, the cutaneous involvement is usually limited to acral areas (hands, feet, face, and forearms).
- Patients with progressive systemic sclerosis often have widespread, progressive disease.

CLINICAL MANIFESTATIONS

- Morphea *(localized scleroderma)* is generally asymptomatic, usually "burns out" spontaneously, and leaves a scar.
- CREST syndrome consists of the following:
  - *C*alcinosis cutis, most commonly occurring on the palms, fingertips, and bony prominences
  - *R*aynaud's phenomenon
  - *E*sophageal dysfunction
  - *S*clerodactyly ("claw deformity")
  - *T*elangiectasia (macular lesions) on the face, lips, palms, back of hands, and trunk
- Manifestations of progressive systemic sclerosis include the following:
  - Raynaud's phenomenon, often an early symptom, consisting of pain and a characteristic sequence of color changes of the distal fingers from white to purple to red in response to cold exposure
  - Diffuse involvement and symptoms secondary to the tightening of the skin, with difficulty in opening the mouth and loss of manual dexterity; later, contractures of the hands, painful fingertip ulcers resulting from vasculitis, and shortening of fingers resulting from distal bone resorption (Figure 25.40)
  - Esophageal dysfunction, dysphagia, bloating, and diarrhea
  - Systemic symptoms including shortness of breath, difficulty in swallowing, and arthralgia
  - Masklike facies
  - Possibly, rapid progression of kidney disease, reduced breathing capacity, cardiac disease, and renal failure

DIAGNOSIS

Morphea

- The diagnosis is generally made on clinical grounds and skin biopsy.
- The serologic examination is generally negative.

CREST Syndrome

- The diagnosis is generally made on clinical grounds.
- Positive anticentromere antibody is seen in 70% of patients.

Progressive Systemic Sclerosis
- The diagnosis is generally made on clinical grounds.
- Scl-70 is present in approximately 30% of patients.

 DIFFERENTIAL DIAGNOSIS

- Other connective tissue diseases
- Mixed connective tissue disease
- Overlap syndromes
- Lichen sclerosis

 MANAGEMENT

Localized Scleroderma
- Topical, intralesional, and systemic steroids may be helpful in the early inflammatory stage.
- Vitamin D analogues (calcitriol, calcipotriene), ultraviolet A, and methotrexate may also be of some benefit.

CREST Syndrome and Progressive Systemic Sclerosis
These conditions are difficult to treat and remain a great challenge. The following agents and approaches have been used with minimal success:

- The following drugs are currently under investigation for this indication: nifedipine, angiotensin-converting enzyme inhibitors, prostaglandins, immunosuppressive agents, D-penicillamine, colchicine, interferon-γ, and relaxin.
- Systemic steroids, minocycline, psoralen-ultraviolet A (PUVA), lung transplantation, autologous stem cell transplantation, etanercept, and thalidomide have also been used.

 POINT TO REMEMBER

- CREST syndrome has a more favorable prognosis than progressive systemic sclerosis, although visceral involvement may occur late in the course of the disease.

 HELPFUL HINTS

- Therapy of systemic scleroderma should include full range-of-motion exercises.
- Some evidence suggests that some European cases of morphea may result from *Borrelia burgdorferi* infection. This connection has not been demonstrated in the United States.

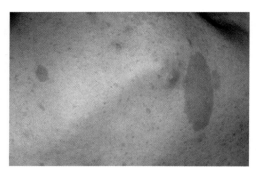

FIGURE 25.41 Neurofibromatosis 1. The multiple light brown, macules are *café au lait spots.*

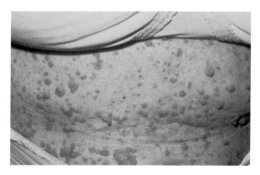

FIGURE 25.42 Neurofibromas 1. Soft, rubbery, flesh-colored papules and nodules are seen.

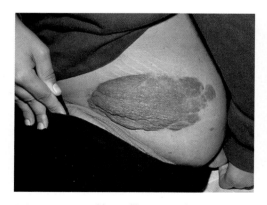

FIGURE 25.43 Neurofibromatosis 1. This plexiform neuroma feels like a "bag of worms."

Overview

Neurocutaneous diseases are genetically determined disorders showing both cutaneous and neurologic involvement.

NEUROFIBROMATOSIS

BASICS

- Neurofibromatosis (NF), or von Recklinghausen's disease, is an autosomally inherited disease in which macular pigmented skin lesions (*café au lait* spots) and skin tumors (neurofibromas) occur in patients in whom a wide range of CNS or spinal cord lesions may ultimately develop.
- The incidence of NF is 4 per 10,000 births. Fifty percent of cases are thought to be inherited in an autosomal dominant fashion; the remaining cases are the result of spontaneous new mutations.

There are two genetic types of NF:

- NF1 is caused by a mutation in a gene on chromosome 17q11.2. This gene has been isolated and encodes neurofibromin. This protein may act as a tumor-suppressor gene by binding to Ras protein.
- NF2, which is localized to chromosome 22q11, is characterized by bilateral acoustic neuromas and fewer skin manifestations. The protein for this gene has not been isolated, but it may also act as a tumor-suppressor gene.

DESCRIPTION OF LESIONS

- *Café au lait* spots are multiple, light brown, macules that are greater than 1 cm in diameter (Figure 25.41).
- Cutaneous neurofibromas are soft, rubbery, skin-colored, or tan, papules and nodules (Figure 25.42).
- Plexiform neuromas, manifesting as large, drooping tumors, which on palpation feel like a "bag of worms" (Figure 25.43).
- Axillary or inguinal freckling (Crowe's sign), consisting of small pigmented macules in some patients, is considered to be pathognomonic for NF1 (Figure 25.44).

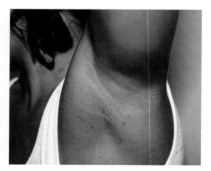

FIGURE 25.44 Neurofibromatosis 1. Crowe's sign (axillary "freckles") is considered pathognomonic for the disease.

DISTRIBUTION OF LESIONS

- *Café au lait* spots most often appear on the trunk and extremities.
- Neurofibromas may appear on the face, trunk, and extremities.

CLINICAL MANIFESTATIONS

- *Café au lait* spots are usually present at birth or shortly thereafter.
- Cutaneous neurofibromas may first develop in adolescence, and new lesions may continue to emerge during the patient's lifetime. Up to 5% of skin tumors may develop into neurofibrosarcomas.
- Ocular lesions *(Lisch nodules)* are asymptomatic, pigmented iris hamartomas seen in 80% of patients with NF.
- CNS tumors, optic gliomas, and spinal cord tumors may develop at any age.
- CNS involvement usually consists of benign lesions such as optic gliomas, acoustic neuromas, and meningiomas. CNS lesions may become astrocytomas.
- CNS involvement may occur in up to 10% of patients with NF.
- Spinal cord tumors may produce spinal cord damage and paraplegia.
- Many patients with NF have seizure disorders and mental retardation.
- Macrocephaly may be present in up to 16% of patients.
- Musculoskeletal disorders are uncommon, but pseudoarthrosis of the tibia and kyphoscoliosis may be diagnostic in some patients with NF.
- Gastrointestinal symptoms may occur in some patients in whom intussusception and obstruction of the small intestine develop from intraabdominal neurofibromas.
- Endocrine disorders occur; 3% to 5% of affected children have sexual precocity associated with short stature.
- Pheochromocytomas characterized by life-threatening severe hypertension occur in less than 1% of patients with NF.

DIAGNOSIS

- NF1: *Café au lait* spots are seen in 10% to 20% of the general population; however, six or more *café au lait* spots that are greater than 0.5 cm in diameter in infants or greater than 1 cm in diameter in adults are supportive of the diagnosis of NF1.
- A first-degree relative with NF1 supports the diagnosis.

Other findings that are supportive of the diagnosis include the following:

Neurofibromatosis 1
- Crowe's sign
- Lisch nodules
- Distinctive osseous lesions such as sphenoid dysplasia or thinning of long bone cortex

Neurofibromatosis 2
- Bilateral masses of the eighth cranial nerve (acoustic neuromas)
- A first-degree relative with NF2

Laboratory Evaluations

- Skin biopsies of *café au lait* macules may show macromelanosomes on electron microscopy, but these findings are not diagnostic.
- Biopsies of neurofibromas show characteristic Schwann cells and neuronal cells.
- Magnetic resonance imaging studies of the brain and cervical spine may be helpful in NF1 patients with symptoms of CNS disease and in patients with suspected NF2 disease.

 DIFFERENTIAL DIAGNOSIS

Segmental Neurofibromatosis

- *Café au lait* macules localized to one area of the body
- Cutaneous localized neurofibromas
- Absence of CNS tumors
- Lack of inheritance (somatic mutation)

McCune–Albright Syndrome

- Pigmented macular lesions
- Polyostotic fibrous dysplasia
- Precocious puberty

 MANAGEMENT

- Surgical removal of symptomatic or disfiguring neurofibromas
- Follow-up for the development of neurofibrosarcomas, optic gliomas, acoustic neuromas, and pheochromocytomas
- Genetic counseling for patients and their families

TUBEROUS SCLEROSIS

BASICS

Tuberous sclerosis (TS; *Bourneville's disease*) is a disease in which cutaneous lesions may be seen in association with hamartomatous tumors of the CNS as well as other organs. The classic triad of TS includes the following:

- Adenoma sebaceum
- Epilepsy
- Mental retardation, although at least 50% of affected persons show no evidence of mental retardation

TS, which is inherited in an autosomal dominant fashion, is found in less than 1 per 10,000 births. Two genetic loci have been identified. The first gene *(TSC1)* is on chromosome q34 and produces tuberin. The second gene *(TSC2)* is on chromosome 16p13 and produces a second protein, hamartin. Tuberin and hamartin are thought to act together to regulate cell differentiation and proliferation. Defects in these gene products may result in the growth of multiple hamartomas in TS.

DESCRIPTION OF LESIONS

- Ash-leaf macules are hypopigmented, characteristically oval, and sometimes linear or "confetti-shaped" macular lesions.
- So-called adenoma sebaceum (actually angiofibromas) are pink to reddish brown, dome-shaped papules (Figure 25.45).
- Periungual fibromas *(Koenen's tumors)* are smooth, firm, skin-colored papules.
- A pebbly, skin-colored *"peau d'orange"* or "pigskinlike" dermal plaque ("shagreen patch") has fine hypopigmentation resembling confetti.

DISTRIBUTION OF LESIONS

- Ash-leaf spots are more common on the trunk and proximal extremities.
- Adenoma sebaceum papules are symmetric in distribution and are most commonly located on the nose, nasolabial folds, and cheeks. More widespread distribution involves the forehead, ears, and scalp.
- Periungual fibromas occur around and under the nails on the periungual areas of the fingers and toes (Figure 25.46).
- "Shagreen patches" appear on the trunk, most often in the lumbosacral region.

CLINICAL MANIFESTATIONS

- Ash-leaf macules and "shagreen patches" are usually present at birth.
- Adenoma sebaceum may begin to develop in late childhood and adolescence.

Central Nervous System Lesions
- Gliomatous brain tumors (tubers), which may calcify in 50% of patients
- Seizure disorders in 60% to 70% of patients, with less than 50% showing evidence of mental retardation
- Retinal and optic nerve gliomas

Other Findings
- In 50% to 60% of patients, cardiac rhabdomyomas of the atrium, which rarely cause cardiac obstructive disease
- Renal hamartomas
- In about 15% of patients, renal tumors (angiomyolipomas) and polycystic kidneys, which must be differentiated from renal carcinoma
- Gastrointestinal tumors with microhamartomatous polyps of the rectum
- Possible bone cyst formation and periosteal new bone growth and sclerosis

DIAGNOSIS

Two major or one major and two minor criteria are necessary for a definite diagnosis of TS.

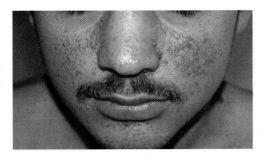

FIGURE 25.45 Tuberous sclerosis. This patient has adenoma sebaceum (angiofibromas). Note the similarity to acne lesions.

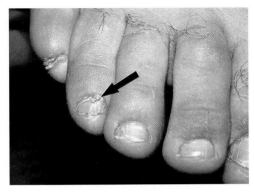

FIGURE 25.46 Tuberous sclerosis. Periungual fibromas (Koenen's tumors) are noted.

Major Diagnostic Criteria

1. Adenoma sebaceum
2. Hypopigmented ash-leaf macules (three or more)
3. Shagreen patch
4. Periungual fibroma
5. Cortical tuber
6. Cardiac rhabdomyosarcoma
7. Subependymal nodule
8. Subependymal giant cell astrocytoma
9. Lymphangiomatosis
10. Renal angiolipoma

Laboratory Evaluations

- Cranial magnetic resonance imaging
- Posteroanterior and lateral skull films (for adults) to demonstrate calcifications of gliomas of the brain
- Echocardiography for rhabdomyomas
- Renal ultrasonograms to search for tumors
- Skin biopsy of cutaneous lesions

Minor Diagnostic Criteria

1. Multiple dental enamel pits
2. Hamartomatous rectal polyp
3. Bone cyst
4. Gingival fibroma
5. Nonrenal hamartoma
6. Retinal achromic patch
7. Confetti skin lesions: fine, hypopigmented macules (2 to 4 mm) that look as though they are "sprinkled" on the lower legs
8. Multiple renal cysts

 DIFFERENTIAL DIAGNOSIS OF ADENOMA SEBACEUM

Acneiform Papules

- They often resemble adenoma sebaceum.
- Acne has a waxing and waning course.
- A skin biopsy is necessary only if the diagnosis is in doubt.

MANAGEMENT

- Follow-up of infants with ash-leaf spots to monitor the development of seizure disorder or mental retardation
- Follow-up of patients with TS to monitor the development of cardiac or renal lesions
- Removal of cosmetically objectionable or disfiguring adenoma sebaceum by excision, electrocautery, dermabrasion, or laser resurfacing
- Surgical removal of painful periungual fibromas
- Genetic counseling of patients with TS and their families after computed tomographic scanning is performed on the parents and siblings of the affected patient (these studies have demonstrated CNS lesions in asymptomatic parents of TS patients)

PART THREE
Dermatologic Procedures

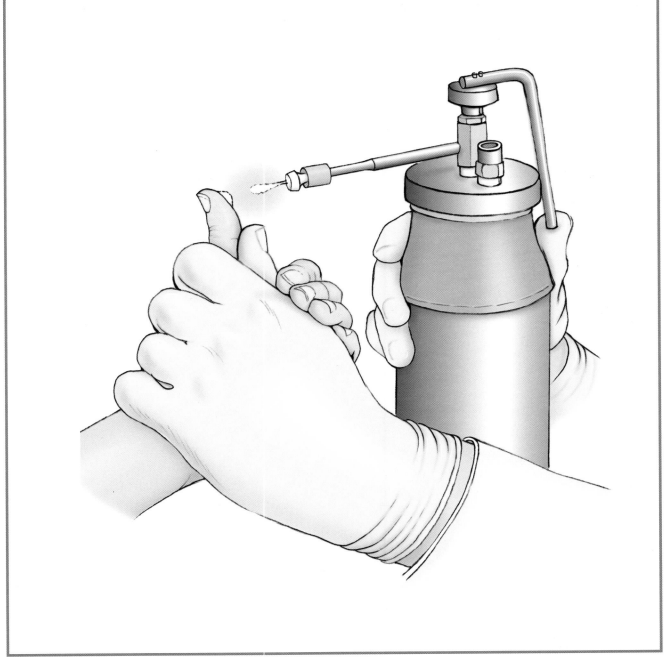

Basic Dermatologic Procedures

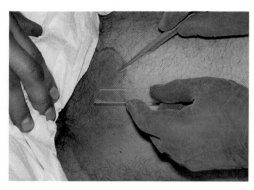

FIGURE 26.1 Potassium hydroxide examination. Collection of scale from the "active" border of a lesion.

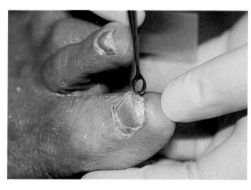

FIGURE 26.2 Potassium hydroxide examination. Collection of scale from under the nail after trimming.

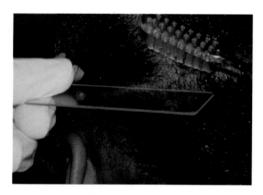

FIGURE 26.3 Potassium hydroxide examination. Collection of scale from the scalp of a child using a toothbrush.

BASICS

- The potassium hydroxide (KOH) examination has the advantage of providing an immediate diagnosis of a superficial fungal infection, rather than waiting weeks for the results of a fungal culture.
- It is a simple, rapid method to detect fungal elements from skin, nails, and hair.

HOW TO PERFORM A KOH TEST

Collection of Specimen
- Collection is optimally performed when no surface artifacts (e.g., topical medications) are present.

Skin
Gently scrape scale from the "active border" with a No. 15 scalpel blade (Figure 26.1).

Nails
Trim the nail. Use a No. 15 scalpel blade or a 1- to 2-mm curette (Figure 26.2) under the nail surface to obtain scale.

Hair
Pluck broken hairs with forceps or use a toothbrush to obtain scale and hairs (Figure 26.3).

Preparation
- A KOH solution such as Swartz–Lamkins Fungal Stain or a KOH solution with dimethyl sulfoxide is used.
- A thin layer of scale or scale plus hair is gathered on the slide and is covered with a coverslip.
- With an eyedropper, a single drop of a KOH solution is placed at the edge of the coverslip and is allowed to spread under the coverslip by capillary action (Figure 26.4).
- The under surface of the slide is heated gently with a lighter or a match until bubbling begins.
- Excess KOH solution is blotted with tissue paper held at the edge of the coverslip.

Observation
- Examine under low light intensity (condenser down).
- Begin with a low-power scan to identify scale and possibly hyphae.
- Become aware of artifacts that are easily confused with hyphae and spores, such as hairs, clothing fibers, keratinocyte cell borders, and air bubbles (Figure 26.5).
- Use high power to confirm the presence of hyphae or spores (Figures 26.6 to 26.11).

Culture
- Fungal cultures are placed on Sabouraud's agar or on Dermatophyte Test Medium and are incubated for 1 to 4 weeks (Figure 26.12).
- Clinical Laboratory Improvement Act guidelines may require the practitioner to use outside laboratory facilities for conducting fungal cultures.

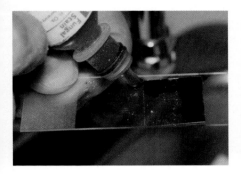

FIGURE 26.4 Potassium hydroxide examination. A single drop of a KOH solution is placed at the edge of the coverslip.

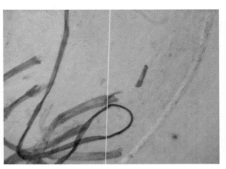

FIGURE 26.5 Potassium hydroxide examination. Artifacts. Note the clothing fibers on the *left* and the single hair shaft on the *right*.

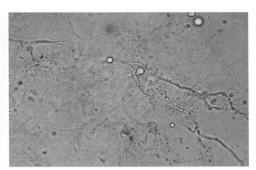

FIGURE 26.6 Potassium hydroxide examination. Dermatophyte. Note the wavy-branched hyphae with uniform widths coursing over cell borders.

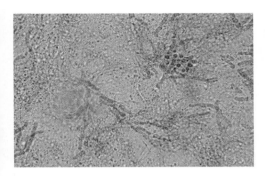

FIGURE 26.7 Potassium hydroxide examination. Tinea versicolor. Note the short, stubby hyphae ("spaghetti") and the clusters of spores ("meatballs").

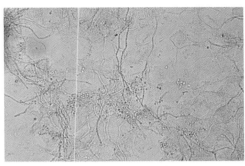

FIGURE 26.8 Potassium hydroxide examination. *Candida.* Spores and pseudohyphae (spores lack septae).

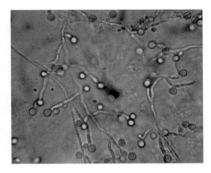

FIGURE 26.9 Potassium hydroxide examination. *Candida.* Pseudohyphae with budding spores (higher magnification).

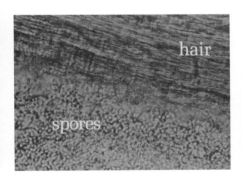

FIGURE 26.10 Potassium hydroxide examination. Ectothrix. Note the spores *outside* the hair shaft.

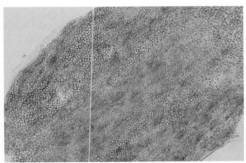

FIGURE 26.11 Potassium hydroxide examination. Endothrix. Note spores inside the hair shaft ("sack of marbles").

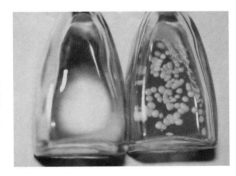

FIGURE 26.12 Fungal culture using the Dermatophyte Test Medium. Note the positive result on the *left* as indicated by the color change from yellow to red and the monomorphic colony growth. On the *right* are discrete mucoid growths of a yeast contaminant, despite the false-positive color change to red.

BASICS

- Various skin biopsy techniques are available to the practitioner: shave biopsy, scissor or snip biopsy, punch biopsy, and excisional biopsy. The surgical tools and approaches vary according to size, shape, depth, and site of a lesion.
- Obtaining the appropriate amount of tissue sample that will provide adequate information about the disease is the most important factor to keep in mind when deciding on the proper biopsy technique.
- The biopsy specimen site should not be chosen indiscriminately. The site should be evaluated according to the clinical impression, the lesion's location, the estimated depth of the pathologic process, the planned tissue studies, and the ensuing cosmetic result. The choice of biopsy technique requires some knowledge of where the pathologic process is likely to be located.

Local Anesthesia

Methods to decrease pain caused by injections include the following:

- Use a small, 30-gauge needle.
- Add a buffer (sodium bicarbonate) to the lidocaine.
- Inject very slowly.
- Distract the patient by talking continuously.
- Minimize the number of injection sites by reinjecting into areas that are already numb.

SHAVE BIOPSY AND SHAVE REMOVAL

BASICS

- This is used for the diagnosis and therapeutic removal of superficial (epidermal and upper dermal) skin lesions, such as melanocytic nevi, warts, seborrheic and solar keratoses, pyogenic granulomas, and skin tags, as well as other benign and malignant skin tumors.
- It is used to obtain biopsy specimens to confirm skin disease before a more definitive surgical procedure (e.g., basal or squamous cell carcinoma).
- It is very useful for flattening and diagnosing nevi, particularly in the facial area.

Advantages
- It is fast and economical.
- The technique is easy to learn.
- Wound care is simple.
- Cosmetic results are generally excellent.
- No sutures are used.
- It is useful for difficult to reach sites (e.g., ear canal, orbit of the eye).
- It is useful in areas of poor healing (e.g., the lower leg in elderly or diabetic patients).

Disadvantages
- It is not indicated for lesions that extend into the fat layer.
- It is not indicated when a full-thickness biopsy is necessary (e.g., inflammatory dermatoses).
- It should not be performed on lesions suspected of being melanoma because of the difficulty in clinically determining the maximum thickness or extent of a lesion.

TECHNIQUE

- The area adjacent to the lesion is anesthetized with an injection into the superficial dermis with a 1% plain lidocaine using a 30-gauge needle. If necessary, epinephrine in a 1:100,000 or 1:200,000 dilution can be used. Lidocaine without epinephrine should be used in finger and toe areas, to avoid vascular compromise.
- Local anesthesia with lidocaine creates a wheal and elevates the lesion above the surrounding skin (Figure 26.13).
- Applying traction with the thumb and index finger of the free hand on either side of the lesion stabilizes it.
- A No.15 scalpel blade is placed flat on the skin; used in a slight sawing motion with smooth strokes parallel to the skin surface, the middle of the blade is drawn through the lesion (Figure 26.14).
- Traction is released when the lesion becomes sufficiently free; small forceps with teeth are used to hold and elevate the lesion to complete the "shave" and then to deliver it to a bottle of formalin.
- Jagged edges can be "feathered" with electrocautery or further shaving.
- Hemostasis may be rapidly achieved with the use of Monsel's solution (ferric subsulfate) applied with a cotton pledget (Q-Tip). Hemostasis is possible only if the field is wiped dry of blood.
- All pigmented lesions should be sent to a pathologist; nonpigmented skin tags do not need to be sent for pathologic evaluation.

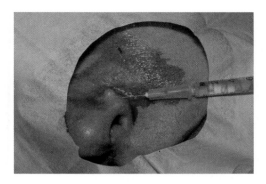

FIGURE 26.13 Shave biopsy. Local anesthesia creates a wheal that elevates the lesion above the surrounding skin.

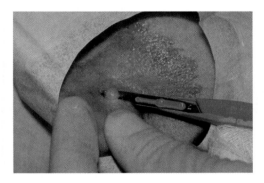

FIGURE 26.14 Shave biopsy. The lesion is stabilized with the free hand; the blade, which is parallel to the skin surface, is drawn through the lesion.

SCISSOR (SNIP) BIOPSY AND SNIP EXCISION

BASICS

- Various lesions can be removed from the skin in a short period of time.
- Certain elevated or pedunculated lesions, such as warts, nevi, seborrheic keratoses, and skin tags, are ideally suited for removal with scissors. Many can be precisely removed level to the skin.

Advantages
- It is fast, many lesions can be removed in one visit, and it is economical.
- It frequently can be done without anesthesia.

Disadvantages
- None exist, except for the possibility of obtaining an inadequate amount of tissue if a specimen is to be sent for histopathologic examination.

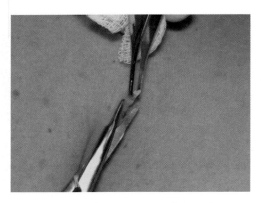

FIGURE 26.15 Snip excision. This filiform wart is snipped off after having been anesthetized with lidocaine.

TECHNIQUE

- Thin, small lesions may be snipped off without any anesthesia; larger lesions require the administration of local anesthesia. The area of larger lesions may be anesthetized in the same manner as for scalpel shave excisions.
- The lesion is gently held with small forceps without teeth and is pulled to cause slight tenting of the epidermis and upper dermis (Figure 26.15).
- Straight or curved sharp iris scissors with fine points may be used to snip off the lesion.
- The base of the lesion may be lightly electrodesiccated, or a styptic (e.g., Monsel's solution) may be applied to cause hemostasis (stinging or burning may result if lesion has not been anesthetized). Local pressure also is effective in preventing blood flow.
- A slight elevation or irregularity of the margin is easily trimmed away with scissors.

PUNCH BIOPSY

BASICS

- A punch biopsy is performed by using a 3- to 5-mm cylindric cutting instrument ("punch") to remove all or part of a lesion.
- This method is most useful for biopsy of relatively flat, inflammatory lesions such as seen in psoriasis, lichen planus, and vasculitis.

Advantages
- The specimen obtained is uniform.
- This is an effective method to evaluate inflammatory skin diseases.
- It is an efficient biopsy method for full-thickness skin.
- The operative site heals rapidly.
- Skin closure establishes a barrier to infection almost immediately after the procedure.

Disadvantages
- The sample may not adequately show the entire lesion; a second technique (i.e., an elliptic biopsy) may be necessary for adequate demonstration of tumor architecture.
- It is not suited for lesions primarily located in the subcutaneous tissue.
- Areas to be avoided are the digits, around the facial nerve, or in any region where the operator is unfamiliar with the underlying anatomy.

TECHNIQUE

- In contrast to shave biopsy, a more thorough approach to sterile technique is necessary.
- The lesion and surrounding skin is cleansed with 70% isopropyl alcohol, povidone-iodine (Betadine), or chlorhexidine (Hibiclens).
- The area is then anesthetized with an injection into the deep dermis with 1% plain lidocaine using a 30-gauge needle. If necessary, epinephrine in a 1:100,000 or 1:200,000 dilution can be used (Figure 26.16).
- With the fingers of the nondominant hand, the skin is stretched at a 90° angle to the natural wrinkle lines.

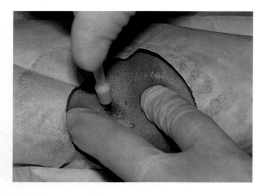

FIGURE 26.16 Punch biopsy. Traction of surrounding skin is performed with fingers while the punch is rotated.

- The punch is held between the thumb and forefinger.
- The punch is then gently pushed downward into the dermis, while being advanced slowly and twirled back and forth until it "gives." Caution should be used over thin tissue or over vital structures.
- It is important to push the punch deep enough to obtain underlying fat tissue for an adequate sample.
- The punch is then withdrawn along with the tissue sample. If the sample does not come out with the punch, it may be cut at the base while depressing the surrounding skin.
- The tissue specimen is removed with forceps with teeth and then the specimen is cut, if necessary, with iris scissors. Care must be taken to avoid crushing the specimen and distorting the tissue sample.
- Firm pressure is placed on the circular skin wound to curtail bleeding.
- A single suture for closure is all that is usually necessary.

SIMPLE PUNCH BIOPSY METHOD TO REMOVE CYSTS

A large lesion such as an epidermoid or pilar cyst can be removed through a small hole and heals with excellent aesthetic results. If the results of this procedure are not completely satisfactory, a standard excision can be performed at a future date.

TECHNIQUE

- Local anesthesia is administered superficially over the cyst (Figure 26.17A).
- The center of the cyst (the "pore") is punched with a 4-, 6-, or 8-mm disposable punch (Figure 26.17B).
- The cyst wall is dissected using forceps, iris scissors, and manual pressure around the cyst (Figure 26.17C and D).
- The defect is closed with a 4-0 nylon stitch.

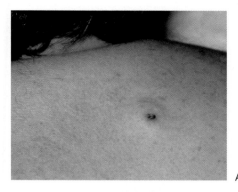

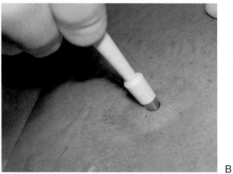

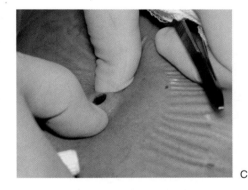

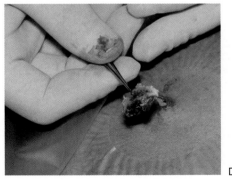

FIGURE 26.17 *A:* Punch biopsy removal of a cyst. This epidermoid cyst has a central "pore." *B:* A 6-mm disposable punch creates an opening. *C:* After dissection with iris scissors, pressure is exerted with the operator's thumbs. *D:* The cyst wall is extracted.

BASICS

- **Excisions** are used for obtaining tissue samples for biopsy specimens and for the removal of many benign and cancerous lesions.
- Excisional biopsies may be performed on discrete lesions, such as cysts, basal or squamous cell carcinoma, malignant melanoma, or other solitary tumors and nevi.
- An **incisional biopsy** is the incomplete or partial removal of a lesion that may be too big or poorly located to perform a complete excision (e.g., a suspected melanoma that is too large to remove).

Advantages
- It provides a more extensive tissue sample of a lesion that is too large for a shave or a punch biopsy.
- The margins of submitted tissue can be examined for possible involvement (e.g., basal cell carcinoma, squamous cell carcinoma and melanoma).
- It often affords a definitive cure for many benign and malignant lesions.

Disadvantages
- It is time-consuming and is less economical than shaves or snips.
- It usually requires a return visit for suture removal.

TECHNIQUE

- The operator should be familiar with the underlying and surrounding anatomy.
- A thorough approach to sterile technique is necessary: sterile gloves and sterile drapes should be used.
- The best cosmetic results are achieved by placing the lines of incision in or parallel to the relaxed skin tension lines. This placement is demonstrated by observing wrinkle lines and the effect of pinching the skin.
- Once a direction for the long axis of the ellipse is decided, the ellipse should be drawn around the lesion before a local anesthetic is administered. This approach minimizes tissue distortion, which may cause difficulty in subsequent planning of the ellipse. A gentian violet or surgical skin marker can be used to mark the skin.
- The excision should have a length-to-width ratio of at least 3:1, and the apices should have a 30° angle.
- The area is anesthetized by local infiltration with lidocaine and epinephrine 1:100,000.
- A No. 15 scalpel blade can be used to make the incision. The scalpel is held in the clinician's dominant hand with the index finger and thumb of the other hand placed on either side of the incision. This pushes the skin under tension downward and away from the scalpel (Figure 26.18A).
- The incision should be started using the point of the scalpel, held in a vertical position, at the apex of the ellipse (Figure 26.18B). The belly of the scalpel then should be used along the side of the ellipse as the incision is elongated.
- The scalpel should cut through the full thickness of the skin, including the upper subcutaneous fat, to obtain an optimal tissue sample for histologic examination.

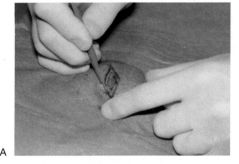

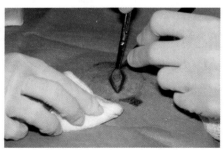

FIGURE 26.18 *A:* Excision. The incision is started using the point of the scalpel, held in a vertical position, at the apex of the lesion. Traction is accomplished with the nondominant hand. *B:* The tissue is dissected free of the underlying fat. Forceps are used to hold the apex of the skin being removed.

- The tissue is dissected free of the underlying fat after incisions have been made on both sides of the ellipse. Forceps with teeth can be used to hold the apex of the skin being removed.
- If the defect is large, the ellipse is dissected (undermined) by using curved, blunt-tipped scissors (e.g., Steven's tenectomy or Gradle scissors), making certain that the plane of the dissection is at the same level throughout. Undermining allows for the mobilization of tissue so that it can be advanced to close the defect; it also allows skin edges to come together with less tension and allows eversion of the wound edges with suturing.

UNDERMINING TECHNIQUE (FIGURE 26.18C)

- Undermining is performed using blunt-tipped scissors while the skin edge is elevated by forceps with teeth or a skin hook.
- Scissors are advanced to the desired degree and are opened to stretch the underlying skin. If necessary, this procedure is repeated several times to achieve the desired skin mobility for wound closure.
- Any remaining tissue septa should be removed using the open blades of the scissors.
- Undermining is most effective when performed at the level of superficial fat tissue. This reduces the possibility of injury to nerves and blood vessels in the facial and neck areas.
- Wound repair is facilitated if an adequate ellipse has been formed and the edges are perpendicular to the skin and skin lines are followed.
- Meticulous hemostasis must result after undermining. This is achieved by direct pressure or electrocoagulation (Figure 26.18D).
- Subcutaneous sutures may be placed after undermining, to allow the edges of the wound to be approximated to close the wound (Figure 26.18E).

WOUND CLOSURE

- Wounds should be closed in layers.
- The closure of dead space is necessary when large, subcutaneous vacuities have been created, such as after removal of subcutaneous cysts.
- Dermal, buried sutures are important on areas of the body that overlie large muscle groups, such as the upper trunk.

Suture Material
- Hemostasis (a "dry field") should be obtained before initiating wound closure.
- Choice of suture material depends on the size and degree of tension on the wound and the area of placement.
- For facial or limb areas, Vicryl or Dexon sutures are suitable for proper wound closure; 5-0 or 6-0 synthetic (Prolene or Ethilon) sutures are recommended for the face.
- On the upper trunk, greater skin support is required for proper wound closure. Therefore, Maxon or PDS sutures are recommended; 3-0 or 4-0 are preferred.

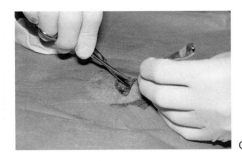

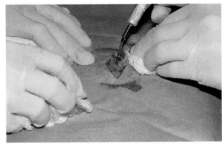

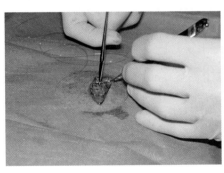

FIGURE 26.18 *C:* Undermining is performed using blunt-tipped scissors while the skin edge is elevated by forceps. *D:* Hemostasis is achieved with an electrocautery device. *E:* Deeper, nonabsorbable sutures are used to approximate the wound edges.

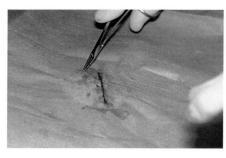

F

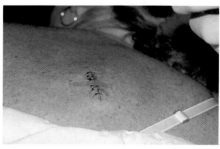

G

FIGURE 26.18 *F:* Closure. Interrupted skin sutures are placed using the method of "halving." The first suture was placed in the center of the ellipse. *G:* Dressing. A transparent dressing overlying Steri-Strips allows for visualization of the wound as it heals.

Suturing

- Simple, interrupted skin sutures are most commonly used in this procedure.
- The method of "halving" is the most effective technique for wound closure. "Halving" allows for equal distribution of wound tension (Figure 26.18F).
- The first suture is placed in the center of the ellipse.
- The second and third sutures are placed in the centers of the remaining wound lengths.
- This procedure is repeated until the wound is completely closed.
- Suture removal depends on wound tension, area of location, and depth of placement.
- Generally, facial sutures may be removed in 5 days; sutures in the trunk and extremities are removed in 1 to 2 weeks.

WOUND CARE AND HEALING

- Infections after simple skin surgery are unusual.
- Administration of systemic antibiotics is generally unnecessary.
- Meticulous hemostasis during surgery is essential.
- Small amounts of necrosis normally occur in wound healing.
- Hemostasis induced by electrosurgery, suture ligature, or cautery always produces tissue necrosis.
- Wound healing is delayed when necrosis is extensive.
- Hemostasis can be achieved with a pressure dressing, which is applied for 24 hours.
- When wounds are closed with a considerable amount of tension or if the patient has been taking steroids, the wound should be closed with sutures that are nonabsorbable and buried (nylon or Prolene) or have prolonged tensile strength (PDS, Dexon, Vicryl). Under the former conditions, skin sutures may be left in place for longer periods of time.
- External splinting using tape provides additional support until the tensile strength of the wound increases after suture removal.
- Exercise that stretches the skin should be avoided to minimize spreading of the scar.

DRESSINGS AND WOUND MANAGEMENT

- For small ellipses, dry, sterile gauze covered with paper tape may be all that is necessary.
- An occlusive dressing (a perforated plastic film or sheet with an absorbable pad) or pressure dressing should be applied, if necessary, to prevent postoperative bleeding (Figure 26.18G.)
- After 24 hours, the patient can remove the dressing and compress the wound with tap water or hydrogen peroxide. The hydrogen peroxide mechanically softens the wound and removes any debris.
- A topical antibiotic such as bacitracin is applied to the surface of the wound before applying a clean, occlusive dressing.
- Patients repeat this procedure daily at home until the wound is covered with fresh epidermis.
- Patients are advised to return for follow-up if there is any pain, swelling, tenderness, purulent drainage, discharge, or bleeding of the wound.
- Postoperative pain usually is negligible, and patients are advised to call the surgeon should any pain occur.

BASICS

- Electrodesiccation and curettage is a method to remove or destroy many types of benign superficial skin lesions such as warts, seborrheic keratoses, solar keratoses, pyogenic granulomas, and skin tags. In experienced hands, it is often used as a method to treat skin cancers such as small basal cell and squamous cell carcinomas.
- Electrodesiccation uses monopolar high-frequency electric currents to destroy lesions; curettage is a scraping or scooping technique performed with a dermal curette, which has a round or oval sharp ring.
- Electrodesiccation without curettage (as an alternative to shave procedures) is often used to eliminate warts, skin tags, and spider angiomas and to flatten lesions (e.g., melanocytic nevi).
- Conversely, curettage without electrodesiccation may also be used to remove many of these epidermal lesions.
- Curettage is a blind technique in which the specimen cannot be examined for margin control.

Advantages
- It is fast and economical.
- It is useful for difficult-to-reach sites—ear canal, orbit of the eye.
- It is useful in areas of poor healing—the lower leg in elderly or diabetic patients.
- Secondary infection is uncommon.

Disadvantages
- The procedure is "blind"; margins of lesions can only be guessed.
- Cosmetic results are unpredictable; hypopigmentation and scarring may result.
- Healing is by secondary intention and takes 2 to 3 weeks, which is longer than healing after an excisional procedure.
- Biopsy specimens obtained from curettage are discouraged.

CURETTAGE

TECHNIQUE

- The area to be biopsied is anesthetized in a similar manner described earlier (see "Shave Biopsy and Shave Removal").
- The local anesthetic creates a wheal and elevates the lesion above the surrounding skin.
- Applying traction with the thumb and index finger of the free hand on either side of the lesion stabilizes it and keeps it taut.
- A sharp curette is held like a pencil and is drawn through the tissue with strokes pushed away from the surgeon with the thumb until an adequate amount of tissue is removed (usually when the dermis is reached) (Figure 26.19).
- Hemostasis is obtained with the use of Monsel's solution after wiping the field dry of blood.

ELECTRODESICCATION

Electrodesiccation may be used before or after curettage or used alone. It causes superficial destruction with a charring of the skin.

TECHNIQUE

- This procedure is performed after local anesthesia has been administered.
- The lowest possible setting should be used to prevent unnecessary tissue destruction.

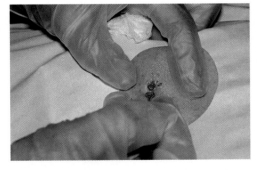

FIGURE 26.19 Curettage. Note the traction exerted by the operator's fingers.

BASICS

- Cryosurgery entails the destruction of tissue by freezing in a controlled manner, to produce sharply circumscribed necrosis. Tissue destruction results from intercellular and extracellular ice formation, denaturing liquid protein complexes, and cell dehydration. A repeat freeze–thaw cycle results in more cellular damage than a single cycle.
- Liquid nitrogen (LN_2) at $-195.8°C$ is the standard agent that is used. It is applied with a cotton swab, a cryospray gun, or a cryoprobe, and it is stored in a special vacuum container.
- Cryosurgery should be used only when a confident, clinical diagnosis is made.
- It is most commonly used on warts and solar keratoses.

Advantages

- Cryosurgery is an inexpensive, rapid, and simple technique that does not require complicated apparatus.
- Anesthesia is usually not necessary.
- Postoperative pain is minimal.
- Bleeding is not a problem during or after treatment.
- Sutures are not necessary, and scarring is generally minimal or absent.
- It is a relatively risk-free treatment for the cryosurgeon who treats some skin conditions in patients who are human immunodeficiency virus positive. These include patients with molluscum contagiosum, condylomata acuminatum, Kaposi's sarcoma, and warts.

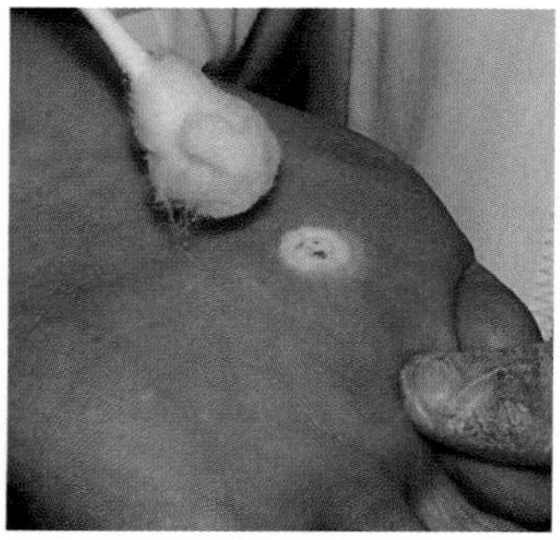

Disadvantages

- Cryosurgery is not well tolerated by very young children.
- Scarring may occur, particularly if lesions are overzealously frozen or if the patient tends to heal with hypertrophic scars or keloids.
- Postinflammatory pigmentary alterations may occur; more often, hypopigmentation will result because of the destruction of melanocytes.

TECHNIQUE

Cotton Tip Applicator Technique

- Place LN_2 in a Styrofoam cup.
- Dip a cotton swab into the cup.
- Touch the lesion with the saturated cotton-tipped applicator, with a minimal amount of pressure, and create a 2- to 3-mm zone of freeze around the lesion for a total of 4 to 5 seconds (Figure 26.20).
- The skin will turn white. Care must be taken to avoid dripping onto surrounding, normal skin.

Cryospray Technique

- A handheld cryogun, which operates under a working pressure of approximately 6 psi, is the standard instrument. Nozzle attachments with apertures of varying diameter for spray application are available (the "A" nozzle applies the greatest amount of spray; the "D" has the least amount for delicate work) (Figure 26.21).
- Local anesthesia is generally not required.

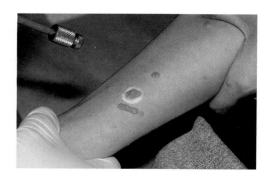

FIGURE 26.20 Cryosurgery. Liquid nitrogen is applied with a cotton pledget.

FIGURE 26.21 Cryosurgery. Here liquid nitrogen is delivered with a cryospray gun. Note the 2- to 3-mm zone of freeze around the lesion.

- For smaller lesions, this procedure is done by treating the center of the lesion and allowing the freeze to spread laterally.
- The time of application varies, depending on the thickness of the lesion.
- Standardization of freeze times is difficult to categorize for the treatment of benign and premalignant lesions. The goal is to produce, with either the swab or spray technique, a solid ice ball that extends 2 mm onto normal skin.

Postoperative Course and Wound Care
- Mild to moderate swelling may develop at the lesion site.
- A blister or blood blister may form within 24 hours and resolves in 2 to 7 days (Figure 26.22)
- The lesion site may be cleansed with soap and water during the exudative stage.
- The lesion site starts to dry at the end of the exudative stage and will then slough.
- A crust, which loosens spontaneously, commonly occurs.

HELPFUL HINTS

- It is best to underfreeze lesions; they can be retreated at a later date.
- For anxious children, a topical anesthetic such as EMLA cream (eutectic mixture of local anesthetics) can be applied under occlusion 1 hour before cryosurgery to decrease the discomfort associated with the procedure.
- Alternative delivery methods that can help to minimize pain are shown in Figures 26.23 and 26.24.

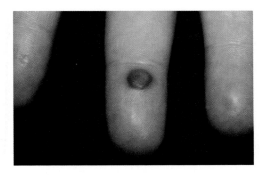

FIGURE 26.22 Cryosurgery. Note the wart on the surface of a hemorrhagic blister that appeared 24 hours after treatment.

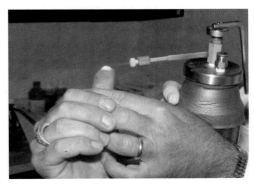

FIGURE 26.23 Cryosurgery. Application with a cryogun apparatus (freezing the lesion at a right angle may lessen the pain).

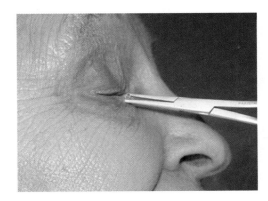

FIGURE 26.24 Cryosurgery. Treatment of a cutaneous horn with a hemostat that has been immersed for 30 seconds in liquid nitrogen. This simple, relatively painless procedure causes very little collateral damage to the surrounding skin.

Patient Handouts

Appendix A provides patient handouts in English and Spanish. The Spanish translation of the English patient handout is located on the back of the English version. English headings are boxed in red, and Spanish headings are boxed in green.

Apéndice A provee informes para el paciente en inglés y en español. La traducción en español se encuentra al reverso del inglés. Los capítulos españoles se dibujan en cajas verdes y los capítulos ingleses se dibujan en cajas rojas.

The patient handouts may be photocopied directly from the book and given to individual patients as necessary.

INFORMATION AND INSTRUCTIONS FOR ACNE PATIENTS

- Acne is the most common skin problem for teenagers; however, it is not limited to that age group. Acne can begin before adolescence in both boys and girls, or it can begin in adulthood (especially in women).
- Acne usually runs in families. It is caused by the reaction of the skin's oil glands to sex hormones. Patients with acne usually have normal levels of these hormones. However, their oil glands are more sensitive to those hormones, and this sensitivity sometimes causes increased amounts of oil. Also, certain bacteria beneath the skin that act on the oil form irritating substances. When the openings to the oil glands become clogged, these irritating substances lead to the formation of blackheads, whiteheads, pimples, or acne cysts.
- Acne can be aggravated by numerous things. Emotional stress may worsen acne, and women often "break out" before their menstrual cycle.
- Picking or squeezing of pimples is damaging and can lead to scars.

ACNE MYTHS AND ACNE FACTS

Myth: Frequent facials are beneficial.

Fact: Professional facials and at-home scrubs, astringents, and masks are generally not recommended because they tend to aggravate acne.

Myth: Cosmetics, particularly oil-based preparations, "clog pores" and cause acne.

Fact: Cosmetics probably pose much less of a problem to women's skin than previously thought. Cosmetic use, rarely, if ever, causes acne. More commonly, however, cosmetics can be irritants and may cause contact dermatitis.

Myth: Acne should disappear by the end of adolescence.

Fact: Some people have acne that persists well beyond their adolescence. Some women may even develop their first bout of acne in their 20s or 30s.

Myth: Acne is caused or worsened by certain foods, such as chocolate, sweets, and greasy junk food.

Fact: Despite myths, acne is probably not significantly influenced by diet.

Myth: Oily skin causes acne.

Fact: Oily skin is more often a result of acne, which increases oil gland activity, rather than the main cause of acne.

Myth: A dirty face worsens acne; therefore, scrubbing the face daily will help to clear it up.

Fact: Scrubbing and rubbing a face that has acne, particularly inflammatory acne, will only serve to irritate and redden an already inflamed complexion. Instead, the face should be washed daily with a gentle cleanser.

The treatments described on the next page are used to **control** acne, not cure it! Be patient . . . and don't expect results overnight!

- Acné es el problema de piel más común en adolescentes; sin embargo, no solo se observa en este grupo. El acné puede comenzar antes de la adolescencia en varones y hembras, o puede comenzar en edad adulta (especialmente en mujeres).
- El acné se ve usualmente en varios miembros de una familia. Es causado por la reacción de las glándulas sebaceas de la piel ante las hormonas sexuales. Los pacientes con acné usualmente tienen niveles normales de dichas hormonas. Sin embargo, las glandulas sebáceas son más sensibles a dichas hormonas lo cual resulta en excesiva producción de sebo. Asi mismo, bacterias de la piel actúan sobre el sebo produciendo substancias irritantes. Cuando los poros de las glándulas sebáceas se ocluyen, estas substancias irritantes conducen a la formación de espinillas, granos y quistes.
- El acné se agrava por varias causas. El estrés emocional puede empeorar el acné, y muchas mujeres notan aparición de acné antes de su período menstrual.
- Tratar de exprimir o remover con las manos lesiones de acné es prejudicial y puede resultar en cicatrices.

MITOS Y REALIDADES DEL ACNÉ

Mito: Frecuentes tratamientos faciales son beneficiosos.

Realidad: Tratamientos profesionales incluyendo astringentes, máscaras faciales, y otros no son recomendados porque tienden a agravar el acné.

Mito: Cosméticos con ingredientes grasosos ocluyen los poros y causan acné.

Realidad: Los cosméticos son mucho menos problemáticos para la mujer que lo que antes se pensaba. El uso de cosméticos, muy rara vez, si acaso, causa acné. Más comunmente, los cosméticos pueden ser irritantes y causar dermatitis por contacto.

Mito: El acné desaparece al final de la adolescencia.

Realidad: Algunas personas padecen de acné largo tiempo después de la adolescencia. Algunas mujeres desarrollan su primer episodio de acné a los 20-30 años.

Mito: Algunos alimentos como el chocolate, los dulces, o comidas grasosas causan o empeoran el acné.

Realidad: Independientemente de las creencias, las dietas influyen poco en el acné.

Mito: La piel grasosa causa acné.

Realidad: La piel grasosa es consecuencia del acné, el cual incrementa la producción de sebo de las glándulas sebáceas. La piel grasosa por lo tanto no es la causa del acné.

Mito: La suciedad en la cara produce acné, y por lo tanto una limpieza excesiva ayuda a controlar el acné.

Realidad: La limpieza excesiva y la intensa fricción del cutis con acné, especialmente del tipo inflamatorio, puede irritar y enrojecer la piel. Lo que se recomienda es el lavado diario de la cara con un jabón delicado.

Los tratamientos descritos en la próxima página son utilizados para **controlar** el acné, pero no curarlo!

Sea paciente, y no espere resultados inmediatos!

TREATMENT	HOW THEY WORK	HOW TO USE THEM	POSSIBLE SIDE EFFECTS
BENZOYL PEROXIDE	Benzoyl peroxide agents such as Oxy 5, Clearsil, Desquam-X, and Fostex cause the skin to dry and peel. Benzoyl peroxide destroys the bacteria that help cause acne.	Apply once or twice daily, or as directed	Redness, scaling, itching: These side effects may occur in the first few weeks and gradually lessen. Benzoyl peroxide may bleach clothing. **STOP** using the preparation and contact your health care provider if excessive redness, burning, or irritation develops.
TOPICAL RETINOIDS	Differin, tretinoin, Retin-A, and Tazorac dry and peel the outer layer of skin to loosen blackheads and whiteheads. They also help to clear the red pimples and white pustules. Improvement of acne may take up to 2 to 3 months, and in the first few weeks, the condition may actually appear to worsen. This does not mean that the preparation is not working, and it should not be discontinued. The apparent worsening results from deeper acne coming to the surface; the acne will eventually clear.	Use a pea-size amount of the preparations once nightly at bedtime. Apply to the entire face from the hairline to the jaw line, avoiding the areas around the corners of the eyes and mouth. People with fair, sensitive, or dry skin, especially in winter, can begin using it every other night, and gradually increase the frequency after 2 to 3 weeks.	Burning, stinging, irritation: These side effects may occur in the first 2 to 3 weeks. A mild soap such as Dove may be used for a routine facial washing, but avoid too much washing. A moisturizer may be used as necessary. Excessive sun exposure should be avoided. If you plan to be out in the sun, especially if you are fair skinned, a sunscreen should be applied beforehand. It is advised not to apply topical retinoids during pregnancy, even though there have been no proven problems with their use. If excessive redness, burning, or irritation develops, **STOP** using the preparation and contact your health care provider.
TOPICAL ANTIBIOTICS	Clindamycin (Cleocin T Lotion, Gel, and Solution), as well as topical, erythromycins, such as A/T/S, Eryderm, Erygel, Emgel, etc., are topical antibiotic preparations. They act primarily by reducing the inflammatory lesions (red pimples and pus pimples) of acne.	Apply each morning and evening to the affected areas, as well as to other areas where your acne usually occurs. Gently wash with a mild soap and pat dry before application. Makeup may be used over these preparations.	Redness, peeling, burning, drying: These side effects can occur, especially in patient with sensitive skin and may be controlled by reducing the frequency of application.

(continued on page 441)

TRATAMIENTO	COMO FUNCIONA	COMO SE USA	POSIBLES EFECTOS SECUNDARIOS
PERÓXIDO DE BENZOÍLO	Medicinas a base de peróxido de ben-zoylo tales como Oxy 5, Clearasil, Desquam-X, y Fostex resecan y pro-ducen exfoliación de la piel. También destruyen ciertas bacterias que ayudan a producir acné.	Aplicar una o dos veces al día o como sea indicado.	Enrojecimiento, resequedad, picazón: es-tos efectos ocurren en las primeras se-manas, y luego mejoran progresiva-mente. El peróxido de benzoílo puede manchar la ropa. **Descontinue** el uso de este medicamento y contacte a su doctor si nota enrojecimiento o irritación excesivos.
RETINOIDES TÓPICOS	Differin, tretinoin, Retin-A, y Tazorac secan la piel y exfolian la capa superficial de la piel. Estos productos eliminan gra-nos blancos y espinillas. También ayu-dan a reducir granos rojos y pústulas. La mejoría puede tardar en notarse hasta 2-3 meses, y en las primeras semanas de tratamiento puede incluso empeorar. Esto no significa que el tratamiento no funcione, y no debe descontinuarse. Este aparente empeoramiento se debe a que lesiones profundas de acné han comenzado a alcanzar la superficie de la piel. El acné eventualmente responde a este tratamiento.	Use una pequeña cantidad del producto en la noche antes de acostarse. Aplique en la cara desde la frente hasta las mandíbulas, evitando aplicar en la piel alrededor de la boca y los ojos. Las personas con piel clara, sensible, o reseca, especialmente en el invierno, pueden usar cada 48 horas en la noche, e incrementar la frecuencia de su uso gradualmente después de 2-3 semanas.	Ardor, picazón, irritación: estos efectos secundarios pueden ocurrir en las primeras 2-3 semanas. Un jabón delicado como Dove puede usarse rutinariamente para lavar la cara. Evite el lavado excesivo. Si es necesario, puede utilizar un humec-tante. Debe evitar la exposición exce-siva al sol. Si planea estar expuesto al sol, especialmente si su piel es clara, se recomienda usar protector solar. No se recomienda el uso de retinoides tópicos durante el embarazo, aun cuando no exista evidencia de que su uso durante el embarazo esté asociado a problema alguno. Si usted nota excesiva resequedad o enrojecimiento o irritación, **DESCON-TINUE** el medicamento y contacte a su médico.
ANTIBIOTICOS TOPICOS	La clindamycina (Loción de Cleocin T, Gel y Solución) y las erytromicinas como el A/T/S, Eryderm, Erygel, Emgel, etc., son antibióticos tópicos. Ellos actúan primariamente reduciendo le-siones inflamatorias de acné (granos rojos, pústulas).	Aplíquese en la mañana y en la noche en áreas afectadas, y en áreas donde usualmente usted tiene acné. Lave la piel con agua y jabón suave y seque levemente antes de aplicar. Se pueden usar cosméticos sobre éstos productos.	Enrojecimiento, descamación, ardor, rese-quedad: Estos efectos pueden ocurrir especialmente en pacientes con piel sensible y pueden ser controlados reduciendo la frecuencia de su aplicación.

(continued on page 442)

ONE OR MORE OF THE FOLLOWING MEDICATIONS HAS BEEN PRESCRIBED FOR YOU:

TREATMENT	HOW THEY WORK	HOW TO USE THEM	POSSIBLE SIDE EFFECTS
BENZACLIN GEL AND BENZAMYCIN GEL	BenzaClin gel and Benzamycin gel combine benzoyl peroxide with the topical antibiotic clindamycin or erythromycin.	BenzaClin gel does not have to be refrigerated. Benzamycin should be refrigerated to maintain potency. Both are applied once or twice per day, as tolerated.	As with benzoyl peroxide and topical antibiotics, mild to moderate irritation may occur. These preparations may also bleach clothing.
ORAL ANTIBIOTICS	Antibiotics, such as tetracycline, minocycline, doxycycline, and erythromycin, are used to kill the bacteria that form irritating products from the oil made in oil glands. They also lessen the inflammation of acne.	Plain tetracycline should be taken on an empty stomach. Minocycline and doxycycline are also types of tetracycline, but they can be taken with food. They **should not** be taken by pregnant women. Tetracycline and erythromycin may interact with birth control pills. If you are taking or planning to take oral contraceptives, tell your doctor. Erythromycin may be taken with meals.	In sun-sensitive individuals, doxycycline can cause a faster and more severe sunburn in some instances. At high doses, minocycline and doxycycline may cause dizziness. Erythromycin can cause gastrointestinal upset and diarrhea. Long-term use of these antibiotics in some women may result in "yeast infections."

UNO O MÁS DE LOS SIGUIENTES MEDICAMENTOS LE HAN SIDO INDICADOS PARA USTED:

TRATAMIENTO	COMO FUNCIONA	COMO SE USA	POSIBLES EFECTOS SECUNDARIOS
BENZACLIN GEL Y BENZAMYCIN GEL	BenzaClin gel y Benzamycin gel son combinaciones de peróxido de benzoilo con el antibiótico erytromycina.	BenzaClin gel no necesita ser refrigerado. Benzamycin gel debe refrigerarse para mantener su actividad. Ambos se aplican una o dos veces al día como sea tolerado.	Asi como ocurre con el peróxido de benzoilo y con los antibióticos tópicos, usted puede desarrollar irritación leve a moderada. Estos productos pueden desteñir su ropa.
ANTIBIÓTICOS ORALES	Los antibióticos, tales como la tetracyclina, minocyclina, doxycyclina, y erytromycina, son usados para eliminar bacterias que generan productos irritantes derivados del sebo producido en las glándulas sebáceas. También disminuyen la inflamación de ciertas lesiones de acné	La tetracyclina debe tomarse con el estómago vacío. La minocyclina y la doxycyclina, que son un tipo de tetracyclinas, pueden ser tomadas con las comidas. Estas medicinas **no deben** usarse durante el embarazo. La tetracyclina y la erythromycina pueden interactuar con las píldoras anticonceptivas. Si usted está tomando o planea tomar píldoras anticonceptivas, hágaselo saber a su doctor. La erythromycina puede ser tomada con las comidas.	En personas sensibles al sol, la doxycyclina puede causar quemadura solar con mayor facilidad y mayor severidad en ciertos casos. A altas dosis, la minocyclina y la doxycyclina pueden causar mareo. La erythromycina puede causar trastorno gastrointestinal y diarrea. El uso prolongado de estas medicinas en mujeres puede resultar en infecciones (hongos) vaginales.

What is rosacea?
- Rosacea is a disorder that is frequently mistaken for acne. In fact, as recently as the 1980s, rosacea was referred to as *acne rosacea*.
- Rosacea is a common condition with no known cause.

Who gets rosacea?
- Rosacea develops later in life than acne, usually between 30 and 50 years of age.
- Rosacea occurs most commonly in fair-skinned people of northern European ancestry, particularly those of Celtic descent.
- It is unusual among dark-skinned people.

What does rosacea look like?
- Rosacea consists of red pimples (papules), pus pimples (pustules), and small blood vessels (telangiectasias).

Where does rosacea appear?
- Lesions are most typically seen on the forehead, nose, cheeks, and chin (the so-called *flush or blush* areas).

What are the symptoms of rosacea?
- Rosacea is primarily a cosmetic problem.
- It can also sometimes involve the eyes and eyelids.

What makes rosacea worse?
- Sun exposure often exacerbates rosacea.
- Excessive washing of the face aggravates rosacea.
- Irritating cosmetics can worsen rosacea.

In some people, the following factors may aggravate rosacea:
- Excess alcohol ingestion
- Emotional stress
- Spicy foods, smoking, or caffeine

How is rosacea treated?
Topical therapy
- Metronidazole (Noritate) 1% cream is used once daily.
- Twice-daily applications of 0.75% metronidazole (MetroCream), which is also available as a lotion, and gel preparations are also used.
- Other topicals include topical antibiotics as well as other lotions such as Klaron or Sulfacet-R.

Oral therapy
- An oral antibiotic such as a tetracycline or minocycline may be prescribed.

ROSÁCEA

¿Qué es la rosácea?
- Rosácea es una enfermedad que se confunde frecuentemente con el acné. De hecho, hasta hace 20 años, a la rosácea se le conocía como *acné rosácea*.
- Rosácea es una condición común de causa desconocida.

¿A quién afecta la rosácea?
- La rosácea se presenta más tarde que el acné, usualmente entre los 30 y 50 años de edad.
- La rosácea ocurre más comunmente en individuos de piel clara de ascendencia del norte de Europa, particularmente de origen Celta.
- Es inusual en personas de piel oscura.

¿En qué consiste la rosácea?
- La rosácea consiste de granos rojos (pápulas), granos con pus (pústulas), y pequeños vasos sanguineos (telanjiectasias).

¿En dónde aparece la rosácea?
- Típicamente aparece en la frente, nariz, mejillas, and barbilla.

¿Cuáles son los síntomas de la rosácea?
- La rosácea es primordíalmente un problema estético.
- En algunos casos puede afectar los ojos y los párpados.

¿Qué hace que empeore la rosácea?
- La exposición a la luz solar.
- Lavado excesivo de la cara.
- Cosméticos irritantes.

En algunas personas, los siguientes factores pueden agravar la rosácea:
- La ingestión excesiva de alcohol.
- El estrés emocional.
- Comidas condimentadas, picantes, el tabaco, o la cafeína.

¿Cómo se trata la rosácea?
Tratamiento tópico
- 1% crema de metronidazole (Noritate) una vez al día.
- 0.75% crema de metronidazole (MetroCream), la cual también existe en loción, y en gel dos veces al día.
- Otros productos tópicos incluyen antibióticos tópicos y lociones como Klaron o Sulfacet-R.

Tratamiento oral
- Un antibiótico oral como la tetracyclina o la minocyclina puede ser indicado.

What is atopic dermatitis?
- Atopic dermatitis, which is sometimes called atopic eczema or hereditary eczema, is an itchy, sensitive skin condition that runs in certain families.
- It may flare at times of stress or during the change of seasons, or it may just appear for no obvious reason. The problem frequently goes away by itself—in 40% to 50% of children—but it may return in adolescence or adulthood and possibly may be a lifelong problem.

Who gets atopic dermatitis?
- You, your child, or other family members will have one or more of the following symptoms: dry, sensitive skin; allergies to medications, pollen, dust, house dust mites, ragweed, dogs or cats; or other problems such as persistent, runny noses, sinusitis, sneezing attacks, or chronic itchy or irritated eyes. Any one of these symptoms helps to suggest that atopic dermatitis is the cause of a chronic skin rash.
- This tendency may be found in other relatives (aunts, uncles, cousins, and grandparents) who also may have similar symptoms.
- Although most cases begin in childhood (often in infancy), atopic dermatitis may start at any age and has an unpredictable course.

How is atopic dermatitis treated?
Topical steroids
The mainstay of treatment is the application of topical steroids. Topical steroids are safe if used as directed and should be applied only for short periods of time, if possible, and only against active disease (i.e., with itching and redness). Topical steroids should be stopped when the skin is healed, and they should not be used for prevention of future rashes.

Noncortisone topical treatments
Tacrolimus (Protopic) ointment and pimecrolimus (Elidel) cream are medications that contain no steroids and have been shown to reduce the symptoms of atopic dermatitis.

Other treatment measures
- Sometimes oral steroids such as prednisone or prednisolone (Prelone) may be necessary.
- Oral antihistamines such as the over-the-counter diphenhydramine (Benadryl) and chlorpheniramine (Chlor-Trimeton) may reduce itching, but they often work only when they bring about drowsiness or sleep.
- Sun exposure, ideally in the early morning and late afternoon when humidity is lowest, may improve the condition.

Is there a cure for atopic dermatitis?
- There is no cure, but it can be kept under control, and sometimes it clears up by itself for long periods of time.

How is atopic dermatitis prevented?
The following measures may help the patient avoid or reduce exposure to trigger factors such as dry skin, irritants, overheating, sweating, and allergens:

Dryness
- Moisturizers, particularly in the dry winter months, should be applied immediately after bathing, to "trap" water in the skin. Suggested ointments are Vaseline Petroleum Jelly and Aquaphor. Suggested creams and lotions are Eucerin, Cetaphil, Lubriderm, Curel, and Moisturel.

DERMATITIS ATÓPICA

¿Qué es la dermatitis atópica?
- La dermatitis atópica, la cual es también conocida como eczema atópico o eczema hereditario es una condición pruriginosa, caracterizada por piel sensible, que afecta a individuos de ciertas familias.
- Puede empeorar en momentos de estrés o durante cambios climáticos, o puede aparecer sin razón aparente. El problema frecuentemente desaparece espontáneamente en un 40% al 50% de los niños, pero puede recurrir en la adolescencia o en la edad adulta y eventualmente se puede convertir en un problema de por vida.

¿A quién afecta la dermatitis atópica?
- Usted, su hijo, u otro miembro de su familia puede presentar los siguientes síntomas: piel reseca, sensible; alergias a medicamentos, polen, polvo, ácaros, perros o gatos; u otros problemas como congestión nasal persistente, sinusitis, ataques de estornudos, o irritación y picazon crónica de los ojos. Cualquiera de éstos síntomas ayudan a sugerir que la dermatitis atópica es la causa de la erupción de la piel.
- Esta tendencia puede encontrarse en otros familiares (tíos, tías, primos, abuelos) los cuales pueden presentar síntomas similares.
- Aunque la mayoría de los casos comienzan en la niñez (usualmente durante la infancia), la dermatitis atópica puede comenzar a cualquier edad y puede tener un curso impredecible.

¿Cómo se trata la dermatitis atópica?
Esteroides tópicos
El tratamiento fundamental es la aplicación de esteroides tópicos. Los esteroides tópicos son seguros si se emplean como son indicados y si se emplean por cortos períodos de tiempo, si es possible, y solo cuando la enfermedad esté activa (por ejemplo, cuando hay picazón y enrojecimiento). Los esteroides tópicos deben descontinuarse cuando la piel está sana, y no deben utilizarse para prevenir futuros brotes.

Tratamientos tópicos sin cortisona
El unguento tacrolimus (Protopic) y la crema pimecrolimus (Elidel) son medicinas que no contienen esteroides y que han demonstrado reducir los síntomas de la dermatitis atópica.

Otras medidas terapéuticas
- En ciertas ocasiones, esteroides orales como la prednisona o la prednisolona (Prelone) pueden ser necesarios.
- Los antihistamínicos orales tales como la diphenhydramina (Benadryl) y la chlorpheniramina (Chlor-Trimeton) pueden reducir la picazón, pero éstos funcionan únicamente a través de su mecanismo de sedación.
- La exposición al sol, idealmente temprano en la mañana y en la tarde, cuando la humedad es baja, puede mejorar su condición.

¿Existe cura para la dermatitis atópica?
- No existe cura, pero es controlable y a veces se cura por si sola por largos períodos de tiempo.

¿Cómo se puede prevenir la dermatitis atópica?
Las siguientes medidas pueden prevenir la exposición a factores desencadenantes de episodios de dermatitis atópica tales como la piel reseca, irritantes, calor excesivo, sudoración y alergenos:

Resequedad
- Se recomienda el uso de emolientes, particularmente durante el invierno, inmediatamente después del baño, para "atrapar" agua en la piel. Son recomendables el Vaseline Petroleum Jelly y Aquaphor. También se recomienda cremas y lociones como Eucerin, Cetaphil, Lubriderm, Curel y Moisturel.

Irritants
- Nonirritating fabrics, such as cotton, should be worn. Wool clothing may cause itching.

Overheating and sweating
- A bedroom air conditioner may help to avoid the dramatic changes in climate that may trigger outbreaks.
- Humidifiers do not seem to help very much.

Diet and allergens
- Although some foods may provoke attacks, eliminating them will rarely bring a lasting improvement or cure.
- Skin tests and allergy shots may actually bring on attacks of atopic dermatitis.

Bathing
There are many reasons not to restrict frequent bathing:
- Bathing provides pleasure and reduces stress. Bathing removes scabs, irritants, allergens, and bacteria.
- Bathing hydrates the skin and allows better delivery of topical steroids and moisturizers. However, excessive bathing that is not followed immediately by application of a moisturizer tends to dry the skin.

Bathing tips: Mild, moisturizing soaps such as Dove or nonsoap cleansers such as Cetaphil Lotion should be used. Excessive toweling and scrubbing should be avoided. Try to avoid using soap on red or itchy skin (many people are mistakenly led to believe that "good soaps" may actually help red, itchy, inflamed skin).

KEEP IN MIND

- Topical steroid preparations should be applied only to inflamed, itchy skin. They should be stopped when the skin is healed and should not be used to prevent new outbreaks.
- Areas that were darkened or lightened by the rash tend to repigment over time and should not be treated with cortisone preparations.
- Milder topical steroid preparations are recommended for use on the face and eyelids and in skin folds such as the diaper area, groin, and underarms.
- Moisturizers may be applied immediately after bathing to "seal" water in the skin.
- Although some foods may provoke attacks, there is little point in trying to eliminate allergy-causing foods from a child's or an adult's diet in hopes of curing eczema.
- Children's fingernails should be kept short to help minimize damage from scratching.
- Emotional stress in patients or in their families may contribute to atopic dermatitis.
- Teach your children that atopic dermatitis is a common, noncontagious skin condition.
- Inform your child's teacher and the school nurse about his or her condition.
- The National Eczema Association can be contacted at (503) 228-4430 or http://www.eczema-assn.org.

Irritantes
- Como vestimenta se deben utilizar materiales no irritantes como el algodón. La ropa a base de lana puede causar picazón.

Calor excesivo y sudoración
- Un aire acondicionado en el dormitorio ayuda a disminuir cambios intensos de temperatura los cuales pueden desencadenar episodios de la enfermedad.
- El uso de humidificantes no parece ser de mucha ayuda.

Dieta y alergenos
- Aunque algunas comidas pueden desencadenar episodios, su eliminación de la dieta rara vez conduce a una mejoría duradera o cura de la enfermedad.
- Las pruebas de alergias de la piel e inyecciones para tratar alergias pueden desencadenar ataques de dermatitis atópica.

Baño
Existen varias razones por las cuales no se debe restringir la frecuencia del baño:
- El baño es placentero y reduce el estrés. El baño ayuda a remover costras, substancias irritantes, alergenos y bacterias.
- El baño hidrata la piel y ayuda a la penetración más eficiente de medicamentos tales como esteroides tópicos y lubricantes. Sin embargo, el baño excesivo, y en particular si no es seguido por la aplicación de un lubricante inmediatamente después del mismo tiende a producir resequedad de la piel.

Recomendaciones para el baño: Jabones suaves y humectantes como Dove o limpiadores como la loción Cetaphil deben emplearse. Debe evitarse el uso excesivo de la toalla para secar la piel. Evite usar jabón en areas en donde la piel esté roja o con picazón (muchas personas creen equivocadamente que un buen jabón puede ayudar a sanar una piel, roja, irritada y con picazón).

NO OLVIDE QUE

- Los esteroides tópicos deben aplicarse solamente en la piel que esté inflamada y con síntomas de picazón. Los mismos deben ser descontinuados cuando la piel haya curado y no deben utilizarse para prevenir nuevos episodios.
- Ciertas áreas que hayan quedado oscuras o claras como resultado de la erupción tienden a repigmentar con el tiempo y no deben ser tratadas con medicinas a base de cortisona.
- Deben utilizarse preparaciones a base de esteroides con menor potencia en la cara, en los párpados y en areas de la piel como las axilas, el área del pañal y en la ingle.
- Se deben aplicar lubricantes inmediatamente después del baño para "atrapar" agua en la piel.
- Aunque algunos alimentos pueden provocar episodios de dermatitis atópica, no hay razón para eliminar los mismos de la dieta del niño o del adulto con dermatitis atópica ya que rara vez dicha estrategia puede llegar a curar dicha enfermedad.
- Las uñas de los niños deben mantenerse cortas para así minimizar el daño producido por el rascado.
- El estrés emocional en los pacientes o familiares puede contribuir a perpetuar en la dermatitis atópica.
- Enseñe a sus hijos que la dermatitis atópica es una enfermedad de la piel común y no contagiosa.
- En la escuela, informe a los maestros y enfermeras sobre la condición de su hijo o hija.
- La Asociación Nacional del Eczema (The National Eczema Association) puede ser contactada al (503) 228-4430 o http://www.eczema-assn.org.

HAND ECZEMA

What is hand eczema?
- A hand rash (eczema) that is caused by exposure to irritating or allergy-producing substances is called contact dermatitis. This is sometimes called "dishpan hands."
- When there is no evidence of an outside cause of hand eczema, the diagnosis is most likely atopic hand eczema. It is sometimes called *dyshidrotic eczema* when there are small blisters on the fingers or palms.

Who gets hand eczema?
- Some people may develop a hand rash from overexposure to irritating substances (e.g., hairdressers, cement workers), whereas others develop contact dermatitis from an allergic reaction to allergenic substances (e.g., latex gloves in health care personnel).
- Other people who have such hand rashes have inherited this tendency, and other family members sometimes have a similar problem with their hands or other problems such as asthma, hay fever, sinus problems, or other allergies. This is called atopic hand eczema (atopic dermatitis).

What does hand eczema look like?
- Often, the hands are dry, sensitive, scaly, and red.
- The fingers and palms may develop fissures (splits).
- Sometimes, the eczema may consist of blisters that look like little bubbles that eventually dry up.

What are the symptoms of hand eczema?
- The hands can be very itchy.
- Split fingers and palms can be painful and very sensitive to things like citrus fruits.

How is hand eczema diagnosed?
- An evaluation may involve careful history taking and possible patch testing with chemicals or substances that could be the source of the rash.

How is hand eczema treated?
- Usually a prescription topical steroid cream or ointment such as _____ _____ is prescribed to be applied once or twice daily. This medication should not be applied to your face.
- Topical steroids are safe if used as directed and should be applied only for short periods of time, if possible, and only against active disease (i.e., with itching and redness).
- Tacrolimus (Protopic) ointment and pimecrolimus (Elidel) are medications that contain no steroids, and they have been shown to reduce the symptoms of eczema.

What can be done to help prevent hand eczema?
- Use lukewarm water, mild cleansers, or soap substitutes.
- Use only mild, moisturizing soaps such as Dove or nonsoap cleansers such as Cetaphil Lotion.
- Try to avoid using soap on red or itchy skin (many people are mistakenly led to believe that "good soaps" may actually help red, itchy, inflamed skin).
- Avoid latex gloves and use protective vinyl gloves at work and at home.
- Use protective cotton-lined gloves while washing dishes or other similar tasks.
- Use moisturizers often, especially in the cold, dry months.
- Wear gloves in cold weather.
- Band-Aids are helpful in healing fissured (cracked) fingers.

¿Qué es el eczema de las manos?
- Es una erupción en las manos (eczema) que es causado por exposición de las mismas a substancias irritantes o alergénicas, lo cual es llamado dermatitis por contacto.
- Cuando no hay evidencia de una causa externa que explique la aparición del eczema de las manos, el diagnóstico más probable es el de dermatitis atópica de las manos. A veces existen pequeñas ampollas en las manos o en los dedos. A este tipo de eczema se le denomina eczema dishidrótico.

¿A quién afecta el eczema de las manos?
- Algunas personas desarrollan erupciones en las manos debido a la sobre-exposición a substancias irritantes (por ejemplo, peluqueros, trabajadores de la construcción) mientras que otras desarrollan dermatitis por contacto como consecuencia de una reacción alérgica a algún alergeno (por ejemplo, guantes de latex utilizados por profesionales de la salud).
- Otras personas afectadas por estas erupciones en las manos han heredado esta tendencia y otros miembros de la familia pueden presentar un problema similar en las manos otro problema como asma, fiebre del heno, problemas sinusales, u otras alergias. Este último tipo se le denomina dermatitis atópica de las manos (dermatitis atópica).

¿Cómo se manifiesta el eczema de las manos?
- Usualmente, las manos aparecen resecas, sensibles, escamosas y rojas.
- Los dedos y las palmas pueden presentar fisuras.
- A veces, el eczema puede consistir de ampollas que se asemejan a pequeñas burbujas que eventualmente se secan.

¿Cuáles son los síntomas de él?
- Puede haber picazón en las manos.
- Las fisuras en las manos y dedos pueden doler y son muy sensibles a substancias como los jugos cítricos.

¿Cómo se diagnostica el eczema de las manos?
- La evaluación debe incluir una historia médica detallada y debe considerarse una prueba de parche a fin de detectar alergias a diferentes substancias químicas que pueden ser la causa de la erupción.

¿Cómo se trata el eczema de las manos?
- Usualmente se prescribe un esteroide tópico en crema o unguento tales como _____. Estos se deben aplicar una o dos veces al día. Estos no deben aplicarse en la cara.
- Los esteroides tópicos son seguros si se emplean como son indicados y deben ser usados solo por períodos cortos, si es possible, y solamente cuando la erupción está activa (por ejemplo, cuando la piel presenta picazón y enrojecimiento).
- El tacrolimus (Protopic) en unguento y el pimecrolimus (Elidel) en crema son medicinas que no contienen esteroides, y que han demostrado reducir los síntomas del eczema.

¿Qué se puede hacer para prevenir el eczema de las manos?
- Use agua tibia, jabones suaves o substitutos del jabón.
- Use solamente jabones delicados y humectantes como Dove o productos limpiadores como Cetaphil en loción.
- Evite usar jabón en la piel cuando ésta esté roja o con picazón (muchas personas creen equivocadamente que un buen jabón puede ayudar a sanar una piel, roja, irritada y con picazón).
- Evite los guantes de latex y use guantes de vinil en el trabajo y en la casa.
- Use guantes con revestimiento interno de algodón cuando lave los platos o durante actividades similares.
- Use humectantes frecuentemente, especialmente en los meses fríos y secos.
- Utilize guantes durante el invierno.
- Las curitas (Band-Aids) pueden ayudar para las fisuras en los dedos.

What is Burow's solution?
- Burow's solution is a topical antibacterial astringent preparation that helps to dry up and control weeping, oozing, and infected skin conditions.

Where do I get it?
- Purchase a box of Burow's solution (Domeboro, Bluboro, Buropak).
- It is available in most chain pharmacies and does not require a prescription.
- It may come as a powder in packets that must be diluted in water.

How do I use it?
- Dissolve one packet or tablet in an 8-ounce glass of water (about the size of a drinking glass).
- Make a wet compress using a cloth or cotton swab moistened by the solution and leave it in place for 15 to 20 minutes.
- Do this three to four times each day.
- You can apply recommended medications and sterile dressings after soaks.
- Use until all areas are no longer oozing.
- *Cool* water may be more comfortable to use when treating itchy rashes such as poison ivy; *lukewarm* water may be more comfortable for treating wintertime weeping eczema rashes and for drying the blisters of herpes zoster (shingles).

SOLUCIÓN DE BUROW'S

¿Qué es la solución de Burow's?
* La solución de Burow's es una solución tópica astringente y bactericida que ayuda a secar áreas en la piel que presentan exudados o secreción o con signos de infección.

¿Cómo la puedo obtener?
* Usted puede comprar la solución de Burow's (Domeboro, Bluboro, Buropak).
* Se consigue sin prescripción médica en la mayoría de las cadenas de farmacias.
* A veces se consigue en polvo, el cual debe ser diluído en agua antes de ser usado.

¿Cómo lo utilizo?
* Disuelva un sobre o una tableta en 8 onzas de agua (aproximadamente la cantidad de líquido en un vaso de agua).
* Haga compresas de gaza o paño de algodón humedecidas en la solución de Burow's. Aplique sobre el área y déjela reposar en el sitio por 15-20 minutos.
* Repita el procedimiento tres a cuatro veces al día.
* Usted puede usar cualquier medicamento tópico o curas estériles sobre las áreas tratadas después de haber hecho las compresas con la solución.
* Utilize hasta que las áreas estén secas.
* El uso de agua fría puede ser mas confortable cuando usted esté tratando lesiones pruriginosas tales como la hiedra venenosa (poison ivy). Cuando usted esté tratando áreas como el herpes zoster o ciertos eczemas exudativos durante el invierno, es preferible el uso de agua tibia.

What is psoriasis?
- Psoriasis is red and scaly chronic skin condition of unknown cause.

Who gets it?
- About 30% of people with psoriasis have a family history of the condition.
- It affects 1% to 2% of the world's population.
- Psoriasis most frequently begins in the 20s or 30s, but it can first be seen in infants or in elderly persons.

What causes it?
- Psoriasis is now considered to be an immunologic disease.
- The exact cause is unknown; however, we do know that spots (psoriatic lesions) result from an increase in epidermal cell division.

What does it look like, and where on the body does psoriasis occur?
- Thickened, reddened, silvery or whitish scaly patches can vary from only a few small lesions to larger plaques that cover large areas of the body.
- Fortunately, it usually spares the face.
- Lesions are most commonly located on the:
  - Large joints: the elbows, knees, and knuckles
  - Palms and soles
  - Body folds: underarms, under the breasts, anus and genital region, and groin. This body fold type of psoriasis is referred to as **inverse psoriasis.**
  - Trunk: Lesions may be small, teardrop-shaped (guttate) lesions or large plaques.
  - Scalp and ears
  - Nails: Involvement of nails is very common in patients with psoriasis.
- Psoriatic arthritis occurs in about 7% of patients who have psoriasis.

What are the symptoms of psoriasis?
- Psoriasis generally is symptom free, but it can become quite itchy and uncomfortable, particularly during acute flare-ups or when it involves the scalp or skin fold regions.
- A person who has psoriasis is mainly concerned about the appearance of the skin.

What makes psoriasis worse?
- Emotional stress, such as anxiety and depression, is believed to worsen psoriasis.
- Certain drugs and excess alcohol use also aggravate the condition.
- Many patients tend to improve during the summer and worsen in the colder times of the year.
- This fluctuation is probably the result of the positive influence of sunlight on psoriasis.

How is psoriasis diagnosed?
- Dermatologists can usually easily recognize it by simply examining the skin.
- Other helpful diagnostic features include a family history of psoriasis.
- If necessary, other tests, such as a skin biopsy or fungal examination, can be performed to rule out other conditions.

PSORIASIS

¿Qué es la psoriasis?

- La psoriasis es una condición crónica de la piel de causa desconocida caracterizada por lesiones rojas y escamosas.

¿A quién afecta la psoriasis?

- Aproximadamente 30% de las personas con psoriasis tienen historia familiar con ésta condición.
- Afecta al 1% o 2% de la población mundial.
- La psoriasis frecuentemente comienza a los 20 o 30 años, pero puede manifestarse por primera vez en la infancia o en ancianos.

¿Qué la causa?

- La psoriasis se considera como una enfermedad inmunológica.
- La causa exacta es desconocida; sin embargo, se sabe que las lesiones psoriáticas (spots/psoriatic lesions) se deben a un aumento en la division cellular de la capa epidérmica.

¿Cuál es su apariencia y en qué parte del cuerpo ocurre?

- Las lesiones, las cuales consisten de placas gruesas, rojas y con escamas de color plateadas o blancas, pueden variar desde pocas y pequeñas a muy numerosas y que a veces llegan a cubrir extensas áreas del cuerpo.
- Afortunadamente, casi nunca afecta la cara.
- Las lesiones se encuentran comunmente en:
  - Largas articulaciones: los codos, las rodillas, y los nudillos de las manos.
  - Palmas y plantas.
  - Áreas de flexión: debajo de los brazos, debajo de las mamas, ano, y región genital, e ingle. Cuando estas áreas están afectadas, a ésto se le denomina psoriasis inversa.
  - Tronco: las lesiones pueden ser pequeñas, o en forma de gota (psoriasis gutata), o bien placas más grandes.
  - Cuero cabelludo y orejas.
  - Uñas: éstas se ven afectadas frecuentemente en la psoriasis.
- Una forma de artritis (artritis psoriática) puede afectar hasta un 7% de pacientes con psoriasis.

¿Cuáles son los síntomas de la psoriasis?

- La psoriasis es generalmente asintomática, pero puede producir picazón e incomodidad, particularmente durante las exacerbaciones agudas o cuando afecta al cuero cabelludo o areas de flexión.
- A los pacientes con psoriasis les preocupa la apariencia de su piel.

¿Qué hace que la psoriasis empeore?

- Se piensa que el estrés emocional, la depresión y la ansiedad, agravan la psoriasis.
- Ciertos medicamentos y el exceso de alcohol también agravan ésta condición.
- Muchos pacientes notan mejoría durante los meses de verano y empeoramiento durante los meses más fríos del año.
- Esta fluctuación es probablemente el resultado de la influencia positiva de la luz solar en la psoriasis.

¿Cómo se diagnostica la psoriasis?

- Los dermatólogos pueden reconocer fácilmente la psoriasis con un simple examen de piel.
- Una historia familiar de psoriasis ayuda a diagnosticar la enfermedad.
- Si es necesario, otros exámenes tales como biopsia de piel o exámenes para evaluar la presencia de hongos, pueden realizarse a fin de descartar otras enfermedades.

How is psoriasis treated?
• Special diets do not seem to help in any way.

Topical corticosteroids
• The use of a potent topical steroid for a limited period, followed by less potent topical steroids for maintenance, has become a popular method for treating psoriasis.

Topical vitamin D
• Calcipotriene 0.005% ointment, cream, and solution (Dovonex).
• Dovonex is a synthetic vitamin D that is most useful for limited, fairly mild, localized psoriasis.
• It is often used in combination with topical steroids.

Topical retinoids
• Tazarotene 0.05%, 0.1%, cream and gel (Tazorac) is a topical retinoid derivative that is applied once daily.
• It is also used in conjunction with topical steroids.

Topical immunomodulators
• Tacrolimus (Protopic) ointment and pimecrolimus (Elidel) cream are the newest nonsteroidal topical treatments.

Topical tar preparations
• Before the arrival of topical steroids, tar preparations were the mainstay of therapy for most cases of psoriasis. Today, they are used less often.

Ultraviolet light therapy
• Natural sunlight slows the growth of psoriasis.
• People with psoriasis all over their bodies may be treated with light boxes that expose most of the body to ultraviolet light.

Oral treatments, such as methotrexate and Soriatane, may be prescribed when a patient is not responding to topical therapies or ultraviolet light treatment alone.

Newer approaches to psoriasis therapy
• Many new biologic agents are currently being evaluated for the treatment of psoriasis and psoriatic arthritis.

The National Psoriasis Foundation provides information about psoriasis to educate patients, the public, and health care providers. Their address is as follows:

National Psoriasis Foundation
107 Vista del Grande
National Psoriasis Foundation
6600 S.W. 92nd, Suite 300
Portland, OR 97223
(800) 723-9166
www.psoriasis.org

¿Cómo se trata la psoriasis?
- Las dietas especiales no son de ayuda en la psoriasis.

Esteroides tópicos
- Un método popular para tratar la psoriasis incluye el uso de un esteroide tópico potente por un período limitado, seguido por un esteroide tópico de menor potencia como mantenimiento.

Vitamina D tópica
- Unguento, crema y solución de calcipotriene 0.005% (Dovonex).
- Dovonex es un derivado sintético de la vitamina D que ayuda en formas más limitadas y leves de la enfermedad.
- Este medicamento se utiliza frecuentemente en combinación con esteroides tópicos.

Retinoides tópicos
- El tazarotene 0.05%, 0.1%, en crema o gel (Tazorac) es un retinoide tópico que se aplica una vez al día.
- También se utiliza en combinación con esteroides tópicos.

Inmunomoduladores tópicos
- El tacrolimus (Protopic) en unguento y el pimecrolimus (Elidel) en crema son los más nuevos tratamientos no esteroides tópicos.

Derivados de alquitrán tópicos
- Antes de la existencia de los esteroides tópicos, los derivados del alquitrán se utilizaban muy comunmente en la mayoría de los casos de psoriasis. En la actualidad, éstos se usan menos frecuentemente.

Luz ultravioleta
- La luz natural reduce el desarrollo de la psoriasis.
- Las personas con psoriasis en todo el cuerpo pueden ser tratadas a través de unidades especiales que exponen la superficie de la piel a luz ultravioleta.

Tratamientos orales como el methotrexate y el Soriatane pueden prescribirse cuando el paciente no esté respondiendo a los tratamientos tópicos o a la luz ultravioleta.

Nuevos tratamientos de la psoriasis
- Existen muchos nuevos agentes biológicos para el tratamiento de la psoriasis y la artritis psoriática que están siendo evaluados.

La Fundación Nacional de la Psoriasis (National Psoriasis Foundation) provee información para educar a los pacientes con psoriasis, al público en general y a los trabajadores del área de la salud. Su dirección es:

National Psoriasis Foundation
107 Vista del Grande
National Psoriasis Foundation
6600 S.W. 92nd, Suite 300
Portland, OR 97223
(800) 723-9166
www.psoriasis.org

SCALP PSORIASIS

If your health care provider has diagnosed scalp psoriasis, it is often necessary to remove thickened scale to allow the medications to get to where the action is—your scalp. Scale may be removed as often as necessary, usually two to three times per week at the beginning and, later, whenever the scale builds up again.

Here's how:

1. Wash your hair with your favorite shampoo and rinse thoroughly.
2. Then, while your scalp is still damp, apply Keralyt gel (6% salicylic acid in a petrolatum base) only to the thickened scaly areas. (Keralyt gel may be obtained without a prescription).
3. Cover your head with a shower cap and leave it on overnight, or leave it on while you are awake for several hours (whichever is more convenient for you).
4. Shampoo the area again. (You'll note that it is very greasy, and it will take some time to remove the gel.)
5. Other recommended medication(s) such as _____ _____ may now be applied.

PSORIASIS IN HAIRLESS AREAS

1. Soak the area(s) to be treated for 5 minutes.
2. Rub in a thin film of Keralyt gel.
3. Cover the area with plastic wrap (e.g., Saran Wrap, Handi-Wrap) or a plastic bag.
4. Remove the plastic wrap the next morning, and wash the area with soap and water.
5. If irritation occurs, stop the treatment temporarily, and then resume every other night after the irritation clears.
6. Use as necessary when the scale builds up again.
7. Other recommended medication(s) such as _____ _____ may be applied after the scale is cleared away.

PROCEDIMIENTO PARA REMOVER ESCAMAS DE LA PSORIASIS

PSORIASIS DEL CUERO CABELLUDO

Si su médico le ha diagnosticado psoriasis en el cuero cabelludo, es necesario remover las escamas gruesas para así permitir la penetración de los medicamentos tópicos donde está la acción—en el cuero cabelludo. Las escamas pueden ser removidas tan frecuentemente como sea necesario, usualmente dos a tres veces por semana al principio, y luego solo cuando las escamas se vuelvan a acumular.

Cómo:

1. Lave su cabello con su shampoo favorito y enjuage completamente.
2. Luego, mientras su cabello permanece aún húmedo, aplique Keralyt gel (6% ácido salicílico en una base de petrolato) solo en las areas gruesas y escamosas. (Tanto el Keralyt como el Hydrisalic gel pueden ser obtenidos sin prescripción médica.)
3. Cubra su cabeza con un gorro de baño y dejar durante la noche, o durante el día por varias horas mientras esté despierto (lo que le sea más conveniente).
4. Aplique shampoo otra vez. (Ustéd notará que el cabello estará grasoso, y le va a tomar cierto tiempo para poder remover el gel.)
5. Otro(s) medicamento(s) recomendado(s) tal(es) como _____ _____ puede(n) ahora comenzar a aplicarse.

PSORIASIS EN AREAS SIN PELO

1. Empape el area a ser tratada por 5 minutos.
2. Aplique una capa delgada de Keralyt gel.
3. Cubra el área con una capa fina de plástico (por ejemplo, Saran Wrap, Handi-Wrap) o con una bolsa plástica.
4. Remueva el material aplicado el día siguiente, y lave el área con agua y jabón.
5. Si usted nota irritación, suspenda el tratamiento temporalmente, y resuma alternando un día sí y uno no, hasta que la irritación haya desaparecido.
6. Use estos productos cuando las escamas se vuelvan a reacumular.
7. Otro(s) medicamento(s) recomendado(s) tal(es) como _____ _____ puede(n) ahora comenzar a aplicarse.

What is herpes simplex?
- The herpes simplex virus (HSV) causes blisters on almost any part of the body.
- The most common place for blistering to occur is on the edge of the upper or lower lip, where it is often referred to as a "cold sore" or "fever blister."
- After the initial infection (primary infection) heals, the virus retreats to nerve cells, where it slips into a resting phase.
- The virus remains in a resting phase until it is reactivated by a trigger such as sunlight exposure, menstrual cycles, fever, common colds, or emotional stress.

What causes it?
- Herpes simplex is caused by two virus types: HSV-1 and HSV-2.

What are the types of infection caused by HSV?
- HSV-1 and HSV-2 produce small, fluid-filled blisters on a red base.
- The two kinds of infection are primary infection and recurrent infection.

Primary HSV
- The primary infection may go unnoticed (subclinical infection), but when symptoms occur, they are often more severe than in recurrent-type infections. The symptoms may include swollen glands and fever.

Recurrent HSV
- The blisters may reappear in the same area—a recurrent infection.
- Recurrent infections tend to be milder than primary infections.
- Recurrent infections can be set off or reactivated by stress, menses, or sunlight, or lesions may appear for no apparent reason.
- Some people may have recurrent infections that are rare and infrequent, whereas others can have reinfections as often as once a month.
- One or 2 days before the blisters appear, there is often a sensation such as tingling, itching, numbness, or pain in the areas where the blisters will form. This is called the prodrome.
- Over time, recurrences decrease in frequency and eventually often stop altogether.

How is HSV treated?
Treatment of recurrent HSV should begin at the first symptom, the prodrome, because this can often stop the blisters from erupting. This is most effectively accomplished with an oral antiviral medication such as valacyclovir (Valtrex), famciclovir (Famvir), or acyclovir (Zovirax).

Topical therapy
- Using cold compresses on the infected area may relieve some discomfort.
- Topical acyclovir (Zovirax) ointment, penciclovir (Denavir) cream, and docosanol (Abreva) cream are not very effective treatments, but they may help to reduce healing times.

FACTS ABOUT HSV-2

- Condoms may be helpful to prevent the transmission of HSV to sexual partners.
- Many people are not aware that they have the infection, and they may actually be carriers with no symptoms (asymptomatic carriers).
- A pregnant woman who has active HSV lesions may pass the infection on to her infant during delivery.
- A recurrence that arises many years later may be mistaken for a primary episode, and this may lead to unjust accusations about the origin of the HSV infection.

HERPES SIMPLEX

¿Qué es el herpes simplex?
- El virus del herpes simplex (HSV) causa ampollas en casi todas las partes del cuerpo.
- El lugar más común es en el borde del labio superior o inferior de la boca, frecuentemente conocidos como "herpe labial" o "herpe febril."
- Después de que la infección inicial o primaria ha resuelto, el virus se aloja en células del sistema nervioso y pasa a un estadio silente.
- El virus permanece en este estadio hasta que es reactivado por agentes como exposición a la luz solar, menstruación, fiebre, gripes o catarro común o estrés emocional.

¿Qué lo causa?
- El herpes simplex es causado por dos tipos de viruses: el HSV-1 y el HSV-2.

¿Qué tipo de infecciones son causadas por el HSV?
- HSV-1 y HSV-2 producen pequeñas ampollas de fluido sobre una piel roja.
- Los dos tipos de infección son la infección primaria y la infección recurrente.

Infección primaria por HSV
- La infección primaria puede pasar desaperecida (infección subclínica), pero cuando los síntomas ocurren, ellos tienden a ser más severos que en los episodios recurrentes. Los síntomas incluyen fiebre y glándulas linfáticas inflamadas.

Infección recurrente por HSV
- Las ampollas pueden reaparecer en la misma zona—lo cual es una infección recurrente.
- Las infecciones recurrentes son más leves que las infecciones primarias.
- Las infecciones recurrentes pueden desencadenarse o reactivarse por el estrés, menstruaciones, o exposición al sol. A veces ellas pueden reaparecer sin razón aparente.
- Algunas personas pueden padecer de infecciones recurrentes de manera infrecuente, mientras que otras pueden presentar reinfecciones tan frecuentemente como una vez al mes.
- Uno o 2 días antes de que las ampollas aparezcan, existe una sensación de picazón, ardor, o dolor en las areas donde las ampollas van a aparecer. A estos síntomas se les denomina pródromos.
- Con el tiempo, las recurrencias disminuyen de frecuencia y eventualmente pueden desaparecer.

¿Cómo se trata el HSV?
El tratamiento de las recurrencias debe empezar al notarse el primer síntoma, porque ésto puede impedir que las ampollas aparezcan. Esto se logra más efectivamente con medicamentos antivirales orales, tales como el vala-cyclovir (Valtrex), el famciclovir (Famvir), o el acyclovir (Zovirax).

Terapia tópica
- Usted puede aliviar el dolor usando compresas con agua fría.
- El unguento de acyclovir (Zovirax), la crema penciclovir (Denavir) y la crema docosanol (Abreva) no son tratamientos muy efectivos, pero pueden ayudar a reducir la duración de la erupción.

NOTAS SOBRE EL HSV-2

- Los condones pueden prevenir la transmición del HSV a su pareja sexual.
- Muchas personas no saben que tienen la infección, y pueden de hecho ser portadores de la misma sin tener síntomas (portadores asintomáticos).
- Una mujer que presente infección activa por HSV durante el trabajo de parto puede transmitir la infección al bebé durante el parto.
- Un episodio recurrente que ocurra muchos años después puede malinterpretarse como una infección primaria, y ésto puede conllevar a acusaciones injustas sobre el transmisor de la infección por HSV.

What is herpes zoster?

- Herpes zoster (shingles) is caused by the same virus that causes varicella (chickenpox). The varicella-zoster virus first occurs as chickenpox, which is usually seen in childhood; later, it returns as herpes zoster caused by a reactivation of the same virus.
- Reactivation into shingles may be associated with illness, or it may occur with no obvious cause.
- The pain of herpes zoster is thought to result from nerve damage caused by the spread of the virus to the skin.

What does herpes zoster look like?

- Usually, there are blisters in a characteristic pattern that wraps around one side of the body.
- Although it can affect any area of the body, herpes zoster is most commonly found on the side of the chest, on one side of the face, on the lower back, or on an arm or a leg.

How is herpes zoster treated?

Oral antiviral medications

A progressing herpes zoster eruption is sometimes treated with antiviral drugs.

Burow's solution

Burow's solution is a soothing astringent preparation that helps to dry up and control weeping, oozing, and infected skin conditions.

Where do I get Burow's solution?

- Purchase a box of Burow's solution (Domeboro, Bluboro, Buropak).
- It is available in most chain pharmacies and does not require a prescription.
- It may come as a powder in packets or in tablet form that must be diluted.

How do I use Burow's solution?

- Dissolve one packet or tablet in an 8-ounce glass of cool or lukewarm water.
- Make a wet compress using a cloth or cotton swab moistened by the solution, and leave it on the infected area for 15 to 20 minutes.
- Do this three to four times each day.
- Discontinue the soaks when the oozing and any signs of infection are gone.

What should I do if I have pain?

- Over-the-counter pain medications, such as aspirin, acetaminophen (Tylenol), and other nonsteroidal antiinflammatory drugs such as ibuprofen (Motrin and Advil) and naproxen (Aleve) are helpful in mild, self-limited cases.
- If the pain is not controlled by these measures, you may require prescription-strength medications. Discuss this with your health care provider.

HERPES ZOSTER ("HERPES")

¿Qué es el herpes zoster?
- Herpes zoster (herpes) está causado por el mismo virus que causa la varicela (viruela loca.) El virus zoster de la varicela aparece primero como viruela loca, que se ve habitualmente durante el periodo infantil, posteriormente vuelve a presentarse como herpes zoster causado por una reactivación del mismo virus.
- La reactivación del virus como herpes esta tal vez asociado a alguna enfermedad, o puede también ocurrir sin causa evidente.
- El dolor causado por el herpes zoster resulta del daño ocasionado a los nervios debido a la expansión del virus a través de la piel.

¿A qué se parece el herpes zoster?
- Por regla general son vejigas que siguen un determinado patrón situado alrededor de un lado del cuerpo.
- Aunque puede afectar a cualquier área del cuerpo, el herpes zoster suele hallarse con más asiduidad en el lado del pecho, en un lado de la cara, en la parte baja de la espalda, en un brazo o en una pierna.

¿Cómo se trata el herpes zoster?
Con medicamentos antivirales por vía oral
Una erupción progresiva de herpes zoster se suele tratar, en ocasiones con fármacos antivirales.

La solución de Burow
La solución de Burow es un preparado astringente que ayuda a secar y controlar el drenaje, la supuración y las condiciones de infección de la piel.

¿Dónde puedo conseguir la solución de Burow?
- Compre una caja de solución de Burow (Domeboro, Bluboro, Buropak.)
- Puede obtenerlo en cualquier farmacia sin receta médica.
- Puede hallarlo en forma de polvo o en tabletas que deben disolverse.

¿Cómo puedo utilizar la solución de Burow?
- Disuelva un paquete o una tableta en un vaso con ocho onzas de agua fría o templada.
- Prepare una compresa utilizando un trapo o un palillo con punta en forma de algodón, humedézcalo en la solución aplíquelo a la zona infectada y manténgalo por unos 15 ó 20 minutos.
- Efectúe esta operación cuatro veces diarias.
- Cese este procedimiento cuando la supuración y los signos de infección hayan terminado.

¿Qué debo hacer si experimento dolor?
- Los medicamentos que se pueden adquirir sin receta médica, como son la aspirina, el acetaminophen (Tylenol), y otros medicamentos antiinflamatorios sin esteroides, como ibuprofen (Motrin, Advil) y naproxen (Aleve) pueden ayudar en los casos leves y en según que circunstancias.
- Si el dolor no puede controlarse con estas medidas, necesitará medicamentos de doble acción que se obtienen con receta médica. Hable con su asistente de salud a este respecto.

What is molluscum contagiosum?
- Molluscum contagiosum is a common superficial viral infection of the outer layer of skin.

Who gets it?
- Young, healthy children (infants and preschoolers)
- HIV-positive patients
- Young, healthy adults who are sexually active and are not HIV-positive

What causes it?
- It is spread by skin-to-skin contact and is caused by a poxvirus.

What does it look like?
- Molluscum contagiosum consists of dome-shaped, shiny or waxy bumps with a central white core.

Where do they occur?
- Molluscum contagiosum often appears on the face, including the eyelids. It also is seen in the armpits and on the arms and legs.
- They are spread by picking and rubbing.
- Molluscum contagiosum can appear in areas of the skin that are inflamed, such as in arm and leg creases in children.
- They may be seen on the lower abdomen, on the inner thighs, and on the genitalia and pubic area in adults.

How are the lesions treated?
Office treatment
- They may be frozen lightly with liquid nitrogen applied with a cotton swab (Q-Tip) or a "freezing gun."
- A blistering agent, such as cantharidin, may be applied carefully with a toothpick to each bump every 3 to 4 weeks.
- Burning and scraping (electrodesiccation and curettage) may be necessary for stubborn molluscum contagiosum lesions.

Home treatment
- A liquid wart medicine such as salicylic acid (DuoFilm), which can be obtained without a prescription, is applied carefully. It should be applied with a toothpick to only the center of the molluscum.
- The eyelid area should not be treated.
- A little irritation usually occurs. If the area becomes too irritated, stop using the DuoFilm for a day or two and then use it again when the irritation disappears.
- Your health care provider may prescribe other topical medications to try.

Keep in mind
- It is also an option not to treat this condition, especially in very young children, and just wait for them to go away on their own.

¿Qué es el Molusco contagioso?
- El Molusco contagioso en una infección viral superficial de la capa superior de la piel.

¿Quién sufre de ello?
- Niños sanos y jóvenes (niños pequeños y los de edad preescolar.)
- Los pacientes de VIH.
- Adultos sanos y jóvenes sexualmente activos y que no tienen el VIH.

¿Qué causa esta condición?
- Se transmite por el contacto directo con la piel y esta ocasionado por el virus causante de la erupción pustulosa de la piel.

¿Qué aspecto tiene esta condición?
- El Molusco contagioso causa la aparición de pequeñas protuberancias que tienen la apariencia de estar enceradas. Algunas lesiones tienen un centro duro y de color blanco.

¿Dónde suelen aparecer?
- El Molusco contagioso aparece a menudo en la cara, incluyendo las pestañas. También suele verse en las axilas, brazos y piernas.
- Las lesiones se extienden rascándose y frotándose.
- El Molusco contagioso puede aparecer en áreas de la piel que están inflamadas, como en los pliegues de los brazos y las piernas en los niños.
- Las lesiones pueden observarse en la zona inferior del abdomen, en el interior de los muslos y en el área genital, inguinal y en el pubis de los adultos.

¿Cómo son tratadas las lesiones?
Tratamiento en la oficina
- Las lesiones pueden ser congeladas con nitrógeno liquido que se aplicará con la ayuda de un palito de algodón o con una "pistola para congelar."
- Con un agente para levantar ampollas, como el cantharidim, que podrá aplicarse cuidadosamente con la ayuda de un palillo, a cada abultamiento cada 3 o 4 semanas.
- La acción de quemar y raspar (electrodesecación y raspado) son dos tratamientos que tal vez resulten necesarios en los casos de lesiones más intratables.

Tratamiento en la casa
- Un medicamento liquido para verrugas como es el ácido salicílico (DuoFilm), puede conseguirse sin receta médica y debe aplicarse cuidadosamente. Deberá aplicarse con un palillo sólo al centro del molusco.
- El área de las pestañas no deberá tratarse.
- Suele experimentarse una leve irritación. Si la zona sufre de irritación excesiva cese la utilización de DuoFilm por un día o dos y vuelva a utilizarlo una vez que la irritación haya cesado.
- Su consejero de salud podrá recetar otros medicamentos de aplicación tópica para que los ensaye.

Tenga en cuenta
- Que también tiene usted la opción de no utilizar medicamentos para tratar esta condición, en particular en los niños muy jóvenes, puede esperar a que las lesiones desaparezcan por sí mismas.

What are warts?
- Warts are skin growths caused by a viral infection in the outer layer of skin.
- Warts are very common, particularly in children.
- An estimated 20% of school-age children will at some time have at least one wart.
- In children, warts tend to disappear over a period of several months to years.
- In many adults, however, warts often prove difficult to destroy.

What causes them?
- All warts are caused by a type of virus, the human papillomavirus (HPV).

What do warts look like?
- **Common warts** generally grow on the hands and fingers and around the nails. They are frequently seen on the knees and elbows, especially in children. They usually have a bumpy appearance that resembles cauliflower.
- **Plantar warts** are located on the soles of the feet. When they grow in clusters, they are known as *mosaic warts*. Plantar warts often have "black dots."
- **Flat warts** are small, smooth, skin colored, and flat. They are most often seen on the face in children, especially teen-aged girls. In adults, they are seen on the beard area in men and on the legs in women. Shaving tends to spread them.

How are warts treated?
Home treatment
Salicylic acid preparations
- They are available in over-the-counter products such as DuoFilm, Occlusal HP, and Compound W. In addition, 40% salicylic acid plasters that are cut to the size of the wart are available.
- These preparations provide the best treatment for small children, in whom warts disappear on their own.
- For best results, the affected area should be hydrated first by soaking it in warm water for 5 minutes before applying the medication.
- It's also a good method for plantar warts; it's painless and inexpensive, and it does not require office visits.

Office treatment
Freezing (cryotherapy with liquid nitrogen)
- Liquid nitrogen is applied with a cotton swab or with a cryotherapy "freezing gun."
- Freezing is best for warts on the hands.
- It's fast, and many warts can be treated on each visit; however, it can be painful and result in blisters, and it may require many office visits.

Burning and scraping (light electrocautery and blunt dissection)
- This method is best for warts on the knees, elbows, and backs of the hands.

¿Qué son las verrugas?
- Las verrugas son crecimientos causados por una infección viral en la superficie superior de la piel.
- Las verrugas son muy comunes, particularmente en niños.
- Se calcula que un 20% de los niños en edad escolar tendrán en alguna ocasión, al menos una verruga.
- En niños, las verrugas tienden a desaparecer en un periodo de varios meses a un año.
- En muchos adultos, sin embargo, resulta más difícil destruir las verrugas.

¿Qué causa las verrugas?
- Todas las verrugas son causadas por un tipo de virus denominado: el virus del papiloma humano (HPV).

¿A qué se parecen las verrugas?
- **Verrugas comunes** suelen salir por regla general en las manos, en los dedos y alrededor de las uñas. Se ven con frecuencia en las rodillas y en los codos, particularmente en los niños. Tienen una apariencia abultada semejante a la de una coliflor.
- **Verrugas plantares** están localizadas en la planta de los pies. Cuando crecen en racimos se las conoce como *mosaico de verrugas*. Las verrugas plantares tienen con frecuencia "puntos negros."
- **Verrugas planas** son pequeñas, lisas, con el mismo color de la piel y planas. Son vistas con más asiduidad en la cara de los niños, especialmente en niñas adolescentes. En los adultos, suelen verse en la zona de la barba en los hombres y en las piernas en las mujeres. El afeitado tiende a que estas se extiendan.

¿Cómo se tratan las verrugas?
Tratamiento en la casa
Acido salicílico preparationes
- Puede encontrar en la farmacia sin receta médica los productos DuoFilm, Occlusal HP y Compound W. También se hallan disponibles para su uso los emplastos con un 40% de ácido salicílico que se cortan a medida para aplicar directamente sobre la verruga.
- Estas preparaciones ofrecen el mejor tratamiento para los niños pequeños, en los cuales las verrugas desaparecen por si solas.
- Para obtener unos resultados mejores, el área deberá ser hidratada empapándola en agua templada durante unos 5 minutos antes de aplicar el medicamento.
- Es un buen método para tratar las verrugas plantares, es barato, sin dolor y no requiere visitas al doctor.

Tratamiento en la oficina
Procedimiento de congelación (crioterapia con nitrógeno liquido)
- El nitrógeno líquido se aplica con un palillo de algodón o con una pistola de congelación de crioterapia.
- El procedimiento de congelado es el mejor para tratar las verrugas en las manos.
- Resulta rápido y muchas verrugas pueden ser tratadas en una sola visita, sin embargo, puede resultar doloroso, crear ampollas y requerir varias visitas.

Pueden ser quemadas y raspadas (una ligera electrocauterización y brusca disección)
- Este método es mejor para verrugas en las rodillas, los codos y en las palmas de las manos.

Other treatments
- Lasers, blistering chemicals, and acids are just a few of many treatments used in patients with warts.
- There have been reports of the successful use of imiquimod (Aldara) cream on flat warts, some common warts, and plantar warts. Aldara (imiquimod) cream is a potent stimulator of the immune system.

WART FACTS

- As you can see, the numerous treatments used for warts are testimony to the fact that we don't have any definite "cure" for them.
- Treatment of warts can be difficult and multiple treatments may be required.
- More often than not, warts tend to "cure" themselves over time.
- The hero of successful wart treatment is usually the last person to treat the wart or the last person to recommend a treatment before the wart goes away.
- The "wart hero" may be a wart charmer, a dermatologist, a hypnotist, or a person who recommended a folk medicine, such as the application of duct tape, garlic, or aloe vera.

How do I know when the warts are gone?
When they don't come back.

How do you get warts and how do you avoid getting warts?
Never shake hands. Never kiss anyone. Never walk barefoot. Live in a bubble. And . . . you still can get 'em.

Otros tratamientos
- Los láser, los químicos para matar verrugas y diferentes tipos de ácidos son unos pocos de los numerosos tratamientos utilizados en pacientes con verrugas.
- Ha habido resultados muy exitosos con el uso de medicamentos antivirales como el imiquimod (Aldara) en forma de crema en las verrugas planas, en algunas verrugas comunes y en las verrugas plantares. La crema de Aldara (imiquimod) es un poderoso estimulante del sistema inmunológico.

REALIDAD SOBRE LAS VERRUGAS

- Como puede observar, el gran número de tratamientos disponibles para las verrugas son una contundente de que en si, no poseemos una cura para ellas.
- El tratamiento para las verrugas puede ser muy difícil y tal vez se requerirán varios tratamientos.
- Con frecuencia, las verrugas suelen curarse por si solas, con el tiempo.
- El héroe con más éxito en el tratamiento contra las verrugas suele ser la última persona que dio su consejo de cómo tratarlas, justo antes de que desapareciesen las verrugas.
- Ese "héroe de las verrugas" tal vez sea un encantador de verrugas, un dermatólogo, un hipnotizador o una persona que recomendó la medicina folklore, como es la aplicación de ajo o aloe vera.

¿Cómo sabré cuando han desaparecido las verrugas?
Cuando ya no regresen.

¿Cómo se contagian las verrugas y como puedo evitar el tenerlas?
Nunca saludé con un apretón de manos a otra persona. Nunca besé a nadie. Nunca caminé con los pies descalzos. Viva en una burbuja aislado del resto del mundo. Y aun así . . . le aparecerán.

What is tinea versicolor?

- Tinea versicolor is a harmless, noncontagious fungal infection of the skin.
- The rash may last for years. It often becomes more noticeable in the summer because of heat, sun exposure, and tanning of the skin.

Who gets it?

- The fungus that causes it normally lives in small numbers on almost everybody, but in some young adults, it may grow and cause a discolored rash.

What does it look like?

- The color of the rash may vary from white to pink to tan or brown.

How is it treated?

- Sometimes, you can clear the rash on your own by using medications such as Selsun Blue, Head & Shoulders, or miconazole (Micatin) or clotrimazole (Lotrimin) cream or spray (cheaper generically). These preparations are available over the counter without a prescription. Do this for 3 or 4 weeks or:
- Your health care provider may have prescribed selenium sulfide 2.5% shampoo or ketoconazole (Nizoral) shampoo. These shampoos are lathered all over the affected area and are left on for 15 minutes and rinsed off in the shower. Do this for 3 or 4 weeks and:
- A prescription antifungal medication cream may also have been given to you by your health care provider. Apply this cream to all affected spots after showering. Do this for 3 or 4 weeks.
- *It is also a good idea to repeat this routine before the next warm season or before taking a tropical vacation.*
- Sometimes a prescription oral antifungal medication is given for 7 to 10 days to treat stubborn cases.

What can I expect?

- Keep in mind: The scale of this rash will disappear after a few treatments, but it may take months for your skin color to return to normal. This slow return of color is part of the normal healing process and does not mean that the treatment has failed.

¿Qué es la tiña multicolor?
- La tiña multicolor es una infección de hongos de la piel inofensiva y no contagiosa.
- El sarpullido puede durar por años. Con frecuencia suele tener una apariencia más evidente en verano debido al calor, a la exposición al sol y al efecto del bronceado de la piel.

¿Quién suele sufrir de ello?
- El hongo causante de la tiña generalmente vive dentro de cada uno de nosotros, en pequeñas cantidades, pero en algunos jóvenes adultos, puede crecer y causar un sarpullido descolorido.

¿A qué se parece?
- El color del sarpullido puede variar del blanco al rosa, al marrón claro o al marrón oscuro.

¿Cómo se trata?
- En ocasiones el sarpullido puede tratarlo uno mismo utilizando medicamentos como Selsun Blue, Head & Shoulders o cremas de miconazole (Micatin), clotrimazole (Lotrimim) o un vaporizador barato. Estas preparaciones se encuentran disponibles sin receta médica. Utilícelas por 3 ó 4 semanas.
- Su consejero de salud puede recetarle selenium 2.5% (champú) o ketoconazole (Nizoral) que también es un champú. Deberán aplicarse en la zona afectada y mantenerlo por unos 15 minutos antes de enjuagárselo en la ducha. Haga este tratamiento por 3 ó 4 semanas.
- Posiblemente también se le haya recetado un medicamento para combatir los hongos. Aplíquese esta crema en todas las áreas afectadas después de la ducha. Haga esto por 3 ó 4 semanas
- *También es una buena idea repetir este tratamiento de rutina antes de la estación veraniega o antes de emprender sus vacaciones en una zona tropical.*
- En según que situaciones también se suele recetar un tratamiento por vía oral durante 7 u 10 días para los casos más difíciles de erradicar.

¿Qué puede esperar?
- Tenga en cuenta, la escala de este sarpullido desaparecerá después de unos cuantos tratamientos pero puede que tarde meses en recobrar el color normal de su piel. Este lento proceso forma parte del proceso de curación y no significa que el tratamiento haya resultado un fracaso.

What is alopecia areata (AA)?

- AA is a common condition that results in the loss of hair in the scalp and possibly elsewhere.
- Shedding of hair is often first discovered by a family member or a person's hairdresser.

What does AA look like?

- It usually starts with one or more small, smooth, oval or round patches of hair loss.
- Hairless spots are most often found on the scalp, eyebrows, eyelashes, and areas of the face that bear hair, such as the beard or mustache on men.

Who gets it?

- AA most commonly affects young adults and children.
- It also occurs more often in families whose members have had asthma, hay fever, thyroid disease, vitiligo, and pernicious anemia.

What causes it?

- AA is considered to be an autoimmune condition ("self-allergy"), because antibodies appear to be attacking the hair follicles.
- These antibodies that are carried by white cells (T cells) cause the growth of hairs to slow down and to become very small and go into a state resembling hibernation; however, the hairs remain alive below the surface.
- AA is not caused by "nerves."

How is it treated?

- Frequently, hair grows back without any treatment; however, it can fall out again.
- Regrowing hair is initially thin and sometimes white.
- Because mild cases of AA often show spontaneous regrowth, therapy is often unnecessary.
- The daily application of potent topical steroids, such as _____ _____, may speed hair regrowth.
- For increased drug penetration, the topical steroid may be applied and covered with a plastic shower cap that is left on overnight.
- If necessary, steroid injections with diluted cortisone into the bare patches may be given every 6 to 8 weeks.

¿Qué es la alopecia areata (AA)?

- AA es una condición bastante común que se caracteriza por la perdida de pelo en el cráneo y posiblemente en otras áreas.
- La perdida del pello es a menudo descubierta por un miembro de la familia o por el peluquero del paciente.

¿Cómo aparece AA?

- Generalmente empieza con una o más zonas de pequeñas áreas de forma oval o redondeada donde se produce la perdida de pello.
- Las áreas de calvicie son halladas más comúnmente en el cráneo, cejas, pestañas y en las zonas de la cara donde crece vello, como por ejemplo la barba o el bigote en los hombres.

¿Quién resulta afectado?

- AA se produce con más asiduidad en jóvenes adultos y en niños.
- También suele presentarse más asiduamente en familias cuyos miembros han sufrido condiciones de asma, alergia, enfermedades tiroideas, vitíligo y anemia perniciosa.

¿Qué causa dicha condición?

- AA esta considerado como una condición del sistema inmunitario (auto-alergia) ya que los anticuerpos parecen atacar los folículos capilares.
- Estos anticuerpos que son transportados por las células blancas (células T) causan una disminución del crecimiento del pelo reduciéndolo en tamaño y dándole un aspecto de hibernación, sin embargo los pelos permanecen vivos debajo de la superficie.
- AA no es causa alguna para provocar reacciones "nerviosas."

¿Cómo se trata?

- Frecuentemente, el pelo crece sin necesidad de tratamiento alguno, pero puede volver a caerse.
- El pelo que vuelve a crecer es al principio fino y algunas veces blanco.
- Dado que casos moderados de AA presentan con frecuencia crecimiento espontáneo, la aplicación de una terapia se hace innecesaria.
- La aplicación diaria en forma tópica de potentes esteroides, como por ejemplo _____, pueden ayudar al crecimiento del pelo con mayor rapidez.
- Para aumentar la penetración del medicamento, el esteroide tópico puede ser aplicado y cubierto con un plástico, como los que se utilizan para gorros de baño, y mantenerlo de esa forma toda la noche.
- Si resultase necesario, pueden inyectarse inyecciones de esteroides diluidas con cortisona dentro de las áreas afectadas cada 6 u 8 semanas.

What is vitiligo?

Vitiligo is a skin condition of white patches that result from a loss of skin pigment.

Who gets it?

Vitiligo affects 1% to 2% of the world's population. Thirty percent of patients with vitiligo report a family history of the disorder.

What causes it?

Although the cause of vitiligo vulgaris is still unknown, one theory is that it results from the body's immune system attack on the pigment-producing cells of the skin, the melanocytes.

What does it look like?

- Occasionally, the spots may have various shades of color and may include dotlike islands of repigmentation.
- In dark-skinned people, pigmentary loss may be observed at any time of year, whereas in light-skinned people, the lesions may be most obvious in the summer, because the tanning effects of the summer sun can intensify the contrast between the light and dark skin.

How is vitiligo treated?

- Topical corticosteroids are occasionally helpful in promoting repigmentation.
- Recently, the application of Protopic ointment 0.1% twice daily has shown some promising results in repigmentation of vitiligo.
- Special cosmetic makeup that is formulated to match a person's normal skin color (e.g., Dermablend or Covermark) or self-tanning compounds that contain dihydroxyacetone may effectively hide the white patches.
- Sunscreens can be used to avoid deepening the contrast between normal skin and lesions and to protect the light-colored patches, which are sensitive to the sun.

VITÍLIGO

¿Qué es el vitíligo?

Vitíligo es una condición de la piel formada por manchas blancas que resultan debido a una pérdida del pigmento de la piel.

¿Quién resulta afectado?

Vitíligo afecta a un 1%-2% de la población mundial. Treinta por ciento de los pacientes con vitíligo afirman tener antecedentes familiares quienes sufren de dicha condición.

¿Qué causa dicha condición?

A pesar de que la causa del vitíligo vulgaris sigue siendo desconocida, una teoría es que es el resultado de un ataque del sistema inmunológico del cuerpo contra las células productoras del pigmento de la piel, es decir, un ataque de los melanocitos.

¿A qué se parece?

- En ocasiones, las manchas pueden presentarse en diferentes tonalidades de color y pueden incluir algunas en forma de punto creando islas de repigmentación.
- En gente de piel oscura, la pérdida de la pigmentación puede observarse en cualquier época del año, mientras que en personas de piel clara, las lesiones podrán observarse más obviamente durante el verano, debido a que los efectos de bronceado durante el sol del verano puede intensificar el contraste entre la piel clara y la oscura.

¿Cómo se trata el vitíligo?

- Los esteroides de cortisona de índice potente y superpotente de aplicación tópica pueden en ocasiones ayudar a promover la repigmentación de la piel.
- Recientemente, la aplicación de crema de Protopic con una potencia del 0.1% y aplicándose dos veces al día mostrado resultados prometedores en la repigmentación del vitíligo.
- El maquillaje cosmético especial formulado para ser idéntico al color de la piel normal del paciente (como por ejemplo Dermablend o Covermark) o componentes de autobronceado que contengan dihidroxiacetona podrían resultar eficaces en esconder las manchas blancas.
- Las cremas de protección solar pueden utilizarse para evitar aumentar el contraste entre la piel normal y las lesiones al mismo tiempo que protegen las áreas de coloración clara, que son sensibles al sol.

VARIOUS MEASURES TO PREVENT AND TREAT DRY SKIN

- Moisturizers do not add water to the skin, but they do help to retain or "lock in" water that is absorbed while bathing. Therefore, apply a moisturizer when the skin is still damp after a bath to help to seal in the absorbed water.
- Many over-the-counter preparations are available, such as Aquaphor, Curel, Eucerin, Alpha Keri, Lubriderm, Moisturel, and Vaseline Petroleum Jelly.
- Some are in ointment bases, cream bases, or lotions, and others contain alpha-hydroxy acids. The decision about which product to use involves personal choice, ease of application, cost, and effectiveness.
- Ammonium lactate 12% (Lac-Hydrin) lotion or cream, which is available by prescription only, is very effective for scaly skin. AmLactin lotion or cream is a similar preparation that is available over the counter.
- Take less frequent and shorter showers and baths using lukewarm water.
- Use mild soaps such as Dove, Basis, or a soap substitute such as Cetaphil Lotion. Excessive use of any soap is to be avoided, especially on affected areas.
- Band-Aids can be helpful to promote healing of fissures (cracks in fingers).
- If you have dry, sensitive hands, wear lined gloves while washing dishes.
- Protect yourself from outdoor cold exposure by wearing gloves, hats, and so forth.
- The value of room humidifiers is probably overestimated.
- Drinking large amounts of fluid is also of questionable value.

PIEL SECA

VARIAS MEDIDAS PARA PREVENIR Y TRATAR LA PIEL SECA

- Los humectantes no añaden agua a la piel, pero si ayudan a retener o a "atrapar" agua que es absorbida durante el baño. Por ello, aplique un humectante cuando la piel está todavía mojada después del baño para ayudar a atrapar el agua absorbida.
- Existen muchas preparaciones a su disposición sin necesidad de receta medica, tales como Aquaphor, Curel, Eucerin, Alpha Keri, Lubriderm, Moisturel, y Vaselina Petroleum Jelly.
- Algunas contienen como base ungüento, crema o lociones y otras contienen ácidos de alpha-hydrosy. La decisión de cual producto usar responde únicamente a una elección personal, basada en la facilidad para su aplicación, su precio y su efectividad.
- Lactato de amonio con una potencia de 12% (Lac-Hydrin) loción o crema que está disponible con receta medica únicamente, es sumamente efectiva contra la piel escamosa. La loción o la crema de AmLactin es una preparación similar que se encuentra disponible sin receta.
- Tome duchas y baños menos frecuentes usando agua templada.
- Use jabones suaves como Dove, Basis o sustitutivos del jabón como la loción de Cetaphil. Debe evitarse el uso prolongado de cualquier jabón, en particular en las áreas afectadas.
- Tiritas de Band-Aids pueden resultar beneficiosas en el proceso de curación en las fisuras que se producen entre los dedos.
- Si usted tiene sequedad y sensibilidad en las manos, póngase guantes mientras lava los platos.
- Protéjase contra el frío exterior llevando guantes, gorro y cuanto sea necesario para cubrirse.
- El valor de los humidificadores en la habitación es tal vez sobreestimado.
- El beber grandes cantidades de liquido tiene también, tal vez, un valor cuestionable.

What are hives?
- Hives, known medically as *urticaria*, are very common.
- They are reddish, itchy swellings sometimes called "wheals" that last for a few hours before fading away; then new ones may develop as old ones fade away.
- There may be deep swelling (angioedema) around the eyes, lips, and tongue.

Acute hives last for less than 6 weeks.
- There may be an obvious cause such as an acute viral infection, a reaction to a drug, or an insect bite.
- The most common drugs that may cause acute hives are antibiotics (especially penicillin and sulfa drugs), pain medications such as aspirin and ibuprofen, narcotics, radiocontrast dyes, diuretics, and opiates such as codeine.
- The most common foods that are associated with hives are milk, wheat, eggs, chocolate, shellfish, nuts, fish, and strawberries. Food additives and preservatives such as salicylates and benzoates may also be responsible.
- Rarely, a severe, life-threatening reaction known as anaphylaxis can occur and requires immediate medical attention.

Chronic hives are hives that last longer than 6 weeks.
- They are more commonly seen in women.
- The cause is usually unknown; however, chronic hives may, very infrequently, be a sign of an underlying illness.
- In 85% to 90% of patients, the cause is unknown.
- Emotional stress may trigger recurrences.
- Chronic hives also may be caused by physical stimuli such as cold, sunlight, or exercise. Such hives are called physical urticarias.

Who gets hives?
- From 10% to 20% of the population will have one episode of hives in their lifetime.

What should be done to determine the cause?
- Tell your health care provider all the medications (including oral contraceptives) and vitamins that you are taking.
- Routine blood tests are usually of little or no value in determining the cause of chronic hives.
- Allergy testing is expensive, and often tests are positive for allergies that have nothing to do with hives.

What can be done to treat and prevent hives?
- If possible, the cause of the hives should be eliminated.
- The mainstay of treatment for chronic hives is the use of oral antihistamines.
- People with severe reactions should consider wearing a MedicAlert bracelet that describes their problem.
- Aspirin-containing compounds, ibuprofen, and narcotics, which are all histamine-releasing agents, may aggravate both acute and chronic types of hives and should be avoided.
- Tight clothing and hot baths and showers should be avoided, particularly in people who have physical urticaria.

ERUPCIONES

¿Qué son las erupciones?

- Las erupciones, conocidas en términos médicos como *urticaria*, son muy comunes.
- Son rojas, producen comezón acompañada de inflamación que en ocasiones se denominan "granos" o "ronchas" que duran varias horas antes de desaparecer, entonces nuevos brotes suelen aparecer a medida que las otras van desapareciendo.
- También pueden producir una profunda inflamación alrededor de los ojos, boca y lengua denominada angioedema.

Las erupciones agudas *duran menos de 6 semanas.*

- Existe por lo general una causa obvia como una infección viral, reacción a un medicamento o picadura de insecto.
- Las drogas que con más asiduidad producen erupciones agudas son los antibióticos, especialmente la penicilina y los medicamentos que contienen sulfa, los medicamentos contra el dolor como son la aspirina y el ibuprofen, los narcóticos, las tinturas de radiocontraste, los diuréticos, y los derivados del opio como la codeína.
- Los alimentos que más comúnmente están asociados con erupciones son la leche, el trigo, los huevos, el chocolate, los mariscos, los frutos secos (nueces, almendras, nuez de brasil, avellanas) el pescado y las fresas. Los aditivos y conservadores alimenticios como los salicilatos y los benzootes pueden ser responsables de erupciones en la piel.
- Raramente, una reacción de índole severa que pone en peligro la vida del paciente y que se conoce bajo el nombre de anafilaxia puede ocurrir y requiere atención medica inmediata.

Las erupciones crónicas *son urticarias que duran más de 6 semanas.*

- Aparecen con más asiduidad en las mujeres.
- La causa es por lo general desconocida, sin embargo, erupciones crónicas pueden, con poca frecuencia ser un signo de otras enfermedades.
- En un 85% al 90% de los pacientes, la causa es desconocida.
- El estrés emocional puede desencadenar recaídas.
- Las erupciones crónicas pueden ser causadas por un estímulo físico como frío, luz solar o ejercicio. Tales erupciones son denominadas urticarias físicas.

¿Quién sufre de erupciones de la piel?

- De un 10% a un 20% de la población tendrá un episodio de erupciones en su vida.

¿Qué podría hacerse para determinar la causa?

- Dígale a su medico todos los medicamentos, incluyendo las píldoras anticonceptivas y las vitaminas que está tomando.
- Los análisis de sangre rutinarios son por lo general de poco valor en poder determinar la causa de las erupciones crónicas.
- Las pruebas de alergias resultan costosas, y a menudo los resultados son positivos para alergias que no están relacionadas con las erupciones.

¿Qué puede hacerse para tratar y prevenir las erupciones?

- A ser posible la causa de las erupciones debe ser eliminada.
- El método regular de tratamiento contra las erupciones es el uso de antihistamínicos por vía oral.
- Las personas que sufren de reacciones severas deberían de llevar puesto un brazalete de alerta médica que describe el problema.
- Los medicamentos que contienen aspirina, ibuprofen, y los narcóticos, todos ellos tienen agentes antihistamínicos y podrían agravar tanto las erupciones agudas como las crónicas, por ello deben ser evitados.
- Las ropas ajustadas al cuerpo y los baños y duchas calientes deberían ser evitadas, especialmente en personas que sufren de urticaria física.

What are genital warts?

- Genital warts, also known as venereal warts or condyloma acuminatum, characterize a very common sexually transmitted disease.
- The warts are usually smooth or cauliflowerlike growths caused by a virus, the human papilloma virus (HPV).
- The warts are seen in the regions of the penis, vagina, vulva, cervix, and anus.
- They are caused by specific types of HPV and probably are not caused by the same virus that causes the common wart.
- It is thought that most genital warts are spread by sexual contact; however, evidence suggests that nongenital spread of the virus can also occur.
- These warts can infrequently be seen in infants of mothers who have genital HPV infection.
- These warts have a fairly long incubation period and may appear several weeks or even years after sexual contact. Therefore, it is difficult to determine the origin of the infection in people who have had multiple sexual partners. Many infected persons are carriers of the virus and may never develop warts but still can pass them to their sexual partners.

How are genital warts diagnosed?

- The diagnosis of genital warts is often simple; however, when the warts are very small and difficult to see, they may be confused with normal structures of the skin.
- Sometimes, a skin biopsy is performed to confirm the diagnosis.
- Often, careful examination using good lighting and magnification is necessary to see them.
- In women, evidence of the viral infection may be detected during a routine pelvic examination or Pap smear.

How are genital warts treated?

- Treatment is often difficult because there is no specific agent, antibiotic, antiviral, or other alternative that actually destroys the virus.
- The biggest problem is the tendency for the warts to recur, whichever method is used. It is impossible to predict who will have recurrences. Sometimes, the warts disappear without treatment.

Methods that are currently used include the following:

Office treatment
- **Electrodesiccation** uses a direct electric current to destroy the warts after local anesthesia is administered.
- **Cryodestruction** ("freezing") is done with liquid nitrogen.
- **Podophyllum** is a liquid medication applied by health care providers.
- **Bichloroacetic acid** and **trichloroacetic acid** may be applied.
- **Laser therapy** is another method to destroy the warts.

Home treatment
- **Imiquimod (Aldara)** and **podofilox (Condylox)** are medications that may be self-applied.

How are genital warts prevented?

- Spread of warts can be lessened by the use of condoms; however, some warts may not be covered by the condom.

¿Qué son las verrugas genitales?
- Las verrugas genitales también conocidas como verrugas venéreas o condiloma cuminado caracterizan una enfermedad sexual transmisible bastante común.
- Las verrugas son lisas o en forma de coliflor causadas por un virus, el papiloma humano (HPV).
- Las verrugas se ven en las áreas del pene, la vagina, la vulva, la cerviz, y el ano.
- Son causadas por tipos específicos de HPV y muy posiblemente no son causadas por el mismo virus que causa la verruga común.
- Se cree que la mayoría de las verrugas genitales son propagadas por contacto sexual, sin embargo existe evidencia de que también el virus puede propagarse por otra vía que no sea necesariamente la genital.
- Estas verrugas pueden, con poca frecuencia verse en niños, cuyas madres tienen infección de HPV.
- Estas verrugas tienen un largo período de incubación y pueden aparecer varias semanas o incluso años después de haberse realizado el acto sexual. Por ello, es difícil determinar el origen de la infección en gente que tienen varios compañeros o compañeras sexuales. Muchas personas infectadas con portadoras del virus y tal vez nunca les aparezcan las verrugas pero pueden seguir contagiando a sus compañeros o compañeras sexuales.

¿Cómo se diagnostican las verrugas genitales?
- El diagnóstico de verrugas genitales es bastante simple, sin embargo, cuando las verrugas son muy pequeñas y difíciles de ver, pueden confundirse con las estructuras normales de la piel.
- En ocasiones se hace una biopsia de la piel para confirmar el diagnóstico.
- A menudo, un examen minucioso con el uso de buena luz y magnificación es necesario para detectarlas.
- En las mujeres, evidencia de la infección viral puede llegar a detectarse en un examen pélvico de rutina o con el papanicolaou.

¿Cómo son tratadas las verrugas genitales?
- El tratamiento puede resultar difícil porque no existe un agente específico para ello bien sea, antibiótico, antiviral o otra alternativa que destruya el virus.
- El mayor problema es la tendencia de las verrugas a reaparecer, no importa que método se utiliza. Es imposible predecir quien sufrirá de su reaparición. En ocasiones, las verrugas desaparecen sin tratamiento.

Métodos de tratamiento que son utilizados en la actualidad son los siguientes:

Tratamiento en la oficina médica
- **Electrodesecación** utiliza una corriente eléctrica directa para destruir las verrugas bajo la aplicación de anestesia local.
- **Criodestrucción** ("efecto de congelación") se efectúa aplicando liquido de nitrógeno.
- **Pódofilo** es un medicamento en forma liquida que es aplicada por un empleado de la salud.
- **Acido bicloracético** y **ácido tricloracético** puede ser aplicado para tratar las verrugas.
- **Terapia con láser** es otro método disponible para destruir las verrugas.

Tratamiento en la casa
- **Imiquimod (Aldara)** y **podofilox (Condylox)** son medicamentos que pueden ser aplicados por uno mismo.

¿Cómo se pueden prevenir las verrugas?
La propagación puede disminuirse con el uso de los preservativos, sin embargo, algunas verrugas no pueden ser cubiertas por el preservativo.

What is scabies?
- A tiny mite causes an itchy skin condition known as scabies.
- The main symptom of scabies is itching, particularly at night.

Who gets scabies?
- Scabies is almost always caught from another person, usually another family member or someone else with whom you came into close contact.
- It has nothing to do with dirt or poor personal hygiene.

What causes scabies?
- A mite that is very small, about 0.4 mm in length, and can barely be seen by the human eye is the cause.

What does scabies look like?
- The itchy rash of scabies is most often located between the fingers, the sides of the hands and feet, wrists, umbilicus (belly button), waistband area, armpits, ankles, buttocks, and groin.

How is scabies treated?
Permethrin (Elimite and Acticin)
- Elimite and Acticin both contain permethrin cream 5%.
- A prescription is required.

Instructions for use
- After a warm bath, a thin layer of Elimite or Acticin is applied to all skin surfaces from head to toe (including the palms and soles and scalp in small children) and is left on for 8 to 12 hours, usually overnight; it is washed off the next morning. Thirty grams (half a tube) of medication is enough for an adult.
- If instructed by your health care provider, other family members and contacts should be treated at the same time.
- All bed linen and intimate undergarments should be washed in hot water after treatment is completed.
- Generally, only one treatment is necessary; however, a second treatment is often recommended in 4 to 5 days, especially in long-standing cases and in infants with scabies of the palms and soles.

What should I expect after treatment?
- It is normal to continue itching for days or weeks after treatment, but the itching is usually less intense.
- Call your health care provider if you or your child is not better.
- Do not continue to apply the prescription medications unless otherwise instructed.

SARNA

¿Qué es la sarna?
- Un insecto pequeño causa una condición de la piel acompañada de comezón conocida como sarna.
- El síntoma más distintivo de la sarna es la comezón, en particular durante la noche.

¿Quién resulta afectado?
- La sarna es casi siempre adquirida de otra persona, generalmente de otro miembro de la familia o quizás de otra persona con quién se ha tenido contacto directo.
- No tiene nada que ver con la suciedad o con la poca higiene personal.

¿Qué causa la sarna?
- La causa es un pequeño insecto, que mide 0.4 mil y que apenas puede ser distinguido por el ojo humano.

¿A que se parece la sarna?
- El sarpullido con síntomas de comezón aparece más a menudo entre los dedos, los lados de las manos y los pies, las muñecas, el ombligo, el área de la cintura, debajo de las axilas, los tobillos, las nalgas y las ingles.

¿Cómo se trata la sarna?
Permetrin (Elimite y Acticin)
- Elimite y Acticin ambos contienen crema con un 5% de permetrin.
- Es necesario receta médica.

Instrucciones de uso
- Después de darse un baño de agua templada, se aplica una fina capa de Elimite o Acticin en la piel desde la cabeza hasta los dedos de los pies (incluyendo las palmas de los pies y el cráneo en los niños pequeños) y debe guardarlo por un período de 8 a 12 horas, generalmente por la noche, se lavará a la mañana siguiente. Treinta gramos (medio tubo) del medicamento es suficiente para un adulto.
- Si se lo recomienda su consejero de la salud, otros miembros de la familia o otras personas que hayan entrado en contacto con dicha condición, deberán también ponerse el tratamiento.
- Todas las sábanas y ropa íntima deberán lavarse en agua caliente una vez que se haya completado el tratamiento.
- Por regla general un solo tratamiento es suficiente, sin embargo, se suele recomendar un segundo tratamiento en 4 ó 5 días, en particular en casos de larga duración y en niños que tienen sarna en las palmas de los pies.

¿Qué debo esperar después del tratamiento?
- Es normal que la comezón continúe por días o semanas después del tratamiento, pero la comezón suele ser menos intensa.
- Llame a su doctor si usted o su hijo no mejoran.
- No continúe aplicándose el medicamento recetado a no ser que le recomienden lo contrario.

TREATMENT OF HEAD LICE (PEDICULOSIS CAPITIS)

What causes head lice infestations?
- *Pediculus humanus* var *capitis* (the head louse) is the cause.

Who gets head lice?
- Head lice are spread from human to human. Epidemics of head lice are most commonly seen in schoolchildren.
- Head lice occur more often in females than in males. They are unusual in African Americans.

How is a head lice infestation treated?
- Nits are removed with a fine-tooth comb after soaking the hair in a vinegar solution; this helps to soften the cementing substance that attaches the nit to the hair.
- Shaving scalp hair is not necessary to treat a person with lice.

First-line treatments
- Permethrin products such as Nix Creme Rinse, RID, and Acticin may be obtained without a prescription.
- These agents all contain low concentrations of permethrin; they are very effective in killing adult lice and nymphs, but not as effective in killing nits (eggs). There has been growing resistance of head lice to these agents.

How to use them:
- The hair is washed with a nonmedicated shampoo and is towel dried. The agent is then applied as a cream rinse, is allowed to remain in place for 10 minutes, and then is rinsed off thoroughly.
- Because these agents do not destroy nits totally, a second application (using the same technique) often is recommended 7 to 10 days after the first treatment.
- An old-fashioned treatment technique is to use petrolatum such as Vaseline Petroleum Jelly. Petrolatum is quite messy and hard to remove, but it is an inexpensive and sometimes effective method that smothers the lice and nits. It is applied to the entire scalp and is left on under a shower cap overnight.

For resistant cases, your health care provider may prescribe one of the following medications:
- **Ovide (malathion lotion 0.5%)**
- The lotion is applied to **DRY** hair in a quantity sufficient to wet hair and scalp.
- It is then massaged into the scalp and is left on for 8 to 12 hours. Heat (e.g., hairdryers, hot curlers) should not be used to dry the lotion.
- The hair is then rinsed, and nits are removed with a fine-tooth (nit) comb.
- Treatment should be repeated in 7 to 10 days if lice are still present (using the same technique).

Elimite Cream (5% permethrin cream)
- This cream is available as prescription-strength 5% cream. It is left on overnight under a shower cap. Treatment is repeated in 1 week to destroy any remaining eggs.

TRATAMIENTO PARA LOS PIOJOS DE LA CABEZA (PEDICULOSIS CAPITIS)

¿Qué causa infestación de piojos en la cabeza?
- La causa es el *Pediculus humanos var capitis,* denominado comúnmente (el piojo de la cabeza).

¿Quién resulta afectado?
- Los piojos de la cabeza se propagan de humano a humano. Las epidemias de piojos se ven con más frecuencia en los niños de edad escolar.
- Los piojos de la cabeza ocurren más a menudo en mujeres que en hombres. Son poco frecuentes entre los afro americanos.

¿Cómo se trata la infestación de piojos?
- Las liendres se retiran con un peine de dientes finos después de haber mojado en pelo con una solución de vinagre, esto ayuda a reblandecer las sustancias cimentadas que unen las liendres al pelo.
- No es necesario afeitar el cuero cabelludo del paciente para efectuar el tratamiento contra los piojos.

Tratamientos de primera linea
- Los productos de permetrin como la crema de enjuague de Nix y Acticin se pueden obtener sin receta medica.
- Todos estos agentes contienen dosis bajas de permetrin, son muy efectivos en eliminar los piojos adultos y las ninfas, pero no resultan tan efectivos para matar las liendres (huevos) poco a poco ha ido aumentando la resistencia de los piojos contra estos productos.

Como se utilizan:
- Se lava la cabeza con un champú no medicinal y se seca con una toalla. Entonces se aplica el producto como si se tratase de una crema de enjuague, tendrá que permanecer puesto durante 10 minutos, y después deberá enjuagárselo abundantemente.
- Debido a que estos productos no destruyen las liendres en su totalidad, se recomienda una segunda aplicación (utilizando la misma técnica) de 7 a 10 días después del primer tratamiento.
- Un tratamiento con una técnica mas anticuada es el de utilizar petrolatum como la Vaseline Petroleum Jelly. El petroleum ensucia bastante y es difícil de retirar, pero es barato y en según que ocasiones, es un método efectivo que asfixia los piojos y las liendres. Se aplica a la totalidad del cuero cabelludo, se cubre con un gorro de plastico y se deja así toda la noche.

Para casos más resistentes, su consejero de salud podrá recetarle uno de los medicamentos indicados a continuación:
- **Ovide (loción de malathion con un 5% de intensidad)**
- La loción se aplica al pelo seco en una cantidad suficiente para mojar el cuero cabelludo.
- Con la ayuda de masajes se hará penetrar en el cuero cabelludo y se guardará por unas 8 a 12 horas. Las fuentes de calor como (los secadores de pelo, y los rulos calientes) no deberán utilizarse para secar la loción.
- A continuación se enjuagará el pelo, y las liendres se retirarán a la ayuda de un peine de púas finas.
- El tratamiento se repetirá en 7 ó 10 días si aun quedan piojos (utilizando la misma técnica)

Crema de Elimite (5% de potencia crema de permetrin)
- Esta crema se halla disponible con receta medica a un 5% de potencia. Se deberá mantener puesta toda la noche cubriendo el cuero cabelludo con un gorro de plástico. El tratamiento se repetirá en una semana para destruir el resto de las liendres.

What is a solar keratosis?

- Solar keratosis, also known as actinic keratosis, is the most common sun-related skin growth.
- A solar keratosis is benign (premalignant); however, it does, if left untreated, have the potential to develop into a skin cancer, a squamous cell carcinoma.
- The good news is that the invasive carcinomas that develop from these actinic keratoses are a very slow-growing, unaggressive type of skin cancer, and the prognosis is usually excellent. Distant metastasis (spread) is extremely rare.

What does a solar keratosis look like?

- These lesions usually appear as crusty, scaly bumps that are typically rough-textured to the touch.

Where do they appear?

- They are found mainly on sun-exposed areas—the face, especially the nose, the temples and forehead, and the lips.
- They are also commonly noted on the bald areas of the scalp and the tops of ears in men, the top of the forearms and hands, and the sun-exposed areas of the neck.
- They may also occur on any area that is repeatedly exposed to the sun.

Who gets them?

- These lesions are seen in people who are fair-skinned, who burn easily, and who tan poorly.
- They are more common in men, particularly those who work in outdoor occupations, such as farmers, sailors, and gardeners, and those who participate in outdoor sports.

What causes them?

- The development of solar keratoses is directly proportional to sun exposure.

How are they diagnosed?

- Small solar keratoses are better felt than seen. They feel like gritty bumps.
- Larger ones are diagnosed by dermatologists, based on their appearance or a skin biopsy.

How are they treated?

Office treatment

Destructive methods include the following:

- Liquid nitrogen (LN_2) is applied to individual keratoses for 3 to 5 seconds.
- Biopsy is followed by electrocautery of individual keratoses, or electrocautery alone is performed.

Home treatment

- Application of a 5-fluorouracil (5-FU) cream is a method that may be used when solar keratoses are too numerous to treat individually. Topical 5-FU treatment can be likened to a "smart bomb," in which the " bomb"—in this case 5-FU—targets only the "enemy," that is, rapidly growing abnormal cells.

How do I prevent them?

- Prevention begins with limiting sun exposure by using sunscreens and wearing protective clothing.

QUERATOSIS SOLAR

¿Qué es la queratosis solar?
- La queratosis solar, también conocida como queratosis actinica, es el tumor más común de la piel relacionado con el sol.
- La queratosis solar es benigna (pre maligna), pero sin embargo, si se deja sin tratar, existe la posibilidad de que se convierta en un cáncer de la piel, en una célula de carcinoma escamoso.
- Las buenas noticias son que los carcinomas agresivos que se desarrollan de esa queratosis actinica crecen lentamente, se trata de un tipo de cáncer de piel poco agresivo, cuyo pronóstico es generalmente excelente. Las metástasis a largo plazo son muy raras.

¿A que se parece la queratosis solar?
- Estas lesiones tienen la apariencia de costras, con abultamientos en forma de escamas de una consistencia áspera al tacto.

¿Dónde aparecen?
- La queratosis solar suele verse con más frecuencia en pieles expuestas asiduamente a los efectos dañinos del sol.
- Se suelen encontrar exclusivamente en las áreas expuestas al sol, como son la cara, especialmente la nariz, las sienes, la frente y los labios.

¿Quién sufre de ello?
- Estas lesiones se ven en personas de piel clara, que se queman con facilidad y que se broncean con dificultad.
- Estas lesiones son más comunes en hombres, especialmente en aquellos que trabajan en actividades al aire libre, como los granjeros, los marineros, y los jardineros así como en aquellos individuos que realizan actividades deportivas al exterior.

¿Cuales son las causas?
- El desarrollo de la queratosis es directamente proporcional a la cantidad de exposición solar.

¿Cómo se diagnostica?
- Las pequeñas queratosis solares se llegan a notar mejor al tacto que observándolas. Al tocarlas parecen pequeñas protuberancias arenosas.
- Las de mayor tamaño son diagnosticadas por el dermatólogo, basándose en la apariencia o realizando una biopsia de la piel.

¿Cómo son tratadas?
Tratamiento en la oficina

Entre los métodos para destruir las queratosis se incluyen los siguientes:
- El nitrógeno liquido (LN) se aplica a las queratosis actinica individuales por 3 ó 5 segundos.
- Una biopsia es seguida por la electrocauterización de las queratosis actinica individuales, o simplemente se hace solo la electrocauterización.

Tratamiento en la casa
- Cuando la queratosis esta muy extendida y es difícil hacer un tratamiento de las lesiones individuales, se puede aplicar una crema de 5-fluorouracil (5-FU) como tratamiento. El uso tópico de 5-FU se puede considerar como un tratamiento comparable a una "bomba inteligente" con la cual se tratarían únicamente las zonas enemigas, en este caso corresponderían a las células que crecen anormalmente.

¿Cómo puede prevenirlas?
- Para empezar a prevenir lo primero que hay que hacer es limitar la exposición solar utilizando cremas de protección y llevando ropa protectora.

What is a basal cell carcinoma (BCC)?
- A BCC is a skin cancer that is easily treated and cured in most cases.
- Although BCC qualifies as a cancer, its harmful effects, if recognized and treated early, are usually minor.
- BCC is usually very slow growing and rarely spreads (metastasizes), but it can cause serious local invasion and destruction if it is ignored or treated inadequately.

Who gets BCC?
- A light complexion with poor tanning ability is a risk factor.
- Patients have a history of long-term sun exposure.
- Other family members have a history of BCC.

What does a BCC look like?
- A BCC resembles a shiny "pimple" or sore that does not heal.
- A BCC is usually a dome-shaped bump that has a pearly appearance.
- It may have a small scab on its surface.

How is a BCC diagnosed?
- Diagnosis is generally made by shave or excisional biopsy.

How is a BCC treated?
- Most often, a simple minor office procedure called electrodesiccation and curettage is performed for small growths and for very superficial BCCs.
- Surgical excision is the preferred method for larger tumors.
- Micrographic (Mohs') surgery may be the preferred method for recurrent or very large lesions. Mohs' micrographic surgery is a microscopically controlled method of removing skin cancers that allows for controlled removal and maximum preservation of normal skin. Excisions (removals) are repeated in the areas proven to be cancerous until a completely cancer-free specimen is reached. The Mohs technique has a high cure rate, but it is not required for all BCCs.

Other treatment methods include the following:
- **Cryosurgery** ("freezing") with liquid nitrogen is a treatment option.
- **Radiation therapy** is used for those patients who are physically debilitated or who are unable to undergo excisional surgery.

How do I prevent getting BCCs in the future?
- Avoid exposure to sun exposure.
- Carefully plan outdoor activities before 10 a.m. and after 4 p.m., wear a broad-brimmed hat during outdoor activities, and use a sunscreen with a sun protection factor (SPF) of 15 or greater.
- Learn skin self-examination, and have annual skin examinations performed by your dermatologist.

CARCINOMA DE CÉLULA BASAL

¿Qué es el carcinoma de célula basal (BCC)?
- Un BCC es un cáncer de la piel que en la mayoría de los casos es altamente tratable y curable.
- A pesar de que BCC está calificado como cáncer, sus efectos dañinos resultan generalmente menores, si son reconocidos y tratados a tiempo.
- El BCC, en términos generales, suele tener un crecimiento lento y raramente se extiende (metástasis) pero puede causar invasión y destrucción local de índole seria, si se ignora su presencia o no se trata adecuadamente.

¿Quién resulta afectado por BCC?
- Una complexión de piel clara que broncea con dificultad representa un factor de riesgo.
- Los pacientes que han estado expuestos a los rayos solares por largo tiempo.
- Si existen otros miembros de la familia que sufren de BCC.

¿A qué se parece un BCC?
- Un BCC asemeja a un grano brillante o llaga que no se cura.
- Un BCC aparece como una protuberancia en forma de cima similar a una perla.
- La lesión puede tener una pequeña costra en su superficie.

¿Cómo se diagnostica un BCC?
- Un diagnostico se hace afeitando el área o efectuando una biopsia.

¿Cómo se trata un BCC?
- A menudo, para extirpar los pequeños tumores y en los casos más superficiales de BCC, se suele efectuar un pequeño procedimiento en la oficina del doctor, denominado electrodesecación y raspado.
- La extirpación quirúrgica es el método preferido para combatir los tumores de mayor tamaño.
- La cirugía micrográfica (Mohs') tal vez sea el mejor método para eliminar lesiones recurrentes o de gran tamaño. La cirugía micrográfica de Mohs' es un método controlado microscópicamente para poder remover canceres de piel de forma tal que sea posible preservar la mayor parte de la piel normal. Las extirpaciones se repetirán en las áreas cancerigenas hasta que estas estén totalmente libres del cáncer. La técnica de Mohs tiene un índice de curación muy alto, pero no es requerida para todos los casos de BCCs.

Otros métodos de tratamiento incluyen lo siguiente:
- **Criocirugía** ("método de congelación") que se efectúa con nitrógeno liquido.
- **Terapia de radiación** se utiliza para aquellos pacientes que están físicamente debilitados o para los que es imposible someterse a una cirugía de extirpación.

¿Como prevenir BCCs en el futuro?
- Evitando la exposición solar.
- Tratando de realizar actividades al aire libre antes de las 10 de la mañana y después de las 4 de la tarde, póngase un sombrero de ala ancha cuando haga actividades al exterior, y utilice crema de protección solar con un índice 15 o mayor.
- Aprendiendo a auto examinarse la piel y realizando exámenes anuales de la piel en un consultorio dermatológico.

What is a squamous cell carcinoma (SCC)?
- SCCs are the second most common type of skin cancer.

What does an SCC look like?
- An SCC usually looks like a scaly or crusty bump.
- It also can appear as a nonhealing sore or ulcer.

Where do they appear?
- SCCs are most often seen on a background of sun-damaged skin.
- They are found mainly on sun-exposed areas—the face, especially the nose, the temples and forehead, and the lips.
- They are also commonly noted on the bald areas of the scalp and the tops of ears in men, the top of the forearms and hands, and the sun-exposed areas of the neck.
- They may also occur on any area that is repeatedly exposed to the sun.
- SCCs may occur on the legs in women.

Who gets SCCs?
- SCC is related to sun exposure and is noted more frequently in those with a greater degree of outdoor activity. It is seen in people who are fair-skinned, burn easily, and tan poorly.
- They are more common in men, particularly those who work in outdoor occupations, such as farmers, sailors, and gardeners, and those who participate in outdoor sports.

Where does SCC come from?
- Most SCCs arise in a solar keratosis, a precancer also known as an actinic keratosis.

How is SCC diagnosed?
- Diagnosis is generally made by shave or excisional biopsy.

How is it treated?
- Most often, a simple minor office procedure called electrodesiccation and curettage is performed for small growths and for very superficial SCCs known as *squamous cell carcinoma in situ.*
- Surgical excision is the preferred method for larger tumors.
- Micrographic (Mohs') surgery may be the preferred method for recurrent or very large lesions, as well as for lesions in "danger zones" (e.g., the nasal area, around the eyes, behind the ears, in the ear canal, and on the scalp). Mohs' micrographic surgery is a microscopically controlled method of removing skin cancers that allows for controlled excision and maximum preservation of normal skin. Excisions are repeated in the areas proven to be cancerous until a completely cancer-free specimen is reached.

Other treatment methods include the following:
- Cryosurgery with liquid nitrogen is a treatment option.
- Radiation therapy is used for those patients who are physically debilitated or who are unable, or refuse, to undergo excisional surgery.

How do I prevent SCC?
- Prevention begins with limiting sun exposure by using sunscreens and wearing protective clothing.

¿Qué es el carcinoma de célula escamosa (SCC)?
- SCCs es el segundo tipo de cáncer de piel más común.

¿A qué se parece un SCC?
- Un SCC se parece a un abultamiento con escamas y costras.
- También puede aparecer como una llaga o ulcera que no cura.

¿Dónde aparecen?
- Los SCCs son vistos más a menudo en pieles con un largo historial de exposición solar.
- Se hallan principalmente en las áreas de la piel más expuestas al sol, como son la cara, especialmente la nariz, las sienes, la frente y los labios.
- También se nota en las áreas de calvicie en el cuero cabelludo y en la parte superior de las orejas en los hombres, la parte superior de los brazos, y los lugares del cuello expuestos al sol.
- También pueden aparecer en cualquier área que está expuesta al sol.
- En las mujeres los SCCs pueden aparecer en las piernas.

¿Quién sufre de SCCs?
- El SCC está relacionado a la exposición solar y se observa más en aquellos individuos que realizan actividades al aire libre. Se suele presentar más en gente de piel clara que se quema con facilidad y que le cuesta broncearse.
- Estas lesiones son más comunes en los hombres, en particular, en aquellos que trabajan en ocupaciones al aire libre, como son los granjeros, marineros, jardineros y aquellos que practican deportes al exterior.

¿De dónde viene el SCC?
- La mayoría de los casos de SCC surgen con la condición de queratosis solar, una lesión cancerigena conocida como queratosis actinica.

¿Cómo se diagnostica el SCC?
- Un diagnostico se hace afeitando el área o efectuando una biopsia.

¿Cómo se trata?
- A menudo un simple procedimiento de oficina denominado electrodesecación y raspado se realiza en los tumores pequeños y también en los SCCs superficiales conocidos como *carcinoma celular escamoso in situ.*
- La excisión quirúrgica es el método preferido en el tratamiento de tumores más grandes.
- La cirugía micrográfica de Mohs tal vez sea el método preferido para tratar lesiones recurrentes, así como para tratar aquellas situadas en "zonas de peligro" (por ejemplo: en el área nasal, alrededor de los ojos, detrás de las orejas, en el canal auditivo y en el cuero cabelludo). La cirugía micrográfica de Mohs es un método controlado microscópicamente para remover los canceres de la piel, que permite excisiones controladas para poder preservar la mayor parte de la piel normal. Las excisiones son efectuadas repetidamente en las áreas de las que se tienen pruebas de ser cancerigenas, hasta que queden libres de cáncer.

Otros métodos de tratamiento incluyen lo siguiente:
- La criocirugía con liquido de nitrógeno es un método de tratamiento.
- La terapia de radiación es utilizada por aquellos pacientes que se encuentran físicamente debilitados, que no pueden o que no desean someterse a una cirugía de excisión.

¿Cómo puedo prevenir SCC?
- La prevención empieza limitando la exposición solar utilizando cremas solares y llevando ropa protectora contra el sol.

SUN PROTECTION ADVICE

Anyone with a personal family history of skin cancer and those who have very fair skin that never tans but always burns should apply a sunscreen. The following are recommendations that are modified from those of the Skin Cancer Foundation:

- Avoid sun exposure during the hours between 10 a.m. and 4 p.m., when the sun is strongest.
- Wear protective headgear such as a hat with a wide brim or a baseball cap; wear long-sleeved shirts and long pants.
- Apply a sunscreen at least 30 minutes before sun exposure.
- Apply sunscreens even on cloudy, hazy days.
- Be aware of reflected light from sand, water, or snow.
- Use a sunscreen with a sun protection factor (SPF) of 15 or greater to prevent burning.
- Apply sunscreens liberally and frequently at least every 2 to 3 hours, as long as you stay in the sun, and reapply after swimming or sweating.
- Choose a waterproof sunscreen.
- Choose a broad-spectrum sunscreen that blocks both ultraviolet B (UVB, the burning rays) and ultraviolet A (UVA, the more penetrating rays that promote wrinkling and aging).
- Excellent choices for babies and young children are Neutrogena Sensitive Skin UVA/UVB SPF 30 and Vanicream (SPF 15). Both are "non-chemical," opaque, physical sunscreens that contain titanium dioxide or zinc oxide. They provide good coverage, are waterproof, and cause fewer allergic reactions than other sunscreens.
- Be aware that moisturizers that contain built-in sunscreens usually have a lower SPF.

Further advice
- Avoid tanning parlors.
- Keep infants out of direct sunlight.
- Teach children sun protection at a young age.
- Wear UV-blocking sunglasses.
- If you tan easily, you may use a lower SPF number.
- Lips are also sun sensitive, so use special lip-coating sunscreens that have a waxy base.
- You can use preparations that dye the skin (self-tanning products), but be aware that they do not offer any sun protection, unless they are combined with a sunscreen.
- Certain drugs can make you more likely to burn, such as tetracycline, diuretics ("water pills"), and certain oral antidiabetic medications.
- Remember, there is no such thing as a healthy tan!

Cualquier persona con antecedentes familiares de cáncer de piel y las de piel muy clara que nunca broncean pero siempre se queman, deberán aplicar crema de protección solar. Las recomendaciones siguientes son una modificación de aquellas ofrecidas por la Fundación del cáncer de piel:

- Evite la exposición solar entre las 10 de la mañana y las 4 de la tarde, cuando el sol es muy intenso.
- Utilice un sombrero de ala ancha o una visera para proteger la cabeza del sol, lleve camisas de mangas largas o pantalones para proteger el resto del cuerpo.
- Aplique cremas de protección solar al menos 30 minutos antes de exponerse al sol.
- Aplíquese crema de protección solar incluso en días nublosos o con niebla.
- Preste atención al reflejo de la luz de la arena, del agua o de la nieve.
- Utilice una crema de protección solar con un índice 15 o mayor para prevenir quemarse.
- Aplique la crema solar generosamente y con frecuencia, al menos cada 2 o 3 horas, por todo el periodo que permanezca al sol, y renueve la aplicación después de nadar o sudar.
- Elija una crema solar resistente al agua.
- Elija una crema solar de largo espectro capaz de bloquear ambos rayos ultravioleta B (UVB, los rayos que causan quemaduras) y los ultravioleta A (UVA, los rayos con capacidad de penetrar más profundo y que promueven las arrugas y el envejecimiento).
- Una elección excelente como crema para los niños y los bebés es la Neutrogena Sensitive Skin UVA/UVB con un índice de protección 30, también la crema Vanicream (SPF 15) ambas no contienen productos químicos, son opacas y contienen dióxido de titanio y oxido de zinc. Son excelentes para cubrirse del sol, son resistentes al agua y causan menos reacciones alérgicas que otras cremas.
- Tenga en cuenta que las cremas humectantes que dicen contener protección solar este es más bajo en SPF.

Otros consejos:
- Evite los centros de bronceado artificiales.
- Mantenga a los niños fuera del alcance de la luz directa solar.
- Enseñe a los niños desde una edad temprana la importancia de protegerse del sol.
- Lleve gafas de sol que bloqueen los UV.
- Si broncea con facilidad, puede utilizar un índice menor de protección solar.
- Los labios también son sensibles al sol, por ello debe utilizar un protector labial con base de cera.
- Puede utilizar preparaciones que tiñen la piel (productos autobronceadores) pero tenga en cuenta que no ofrecen protección solar alguna a no ser, que se combinen con cremas solares de protección.
- Algunas cremas pueden producir una mayor sensibilidad para quemarse por el sol, como por ejemplo: tetraciclina, los diuréticos ("píldoras de agua") y también ciertos medicamentos antidiabéticos.
- Recuerde que no existe en absoluto el concepto de un bronceado sano!

SUNSCREEN RECOMMENDATIONS (SPF 15 OR GREATER)

WATERPROOF SUNSCREENS	FOR OILY SKIN	MOISTURIZER-SUNSCREEN COMBINATION	SPORT SUNSCREENS*	FOR SENSITIVE SKIN†
PreSun (SPF 15, 29, or 46)	Clinique Oil Free (SPF 15)	Neutrogena Moisture (SPF 15)	Coppertone Sport (SPF 15 or 30)	Almay Super-Sensitive (SPF 30) Lotion
Shade (SPF 30 or 45)	Presun Active (SPF 15 or 30)	Oil of Olay Daily UV Protectant (SPF 15)	Neutrogena "No-Stick" Sunscreen (SPF 30)	Clinique Special Defense Sun Block (SPF 25)
Almay (SPF 15, 25, or 30)	Neutrogena (SPF 15)	Eucerin Daily Facial Lotion (SPF 25)		Estee Lauder Advanced Suncare Sunblock (SPF 15 or 25)
Bain de Soleil All Day (SPF 15 or 30)	Presun Facial (SPF 15 or 29)	Almay Moisture Balance Lotion (SPF 15)		Neutrogena Sensitive Skin UVA/UVB Block (SPF 30)
Bullfrog gel For Kids (SPF 36)	Shade Oil Free (SPF 15 or 25)	Basis Protective Facial Moisturizer (SPF 15)		Vanicream (SPF 15)
Sundown (SPF 15, 25, or 30)		Neutrogena Sensitive Skin Sunblocker (SPF 17)		
Coppertone (SPF 15, 25, 30 or 45)				
Neutrogena Sunblock (SPF 15 or 30)				
Solbar (SPF 50)				
BioSun (SPF 15, 30, or 45)				

*Lotion will not run into eyes with sweating.
†"Nonchemical" sunscreens generally contain titanium dioxide or zinc oxide as their sun-blocking agent.

RECOMENDACIONES DE CREMAS SOLARES (SPF 15 O MAYOR)

CREMAS SOLARES RESISTENTES AL AGUA	PARA PIEL GRASA	MOISTURIZER/LAS COMBINACIONES DE SUNSCREEN	SUNSCREEN DEPORTIVO*	PARA LA PIEL SENSIBLE†
Presun (SPF 15, 29 ó 46)	Clinique Oil Free (SPF 15)	Neutrogena Moisture (SPF 15)	Coppertone Sport (SPF 15 ó 30)	Almay Super-Sensitive (SPF 30) Lotion
Shade (SPF 15, 25 o 30)	Presun Active (SPF 15 or 30)	Oil of Olay Daily UV Protectan (SPF 25)	Neutrogena" No-Stick" Sunscreen (SPF 30)	Clinique Special Defense Sun Block (SPF 25)
Bain de Soleil All Day (SPF 15 o 30)	Neutrogena (SPF 15)	Almay Moisture Balance Lotion (SPF 15)		Estee Lauder Advanced Suncare Sunblock (SPF 15 ó 25)
Bullfrog gel For Kids (SPF 36)	Presun Facial (SPF 15 ó 29)	Basis Protective Facial Moisturizer (SPF 15)		Neutrogena Sensitive Skin UVA/UVB Block (SPF 30)
Sundown (SPF 15, 25 ó 30)	Shade Oil Free (SPF 15 ó 25)	Nutrogena Sensitive Skin Sunblock (SPF 17)		Vanicream (SPF 15)
Coppertone (SPF 15, 25, 30 ó 45)				
Neutrogena Sunblock (SPF 15 ó 30)				
Solbar (SPF 50)				
BioSun (SPF 15, 30 ó 45)				

*La loción no penetrará en los ojos al sudar.

†Las cremas "No-químicas" contienen por lo general dióxido de titanium o oxido de zinc como agente protector contra el sol.

Brand Names of Dermatologic Medications in Various Countries

GENERIC NAME	UNITED STATES	FRANCE	GERMANY	UNITED KINGDOM
FOR ACNE AND ROSACEA: ORAL				
Minocycline	Minocin	Mestacine, Mynocine	Skid, Lederderm	Minocin
Doxycycline hyclate	Vibramycin	Vibromycine	Vibramycin	Vibramycin
Erythromycin	E-Mycin	Érythrocyne	Monomycin, Erythrocin	Erythrocin
13-*cis*-retinoic acid	Accutane	Roaccutan	Roaccutan	Roaccutan
FOR ACNE AND ROSACEA: TOPICAL				
Azelaic acid	Azelex	Skinoren	Skinoren	Skinoren
Metronidazole	Noritate, MetroGel, MetroCream	Rosiced, Rozagel	MetroGel	Rozex, MetroGel
Clindamycin	Cleocin T	Dalacine T	Basocin	Dalacin T
Erythromycin	Emgel	Éryacné	Aknemycin, Stiemycine	Erythrocin, Zineryt
Tretinoin	Retin-A	Aberel, Effederm	Eudyna, Airol	Retin-A
Adapalene	Differin	Différine	Differin	Differin
Tazarotene	Tazorac	Zorac	Zorac	Zorac
Benzoyl peroxide	Oxy-5, Oxy-10	Panoxyl, Pannogel Éclaran, Effacné	Benzaknen, PanOxyl	PanOxyl, Acnecide
FOR PSORIASIS: TOPICAL (NONSTEROIDAL)				
Salicylic acid	Keralyt gel	Cold cream salycilé	Squamasol, Psorimed	NA
Calcipotriene	Dovonex	Daivonex	Psorcutan, Daivonex	Dovonex
ANTIFUNGALS: TOPICAL				
Terbinafine	Lamisil	Lamisil	Lamisil	Lamisil
Ketoconazole	Nizoral	Nizoral, Ketoderm	Terzolin	Nizoral
Tolnaftate	Tinactin	Sporilline	Tonaftal	Tinaderm
Econazole	Spectazole	Dermazol	Epi-Pevaryl	Ecostatin, Pevaryl
Ciclopirox	Loprox	Mycoster	Batrafen	NA
ANTIFUNGALS: ORAL				
Griseofulvin	Fulvicin P/G	Fulcine	Likuden, Fulcin	Grisovin
Terbinafine	Lamisil	Lamisil	Lamisil	Lamisil
Itraconazole	Sporanox	Sporanox	Sempera	Sporanox
Fluconazole	Diflucan	Triflucan	Diflucan	Diflucan
ANTIHISTAMINES				
Hydroxyzine	Atarax	Atarax	Atarax, AH3	Atarax
Cyproheptadine	Periactin	Périactine	Peritol	Periactin
Loratadine	Claritin	Clarytine	Lisino	Clarityn
Cetirizine	Zyrtec	Zyrtec	Zyrtec	Zirtek
Doxepin	Sinequan	Quitaxon, Sinquan	Aponal, Sinquan	Sinquan
FOR ALOPECIA				
Minoxidil (topical)	Rogaine	Regaine	Regaine	Regaine
Finasteride (oral)	Propecia	Propécia	Propecia	Propecia
ANTIMITOTIC: TOPICAL				
5-Fluorouracil	Efudex, Carac	Efudix	Efudix	Efudix
SCABACIDES: TOPICAL				
Permethrin	Elimite, Acticin	Nix, Charlieu anti-poux	Infectopedicul	Lyclear
Lindane	Kwell	Aphtiria	Jacutin	Quellada
SCABACIDES: ORAL				
Ivermectin	Stromectol	NA	Stromectol	Mectizan

GENERIC NAME	UNITED STATES	FRANCE	GERMANY	UNITED KINGDOM
Clobetasol propionate	Temovate, Cormax, Clobevate	Dermoval	Emovate	Dermovate
Betamethasone dipropionate	Diprosone	Diprosone	Betadermic	Propaderm (beclomethasone diproprionate)
Amcinonide	Cyclocort	NA	Amciderm	NA
Betamethasone valerate	Valisone	Betneval	Betnesol-V, Soderm	Betnovate
Desoximetasone	Topicort	Topicorte	Topisolon	Stiedex
Fluocinonide	Lidex	Topsyne	Topsym	Metosyn
Halcinonide	Halog	Halog	Halog	Halciderm
Hydrocortisone butyrate	Locoid	Locoid	Pandel	Locoid
Alclometasone	Aclovate	Alclosone	Delonal	Modrasone
Desonide	Tridesilon, DesOwen	Tridesonit, Locapred	Sterax, Topifug (both are 0.1%)	DesOwen
Fluocinolone	Synalar	Synalar	Jellin, Flucinar	Synalar
Triamcinolone acetonide	Kenalog, Aristocort	Kenacort-A	Volon A, Kenalog	Tri-Adcortyl
Mometasone	Elocon	NA	Ecural	Elocon
Hydrocortisone	Hytone, Cortaid, Cortizone	Hydrocortisone Astier	Canesten HC, Hydrozon	Efcortelan, Mildeson lipocream

NA, The brand name of this product was not obtained at time of publication.

Page numbers followed by an *f* refer to figures; page numbers followed by a *t* refer to tables.

Pyogenic adenitis, 295
Pyogenic angioma, 336–337, 336f
Pyogenic granuloma, 2, 229, 229f
   during pregnancy, 364, 364f

Q

Quaternium-15
   allergic contact dermatitis and, 69

R

Radiation therapy, 351
Rapid plasma reagin (RPR), 107
Recurrent herpes simplex virus,
   143, 143f
   treatment of, 146
Reiter's syndrome (RS), 397–399
   basics of, 397–398
   clinical manifestations of, 398
   diagnosis of, 398
   differential diagnosis of, 399
   lesion description of, 398, 398f
   lesion distribution of, 398
   management of, 399
Renal disease, chronic
   pruritus of, 254
Retin-A. See Tretinoin
Retinoids, 40t
   for acne vulgaris, 26–27
   psoriasis and, 88
Rheumatoid nodules, 111
Rhinophyma, 36, 36f
Rhus dermatitis, 44, 44f
   diagnosis of, 68
   lesion description in, 67, 67f
   prevention of, 71
RID, 312
Ringworm. See Tinea capitis;
   Tinea corporis
Rogaine, 203
Rosacea, 25, 32, 74, 407
   acne and, 35
   basics of, 34
   clinical manifestations of, 34, 34f
   clinical variants of, 35–36
   diagnosis of, 35
   differential diagnosis of, 35
   factors of, 34
   folliculitis and, 125, 125f
   lesion description in, 34
   lesion distribution in, 34, 34f
   management of, 37–38
   pathophysiology of, 35
   patient handout for, 443–444
   pityriasis. See Pityriasis rosacea
   points to remember in, 38
   seborrheic dermatitis and, 35, 35f
   systemic lupus erythematosus
     and, 35
   systemic therapy for, 37–38
   topical steroids and, 36, 36f
   topical therapy for, 37
Roseola, 190, 192
Roseola infantum, 187–188
   basics of, 187, 187f
   clinical manifestations of, 187
   diagnosis of, 188
   differential diagnosis of, 188

lesion description of, 187
lesion distribution of, 187
management of, 188
Rubella, 189–190, 192
   basics of, 189
   clinical course of, 189
   diagnosis of, 189
   differential diagnosis of, 190
   lesion description of, 189
   lesion distribution of, 189, 189f
   management of, 190
Rubeola, 191–192
   basics of, 191
   clinical features of, 191–192
   complications of, 192
   diagnosis of, 192
   differential diagnosis of, 192
   lesion description of, 191
   lesion distribution of, 191
   management of, 192
Ruby spots, 335

S

Sabouraud's media, 171
Sarcoidosis, 210, 240, 240f
   cutaneous. See Cutaneous sarcoidosis
Scabicides, 379
Scabies, 49, 62, 68, 256, 299, 305–309
   basics of, 305
   burrow of, 305, 305f
   clinical manifestations of, 306
   clinical variants of, 306–307,
     306f, 307f
   course/secondary lesions of,
     306, 306f
   crusted, 307, 307f
   diagnosis of, 307, 307f
   differential diagnosis of, 307
   etiology of, 305, 305f
   in elderly, 306
   in infants, 306, 306f
   lesion description of, 305, 305f
   lesion distribution of, 306, 306f
   management of, 308
   Norwegian. See Norwegian scabies
   patient handout for, 481–482
Scabs, 5
Scales, 5
Scalp, seborrheic dermatitis of, 73, 73f
Scalp, psoriasis of
   basics of, 94, 94f
   differential diagnosis of, 94
   features of, 94
   management of, 95
Scarlet fever, 188, 190, 192, 194–195,
   195, 197, 199
   basics of, 194
   clinical manifestations of, 195
   diagnosis of, 195
   differential diagnosis of, 195
   etiology of, 194
   lesion description of, 194, 194f
   lesion distribution of, 194
   management of, 195
Scars, hypertrophic, 338, 338f
Sclerosing hemangioma, 334
Schamberg's purpura, 274

Scleredema of Buschke-Löwenstein, 388
Scleroderma, 413–415
Seabather's eruption, 314, 314f
Sebaceous hyperplasia, 329, 329f, 350
Seborrheic dermatitis, 65, 94, 97, 159,
   161, 171, 407
   basics of, 72, 72f
   clinical manifestations of, 74
   clinical variants of, 74
   differential diagnosis of, 74–75
   formulary for, 77
   HIV-associated, 72, 384
   lesion description of, 73
   lesion distribution of, 73–74
   management of, 75–76
   pathogenesis of, 73
   rosacea and, 35, 35f
Seborrheic keratosis, 133, 133f, 323–326,
   342, 350, 354, 354f
   basics of, 323
   clinical variants of, 324–325
   diagnosis of, 325
   differential diagnosis of, 325
   lesion description of, 323, 323f
   lesion distribution of, 324, 324f
   management of, 326
Secondary syphilis, 108, 108f, 289–291
   clinical manifestations of, 290
   diagnosis of, 290
   differential diagnosis of, 291
   lesion description of, 289–290, 289f
   lesion distribution of, 290, 290f
   management of, 291
Selsun, 162
Senile angiomas, 335
Septic vasculitis, 277
Sex hormone binding globulin
   (SHBG), 216
Sexual abuse. See Perianal
   streptococcal dermatitis
Sézary's syndrome, 396
Shaving, 220
Shedding, of hair, 202
Shingles. See Herpes zoster
Sign of Leser-Trélat, 325
Simple elliptical excision, 430–432
   advantages of, 430
   basics of, 430
   disadvantages of, 430
   technique of, 430–431, 430f
   undermining, 431, 431f
   wound closure, 431–432
Skin
   inflammatory disorders of. See
     Inflammatory skin disorders
Skin atrophy, topical steroids and, 14, 14f
Skin biopsy, 426–429
   punch, 428–429, 428f
   shave, 426–427, 427f
   snip, 427–428, 428f
Skin tags, 280
   basics of, 327
   clinical manifestations, 327
   diagnosis of, 327
   differential diagnosis of, 327
   lesion description of, 327, 327f
   management of, 328